PET/CT Imaging in Oncology: Clinical Updates and Perspectives

PET/CT Imaging in Oncology: Clinical Updates and Perspectives

Editors

Arnoldo Piccardo
Francesco Fiz

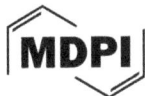

Basel • Beijing • Wuhan • Barcelona • Belgrade • Novi Sad • Cluj • Manchester

Editors
Arnoldo Piccardo
E.O. Ospedali Galliera
Genoa, Italy

Francesco Fiz
E.O. Ospedali Galliera
Genoa, Italy

Editorial Office
MDPI
St. Alban-Anlage 66
4052 Basel, Switzerland

This is a reprint of articles from the Special Issue published online in the open access journal *Journal of Clinical Medicine* (ISSN 2077-0383) (available at: https://www.mdpi.com/journal/jcm/special_issues/PET_CT_Imaging).

For citation purposes, cite each article independently as indicated on the article page online and as indicated below:

Lastname, A.A.; Lastname, B.B. Article Title. *Journal Name* **Year**, *Volume Number*, Page Range.

ISBN 978-3-0365-9450-7 (Hbk)
ISBN 978-3-0365-9451-4 (PDF)
doi.org/10.3390/books978-3-0365-9451-4

© 2023 by the authors. Articles in this book are Open Access and distributed under the Creative Commons Attribution (CC BY) license. The book as a whole is distributed by MDPI under the terms and conditions of the Creative Commons Attribution-NonCommercial-NoDerivs (CC BY-NC-ND) license.

Contents

Francesco Fiz, Gianluca Bottoni, Giorgio Treglia, Pierpaolo Trimboli and Arnoldo Piccardo
Diagnostic and Prognostic Role of ^{18}F-Fluoroestradiol PET in Metastatic Breast Cancer: The Second Youth of an Older Theranostic Concept
Reprinted from: *J. Clin. Med.* **2022**, *11*, 3589, doi:10.3390/jcm11133589 1

Francesco Dondi, Nadia Pasinetti, Roberto Gatta, Domenico Albano, Raffaele Giubbini and Francesco Bertagna
Comparison between Two Different Scanners for the Evaluation of the Role of ^{18}F-FDG PET/CT Semiquantitative Parameters and Radiomics Features in the Prediction of Final Diagnosis of Thyroid Incidentalomas
Reprinted from: *J. Clin. Med.* **2022**, *11*, 615, doi:10.3390/jcm11030615 5

Kgomotso M. G. Mokoala, Ismaheel O. Lawal, Letjie C. Maserumule, Khanyisile N. Hlongwa, Honest Ndlovu, Janet Reed, et al.
A Prospective Investigation of Tumor Hypoxia Imaging with ^{68}Ga-Nitroimidazole PET/CT in Patients with Carcinoma of the Cervix Uteri and Comparison with ^{18}F-FDG PET/CT: Correlation with Immunohistochemistry
Reprinted from: *J. Clin. Med.* **2022**, *11*, 962, doi:10.3390/jcm11040962 23

Domenico Albano, Nadia Pasinetti, Francesco Dondi, Raffaele Giubbini, Alessandra Tucci and Francesco Bertagna
Prognostic Role of Pre-Treatment Metabolic Parameters and Sarcopenia Derived by 2-[^{18}F]-FDG PET/CT in Elderly Mantle Cell Lymphoma
Reprinted from: *J. Clin. Med.* **2022**, *11*, 1210, doi:10.3390/jcm11051210 37

Christian Philipp Reinert, Regine Mariette Perl, Christoph Faul, Claudia Lengerke, Konstantin Nikolaou, Helmut Dittmann, et al.
Value of CT-Textural Features and Volume-Based PET Parameters in Comparison to Serologic Markers for Response Prediction in Patients with Diffuse Large B-Cell Lymphoma Undergoing CD19-CAR-T Cell Therapy
Reprinted from: *J. Clin. Med.* **2022**, *11*, 1522, doi:10.3390/jcm11061522 49

Marta Opalińska, Anna Sowa-Staszczak, Kamil Weżyk, Jeremiasz Jagiełła, Agnieszka Słowik and Alicja Hubalewska-Dydejczyk
Additional Value of [18F]FDG PET/CT in Detection of Suspected Malignancy in Patients with Paraneoplastic Neurological Syndromes Having Negative Results of Conventional Radiological Imaging
Reprinted from: *J. Clin. Med.* **2022**, *11*, 1537, doi:10.3390/jcm11061537 61

Arnoldo Piccardo, Francesco Fiz, Giorgio Treglia, Gianluca Bottoni and Pierpaolo Trimboli
Head-to-Head Comparison between ^{18}F-FES PET/CT and ^{18}F-FDG PET/CT in Oestrogen Receptor-Positive Breast Cancer: A Systematic Review and Meta-Analysis
Reprinted from: *J. Clin. Med.* **2022**, *11*, 1919, doi:10.3390/jcm11071919 71

Christina-Katharina Fodi, Jens Schittenhelm, Jürgen Honegger, Salvador Guillermo Castaneda-Vega and Felix Behling
The Current Role of Peptide Receptor Radionuclide Therapy in Meningiomas
Reprinted from: *J. Clin. Med.* **2022**, *11*, 2364, doi:10.3390/jcm11092364 83

Angela Sardaro, Paolo Mammucci, Antonio Rosario Pisani, Dino Rubini, Anna Giulia Nappi, Lilia Bardoscia and Giuseppe Rubini
Intracranial Solitary Fibrous Tumor: A "New" Challenge for PET Radiopharmaceuticals
Reprinted from: *J. Clin. Med.* **2022**, *11*, 4746, doi:10.3390/jcm11164746 93

Matthias Weissinger, Stefan Kommoss, Johann Jacoby, Stephan Ursprung, Ferdinand Seith, Sascha Hoffmann, et al.
Multiparametric Dual-Time-Point [^{18}F]FDG PET/MRI for Lymph Node Staging in Patients with Untreated FIGO I/II Cervical Carcinoma
Reprinted from: *J. Clin. Med.* **2022**, *11*, 4943, doi:10.3390/jcm11174943 . . . . **103**

Manuela A. Hoffmann, Jonas Müller-Hübenthal, Florian Rosar, Nicolas Fischer, Finn Edler von Eyben, Hans-Georg Buchholz, et al.
Primary Staging of Prostate Cancer Patients with [^{18}F]PSMA-1007 PET/CT Compared with [^{68}Ga]Ga-PSMA-11 PET/CT
Reprinted from: *J. Clin. Med.* **2022**, *11*, 5064, doi:10.3390/jcm11175064 . . . . **115**

Luca Viganò, Egesta Lopci, Luca Di Tommaso, Annarita Destro, Alessio Aghemo, Lorenza Rimassa, et al.
Functional Investigation of the Tumoural Heterogeneity of Intrahepatic Cholangiocarcinoma by In Vivo PET-CT Navigation: A Proof-of-Concept Study
Reprinted from: *J. Clin. Med.* **2022**, *11*, 5451, doi:10.3390/jcm11185451 . . . . **131**

Francesca Tutino, Elisabetta Giovannini, Silvia Chiola, Giampiero Giovacchini and Andrea Ciarmiello
Assessment of Response to Immunotherapy in Patients with Hodgkin Lymphoma: Towards Quantifying Changes in Tumor Burden Using FDG-PET/CT
Reprinted from: *J. Clin. Med.* **2023**, *12*, 3498, doi:10.3390/jcm12103498 . . . . **141**

Matthias Weissinger, Max Atmanspacher, Werner Spengler, Ferdinand Seith, Sebastian Von Beschwitz, Helmut Dittmann, et al.
Diagnostic Performance of Dynamic Whole-Body Patlak [^{18}F]FDG-PET/CT in Patients with Indeterminate Lung Lesions and Lymph Nodes
Reprinted from: *J. Clin. Med.* **2023**, *12*, 3942, doi:10.3390/jcm12123942 . . . . **157**

Editorial

Diagnostic and Prognostic Role of ^{18}F-Fluoroestradiol PET in Metastatic Breast Cancer: The Second Youth of an Older Theranostic Concept

Francesco Fiz [1,*], Gianluca Bottoni [1], Giorgio Treglia [2,3,4], Pierpaolo Trimboli [4,5] and Arnoldo Piccardo [1]

1. Nuclear Medicine Department, E.O. "Ospedali Galliera", 16128 Genoa, Italy; gianluca.bottoni@galliera.it (G.B.); arnoldo.piccardo@galliera.it (A.P.)
2. Clinic of Nuclear Medicine, Imaging Institute of Southern Switzerland, Ente Ospedaliero Cantonale, 6500 Bellinzona, Switzerland; giorgio.treglia@eoc.ch
3. Department of Nuclear Medicine and Molecular Imaging, Lausanne University Hospital, University of Lausanne, 1011 Lausanne, Switzerland
4. Faculty of Biomedical Sciences, Università della Svizzera Italiana, 6900 Lugano, Switzerland; pierpaolo.trimboli@eoc.ch
5. Clinic of Endocrinology and Diabetology, Lugano and Mendrisio Regional Hospital, Ente Ospedaliero Cantonale, 6500 Bellinzona, Switzerland
* Correspondence: francesco.fiz@galliera.it

Since the discovery of the role of female hormones in breast cancer (BC) pathophysiology, in vivo detection of oestrogen receptor (ER) distribution has been one of the major goals of nuclear medicine and molecular imaging [1,2]. Hormone-blockade treatments represent, in fact, a safe and effective way to control ER-positive BC, even in the metastatic setting, and prevent recurrences [3–5]. Such an approach can be attempted in patients with evidence of ER on the clonal cell, which is estimated by biopsy or pathological examination of the primary tumour [6]. However, there is now ample evidence that ER expression might vary across disease sites, and there can be significant differences in this regard between primary tumour and distant metastases [7–9]. Since performing biopsies on remote disease localization might not always be feasible or even advisable, methods to obtain this information non-invasively have been sought after. The initial attempts in developing a molecular imaging tracer for scintigraphy imaging in the late 1970s were not successful, given the limited resolution of the method and the elevated background activity of some organs, such as liver [10,11]. However, some years later, the research group of Katzenellenbogen was able to develop a molecular imaging probe for PET devices, i.e., ^{18}F-fluoroestradiol (FES), which was effectively the first radio-receptor positron-emitting tracer [12]. This tracer showed immediate promise; however, the related PET imaging method was then still in its infancy and, even later, the tracer landscape would continue to be dominated by fluorodeoxyglucose (FDG) for many years to come. It was only towards the end of the second decade of the 21st century that FES gained significant traction, leading to a marked increase of published research papers as well as its official approval, firstly in France (2016) and then in the United States of America (2020) [13].

The approval of FES-PET was grounded on its excellent capability of predicting the actual ER expression status on pathology; in a study by Chae and colleagues, among 37 patients with a positive FES-PET, all of them had oestrogen receptors on immunohistochemistry [14]. These data were recently confirmed by a larger, prospective trial, where FES-PET was able to predict the ER expression with very high sensitivity in the biopsied tumour lesions as well as in remote bone localizations [15]. In turn, the presence of ER is the only factor that can predict the effectiveness of endocrine therapy; tumour sites with poor or absent ER expression do not respond well to this approach [16,17]. Conversely, a widespread and intense FES positivity is linked with well-differentiated, ER-positive tumour forms, which have a significant chance to respond well to the endocrine treatment.

In this sense, FES-PET represents a theranostic approach, directing the patients toward the most suitable therapy, while avoiding the costs and the potential side effects of an inadequate one [18].

It must be highlighted that, understandably, there are some caveats and limitations to this approach. First, the diagnostic potential of the method might vary, since physiological background activity might affect the detectability of tumour lesions; this issue is particularly marked in the liver, which presents the highest density of oestrogen receptors [19]. However, bone is the principal metastatic site of ER$^+$ BC, which has a lower tendency to colonize visceral organs when compared with other BC subtypes [20]. Some factors, such as body mass index and level of sex hormone-binding globulin, may have a mild-to-moderate effect on FES uptake, whereas other factors, such as the menopausal status, do not [21]. Secondly, even if the method is very sensitive in determining the ER expression, this parameter represents a necessary, yet not per se sufficient, condition for the success of the endocrine treatment [16]. In fact, triggering of the ER-dependent intracellular mechanisms in BC can occur despite a pharmacological endocrine blockade, via functional alteration of intracellular domains or crosstalk with other pathways [22,23]. Consequently, even in the case of a positive FES-PET, the real effectiveness of a first-line endocrine treatment could vary across patients. Finally, especially in the metastatic setting, different cellular clones, with varying degrees of biological aggressiveness, might co-exist in the same patients. Particularly, an aggressive disease is signalled by the disappearance of ER on the cell and increased proliferation rate; in such a setting, the switch towards FDG-PET or a dual tracer (FES/FDG) PET is advised [24]. The FDG-positive disease is linked with a poorer prognosis and tends to not respond to endocrine treatment; in the case of mixed FDG- and FES-positive disease, the FDG/FES ratio, i.e., the measure of how prevalent the less differentiated component is, represents an important factor for predicting disease progression and patients' overall survival [25].

Besides the identification of the aggressive clonal component, FDG-PET has an excellent sensitivity at the patient level, which is comparable to the one afforded by FES-PET [26]. However, FES-PET has better lesion-based sensitivity, especially in the restaging setting [26].

In conclusion, considering available evidence-based data [26–28], FES-PET proved to be a valid diagnostic, prognostic, and theranostic approach, which, after many years of preparation, is ready to take the main stage of differentiated cancer identification and treatment.

Conflicts of Interest: The authors declare no conflict of interest.

References

1. Russo, J.; Russo, I.H. The role of estrogen in the initiation of breast cancer. *J. Steroid Biochem. Mol. Biol.* **2006**, *102*, 89–96. [CrossRef]
2. Katzenellenbogen, J.A. The quest for improving the management of breast cancer by functional imaging: The discovery and development of 16α-[(18)F]fluoroestradiol (FES), a PET radiotracer for the estrogen receptor, a historical review. *Nucl. Med. Biol.* **2021**, *92*, 24–37. [CrossRef]
3. Drăgănescu, M.; Carmocan, C. Hormone Therapy in Breast Cancer. *Chirurgia* **2017**, *112*, 413–417. [CrossRef] [PubMed]
4. Diaby, V.; Tawk, R.; Sanogo, V.; Xiao, H.; Montero, A.J. A review of systematic reviews of the cost-effectiveness of hormone therapy, chemotherapy, and targeted therapy for breast cancer. *Breast Cancer Res. Treat.* **2015**, *151*, 27–40. [CrossRef] [PubMed]
5. Dalmau, E.; Armengol-Alonso, A.; Muñoz, M.; Seguí-Palmer, M. Current status of hormone therapy in patients with hormone receptor positive (HR+) advanced breast cancer. *Breast* **2014**, *23*, 710–720. [CrossRef] [PubMed]
6. Jensen, E.V.; Jordan, V.C. The Estrogen Receptor: A Model for Molecular Medicine. *Clin. Cancer Res.* **2003**, *9*, 1980–1989.
7. Walter, V.; Fischer, C.; Deutsch, T.M.; Ersing, C.; Nees, J.; Schütz, F.; Fremd, C.; Grischke, E.M.; Sinn, P.; Brucker, S.Y.; et al. Estrogen, progesterone, and human epidermal growth factor receptor 2 discordance between primary and metastatic breast cancer. *Breast Cancer Res. Treat.* **2020**, *183*, 137–144. [CrossRef]
8. Pusztai, L.; Viale, G.; Kelly, C.M.; Hudis, C.A. Estrogen and HER-2 receptor discordance between primary breast cancer and metastasis. *Oncologist* **2010**, *15*, 1164–1168. [CrossRef]
9. Yeung, C.; Hilton, J.; Clemons, M.; Mazzarello, S.; Hutton, B.; Haggar, F.; Addison, C.L.; Kuchuk, I.; Zhu, X.; Gelmon, K.; et al. Estrogen, progesterone, and HER2/neu receptor discordance between primary and metastatic breast tumours-a review. *Cancer Metastasis Rev.* **2016**, *35*, 427–437. [CrossRef]
10. Hochberg, R.B.; Rosner, W. Interaction of 16 alpha-[125I]iodo-estradiol with estrogen receptor and other steroid-binding proteins. *Proc. Natl. Acad. Sci. USA* **1980**, *77*, 328–332. [CrossRef]

11. Katzenellenbogen, J.A. The development of gamma-emitting hormone analogs as imaging agents for receptor-positive tumors. *Prog. Clin. Biol. Res.* **1981**, *75b*, 313–327. [PubMed]
12. Kiesewetter, D.O.; Kilbourn, M.R.; Landvatter, S.W.; Heiman, D.F.; Katzenellenbogen, J.A.; Welch, M.J. Preparation of four fluorine-18-labeled estrogens and their selective uptakes in target tissues of immature rats. *J. Nucl. Med.* **1984**, *25*, 1212–1221. [PubMed]
13. Pabst, K.M.; Decker, T.; Kersting, D.; Bartel, T.; Sraieb, M.; Herrmann, K.; Seifert, R. The Future Role of PET Imaging in Metastatic Breast Cancer. *Oncol. Res. Treat.* **2022**, *45*, 18–25. [CrossRef] [PubMed]
14. Chae, S.Y.; Ahn, S.H.; Kim, S.B.; Han, S.; Lee, S.H.; Oh, S.J.; Lee, S.J.; Kim, H.J.; Ko, B.S.; Lee, J.W.; et al. Diagnostic accuracy and safety of 16α-[(18)F]fluoro-17β-oestradiol PET-CT for the assessment of oestrogen receptor status in recurrent or metastatic lesions in patients with breast cancer: A prospective cohort study. *Lancet Oncol.* **2019**, *20*, 546–555. [CrossRef]
15. van Geel, J.J.L.; Boers, J.; Elias, S.G.; Glaudemans, A.W.; de Vries, E.F.; Hospers, G.A.; van Kruchten, M.; Kuip, E.J.; Jager, A.; Menke-van der Houven, W.C.; et al. Clinical Validity of 16α-[(18)F]Fluoro-17β-Estradiol Positron Emission Tomography/Computed Tomography to Assess Estrogen Receptor Status in Newly Diagnosed Metastatic Breast Cancer. *J. Clin. Oncol.* **2022**, Jco2200400. [CrossRef] [PubMed]
16. van Kruchten, M.; de Vries, E.G.E.; Brown, M.; de Vries, E.F.; Glaudemans, A.W.; Dierckx, R.A.; Schröder, C.P.; Hospers, G.A. PET imaging of oestrogen receptors in patients with breast cancer. *Lancet Oncol.* **2013**, *14*, e465–e475. [CrossRef]
17. van Kruchten, M.; Glaudemans, A.; de Vries, E.F.J.; Schroder, C.P.; de Vries, E.G.E.; Hospers, G.A.P. Positron emission tomography of tumour [(18)F]fluoroestradiol uptake in patients with acquired hormone-resistant metastatic breast cancer prior to oestradiol therapy. *Eur. J. Nucl. Med. Mol. Imaging* **2015**, *42*, 1674–1681. [CrossRef]
18. Choudhury, S.; Agrawal, A.; Pantvaidya, G.; Shah, S.; Purandare, N.; Puranik, A.; Rangarajan, V. Assessment of the impact of 2015 American Thyroid Association guidelines in management of differentiated thyroid cancer patients. *Eur. J. Nucl. Med. Mol. Imaging* **2020**, *47*, 547–553. [CrossRef]
19. Beauregard, J.M.; Croteau, E.; Ahmed, N.; van Lier, J.E.; Bénard, F. Assessment of human biodistribution and dosimetry of 4-fluoro-11beta-methoxy-16alpha-18F-fluoroestradiol using serial whole-body PET/CT. *J. Nucl. Med.* **2009**, *50*, 100–107. [CrossRef]
20. Lee, S.J.; Park, S.; Ahn, H.K.; Yi, J.H.; Cho, E.Y.; Sun, J.M.; Lee, J.E.; Nam, S.J.; Yang, J.H.; Park, Y.H.; et al. Implications of bone-only metastases in breast cancer: Favorable preference with excellent outcomes of hormone receptor positive breast cancer. *Cancer Res. Treat.* **2011**, *43*, 89–95. [CrossRef]
21. Peterson, L.M.; Kurland, B.F.; Link, J.M.; Schubert, E.K.; Stekhova, S.; Linden, H.M.; Mankoff, D.A. Factors influencing the uptake of 18F-fluoroestradiol in patients with estrogen receptor positive breast cancer. *Nucl. Med. Biol.* **2011**, *38*, 969–978. [CrossRef] [PubMed]
22. Arnesen, S.; Blanchard, Z.; Williams, M.M.; Berrett, K.C.; Li, Z.; Oesterreich, S.; Richer, J.K.; Gertz, J. Estrogen Receptor Alpha Mutations in Breast Cancer Cells Cause Gene Expression Changes through Constant Activity and Secondary Effects. *Cancer Res.* **2021**, *81*, 539–551. [CrossRef]
23. AlFakeeh, A.; Brezden-Masley, C. Overcoming endocrine resistance in hormone receptor-positive breast cancer. *Curr. Oncol.* **2018**, *25*, 18–27. [CrossRef] [PubMed]
24. Paydary, K.; Seraj, S.M.; Zadeh, M.Z.; Emamzadehfard, S.; Shamchi, S.P.; Gholami, S.; Werner, T.J.; Alavi, A. The Evolving Role of FDG-PET/CT in the Diagnosis, Staging, and Treatment of Breast Cancer. *Mol. Imaging Biol.* **2019**, *21*, 1–10. [CrossRef] [PubMed]
25. Bottoni, G.; Piccardo, A.; Fiz, F.; Siri, G.; Matteucci, F.; Rocca, A.; Nanni, O.; Monti, M.; Brain, E.; Alberini, J.L.; et al. Heterogeneity of bone metastases as an important prognostic factor in patients affected by oestrogen receptor-positive breast cancer. The role of combined [18F]Fluoroestradiol PET/CT and [18F]Fluorodeoxyglucose PET/CT. *Eur. J. Radiol.* **2021**, *141*, 109821. [CrossRef]
26. Piccardo, A.; Fiz, F.; Treglia, G.; Bottoni, G.; Trimboli, P. Head-to-Head Comparison between ^{18}F-FES PET/CT and ^{18}F-FDG PET/CT in Oestrogen Receptor-Positive Breast Cancer: A Systematic Review and Meta-Analysis. *J. Clin. Med.* **2022**, *11*, 1919.
27. Kurland, B.F.; Wiggins, J.R.; Coche, A.; Fontan, C.; Bouvet, Y.; Webner, P.; Divgi, C.; Linden, H.M. Whole-Body Characterization of Estrogen Receptor Status in Metastatic Breast Cancer with 16α-18F-Fluoro-17β-Estradiol Positron Emission Tomography: Meta-Analysis and Recommendations for Integration into Clinical Applications. *Oncologist* **2020**, *25*, 835–844. [CrossRef]
28. Mo, J.A. Safety and Effectiveness of F-18 Fluoroestradiol Positron Emission Tomography/Computed Tomography: A Systematic Review and Meta-analysis. *J. Korean Med. Sci.* **2021**, *36*, e271. [CrossRef]

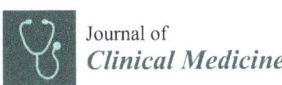

Article

Comparison between Two Different Scanners for the Evaluation of the Role of ^{18}F-FDG PET/CT Semiquantitative Parameters and Radiomics Features in the Prediction of Final Diagnosis of Thyroid Incidentalomas

Francesco Dondi [1,†], Nadia Pasinetti [2,†], Roberto Gatta [3], Domenico Albano [1,*], Raffaele Giubbini [1] and Francesco Bertagna [1]

1. Nuclear Medicine, Università degli Studi di Brescia and ASST Spedali Civili Brescia, 25123 Brescia, Italy; f.dondi@outlook.com (F.D.); raffaele.giubbini@unibs.it (R.G.); francesco.bertagna@unibs.it (F.B.)
2. Radiation Oncology Department, ASST Valcamonica Esine and Università degli Studi di Brescia, 25040 Brescia, Italy; nadia.pasinetti@unibs.it
3. Dipartimento di Scienze Cliniche e Sperimentali dell'Università degli Studi di Brescia, 25123 Brescia, Italy; roberto.gatta@unibs.it
* Correspondence: domenico.albano@unibs.it
† These authors contributed equally to this work.

Abstract: The aim of this study was to compare two different tomographs for the evaluation of the role of semiquantitative PET/CT parameters and radiomics features (RF) in the prediction of thyroid incidentalomas (TIs) at ^{18}F-FDG imaging. A total of 221 patients with the presence of TIs were retrospectively included. After volumetric segmentation of each TI, semiquantitative parameters and RF were extracted. All of the features were tested for significant differences between the two PET scanners. The performances of all of the features in predicting the nature of TIs were analyzed by testing three classes of final logistic regression predictive models, one for each tomograph and one with both scanners together. Some RF resulted significantly different between the two scanners. PET/CT semiquantitative parameters were not able to predict the final diagnosis of TIs while GLCM-related RF (in particular GLCM entropy_log2 e GLCM entropy_log10) together with some GLRLM-related and GLZLM-related features presented the best predictive performances. In particular, GLCM entropy_log2, GLCM entropy_log10, GLZLM SZHGE, GLRLM HGRE and GLRLM HGZE resulted the RF with best performances. Our study enabled the selection of some RF able to predict the final nature of TIs discovered at ^{18}F-FDG PET/CT imaging. Classic semiquantitative and volumetric PET/CT parameters did not reveal these abilities. Furthermore, a good overlap in the extraction of RF between the two scanners was underlined.

Keywords: thyroid incidentalomas; radiomics; texture analysis; ^{18}F-FDG; PET/CT; positron emission tomography; thyroid cancer

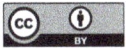

1. Introduction

Differentiated thyroid cancer (DTC) represents about 1% of all malignant tumors; moreover, it is the most frequent form of endocrine carcinoma and is usually characterized by good prognosis [1–4]. In recent years, its incidence has been growing due to the increasing use of needle aspiration and thyroid ultrasound [5–7].

The role of nuclear medicine in the diagnostic and therapeutic work-up of DTC is pivotal. In fact, nowadays, exams performed with 131I are fundamental for the staging, restaging, and the therapy of this carcinoma [4,8].

In recent years, we have been continuously experiencing an increase in the use of positron emission tomography/computed tomography (PET/CT) with ^{18}F-fluorodeoxyglucose (^{18}F-FDG) for the evaluation of various pathologies, both neoplastic and inflammatory. In this context, even in the diagnostic work-up of DTC this hybrid imaging modality has a central role, in particular in the evaluation of patients with no evidence of 131I avid disease but a persistence of elevated thyroglobulin levels [4,9,10].

With the increasing use of ^{18}F-FDG PET/CT in the clinical practice, we have also been experiencing an increase in the detection of thyroid incidentalomas (TI) [11–13]. TIs are defined as thyroid lesions detected at imaging studies performed for non-thyroid pathologies [14,15].

The precise evaluation of TIs is mandatory, given the non-negligible risk of presence of CTD in a high amount of these findings [16–18]. In this context, a lot of authors have tried to clarify the role of ^{18}F-FDG PET/CT for the definition of the precise nature of TIs, in terms of malignancy or benignancy [4]. However, the role of some PET/CT semiquantitative parameters, such as standardized uptake value (SUV), metabolic tumor volume (MTV) and total lesion glycolysis (TLG) has not yet been fully clarified and the results in literature are really heterogeneous [4].

Furthermore, in recent years we have been appreciating an increase in the extraction of specific quantitative features from PET images, called radiomics or texture analysis. In this setting, the use of radiomics for the correct evaluation of every type of incidentalomas is waking increasing interest [19,20]. The case of TIs is not an exception and some works about the use of texture analysis for their correct classification have been produced [21–24]. However, similarly to semiquantitative parameters, the use of radiomics in this setting has given non-clarifying and initial results.

The aim of this retrospective study is to evaluate the role of semiquantitative PET/CT parameters and radiomics features for the correct classification of TIs discovered at ^{18}F-FDG PET/CT scans. Furthermore, the impact of different PET/CT tomographs on texture analysis and on its ability to predict the final outcome is a fundamental part of this work.

2. Materials and Methods

2.1. Patients Selection

We retrospectively analyzed the ^{18}F-FDG PET/CT scans performed in our center between January 2012 and December 2020 in order to find presence of TIs. All of the patients performed PET/CT exams for staging or restaging purpose of various diseases, but no one had a previous history of DTC. Specifically, 82 patients suffered from lymphoma, 19 from carcinomas of the head and neck, 51 from lung cancer, 6 from fever of unknown origin, 12 from vasculitis, 38 from breast cancer, 3 from esophageal cancer, 2 from ovarian cancer, 5 from colorectal cancer and 2 from endocarditis, while 1 patient performed the examination in order to characterize a formation of the right adrenal gland.

Tis were defined as focal uptakes of ^{18}F-FDG inside the thyroid gland with an uptake higher than the background uptakes. Given the fact that diffuse uptakes on thyroid gland are usually expression of benign conditions, they were excluded from the study [4]. Furthermore, other inclusion criteria were the presence of an ultrasound follow-up of at least 1 year for suspected benignant uptakes and the execution of a cytological evaluation and/or histological examination for suspected malignant uptakes. A total of 237 patients were therefore included in the study and data about the lobe of TIs and ultrasound dimension were collected.

2.2. ^{18}F-FDG PET/CT Acquisition and Interpretation

^{18}F-FDG PET/CT scans were acquired after at least 6 h of fasting and with blood glucose levels below 150 mg/dL. An activity of 3.5–4.5 MBq/kg of ^{18}F-FDG was intravenously administrated to the patients 1 hour before images acquisition. Images were acquired from the base of the skull to the mid-thigh. All of the patients were instructed to void before the PET/CT acquisition and no type of oral or intravenous contrast agents were given for the execution of the scan. Similarly, none of the patients had performed any intestinal preparation.

In our study, we made use of 2 different PET/CT tomographs: the first (scanner 1) was a Discovery 690 PET/CT (General Electric Company-Milwaukee, WI, USA) while the second (scanner 2) was a Discovery STE PET/CT (General Electric Company, Milwaukee, WI, USA). On both of them standard acquisition parameters (CT: 80 mA, 120 Kv without contrast; 2.5–4 min per bed- PET-step, axial width 15 cm) and standard reconstruction parameters were used (256 × 256 matrix and 60 cm field of view).

Furthermore, scanner 1 was characterized by the presence of LYSO (cerium-doped lutetium yttrium oxyorthosilicate) scintillator crystals with a decay time of 45 ns, while scanner 2 had BGO (bismuth germanate) scintillator crystals with a decay time of 300 ns. Scanners were not harmonized with a cross-calibration program and all PET/CT scans were acquired at free-breath, instructing the patients to have regular breathing. For both scanners, a low dose CT at free breathing and without contrast agent was acquired in order to perform attenuation correction and for anatomical correlation. In particular, CT acquisition parameters for scanner 1 were: 120 kV, fixed tube current $\approx$ 60 mAs (40–100 mAs), 64 slices × 3.75 mm and 3.27 mm interval, pitch 0.984:1, tube rotation 0.5 s. CT acquisition parameters for scanner 2 were: 120 kV, fixed tube current $\approx$ 73 mAs (40–160 mAs), 4 slices × 3.75 mm and 3.27 mm interval, pitch 1.5:1, tube rotation 0.8 s. Furthermore, on scanner 1 time of flight (TOF) and point spread function (PSF) algorithm were used for the reconstruction of images, with filter cut-off 5 mm, 18 subsets and 3 iterations. Again, on scanner 2, an ordered subset expectation maximization (OSEM) algorithm with filter cut-off 5 mm, 21 subsets and 2 iterations were used.

PET images were visually and semiquantitatively analyzed by a nuclear physician with at least 10 years of experience, measuring parameters of TIs: the maximum standardized uptake value corrected for body weight (SUVmax), mean SUV corrected for body weight (SUVmean), maximum standardized uptake value lean body mass (SUVlbm), maximum standardized uptake value body surface area (SUVbsa), MTV and TLG. SUV-related parameters were measured on a Xeleris 3.1 GE workstation. MTV was calculated by drawing a volume of interest (VOI) on TIs on ^{18}F-FDG PET/CT images corrected for attenuation, using a SUV-based automated contouring program (Advantage Workstation 4.6, GE HealthCare) with an isocounter threshold method based on 41% of the SUVmax, as previously recommended by the European Association of Nuclear Medicine (EANM) because of its high inter-observer reproducibility [25]. TLG values were calculated as the product of the MTV of the VOI for its SUVmean.

2.3. Radiomics Features Extraction

Image features were extracted from PET images by using LIFEx 2.20 software (LIFEx, by the French Alternative Energies and Atomic Energy Commission (CEA), Gif-sur-Yvette, France) (http://www.lifexsoft.org, accessed on 10 September 2021) [26] with the same procedure previously described for SUV-related parameters extraction, with similar VOI and after a new segmentation process.

The extraction of radiomics features (RF) was performed without spatial resampling, with an intensity discretization of 64 grey levels and with a distance from neighbors of 1 voxel for the extraction of GLCM parameters.

A total of 42 RF were generated (Table 1), divided in first-order statistics (histogram-related and shape-related) and second-order statistics: grey level co-occurrence matrix (GLCM) related, grey-level run length matrix (GLRLM) related, neighborhood grey level different matrix (NGLDM) related and grey-level zone length matrix (GLZLM) related.

Table 1. List of semiquantitative parameters and of radiomics features considered in the study.

Semiquantitave Parameters
SUV-related
SUVmax
SUVmean
SUVlbm
SUVbsa
Volumetric parameters
MTV
TLG
Radiomics features
First order features
Histogram related
Histo skewness
Histo kurtosis
Histo excess kurtosis
Histo entropy_log10
Histo entropy_log2
Histo energy
Shape related
Shape volume_mL
Shape volume_vx
Shape sphericity
Shape compacity
Second order features
Grey level co-occurrence matrix (GLCM) related
GLCM homogeneity
GLCM energy
GLCM contrast
GLCM correlation
GLCM entropy_log10
GLCM entropy_log2
GLCM dissimilarity
Grey-level run length matrix (GLRLM) related
GLRLM SRE
GLRLM LRE
GLRLM LGRE
GLRLM HGRE
GLRLM SRLGE
GLRLM SRHGE
GLRLM LRLGE
GLRLM LRHGE

Table 1. Cont.

Semiquantitave Parameters
GLRLM GLNU
GLRLM RLNU
GLRLM RP
Neighborhood grey level different matrix (NGLDM) related
NGLDM coarseness
NGLDM contrast
NGLDM busyness
Grey-level zone length matrix (GLZLM) related
GLZLM SZE
GLZLM LZE
GLZLM LGZE
GLZLM HGZE
GLZLM SZLGE
GLZLM SZHGE
GLZLM LZLGE
GLZLM LZHGE
GLZLM GLNU
GLZLM ZLNU
GLZLM ZP

SUVmax: standardized uptake value body weight max; SUVmean: standardized uptake value body weight mean; SUVlbm: standardized uptake value lean body mass, SUVbsa: standardized uptake value body surface area; MTV: metabolic tumor volume; TLG: total lesion glicolysis; SRE: short-run emphasis; LRE: long-run emphasis; LGRE: Low Gray-level Run Emphasis; HGRE: High Gray-level Run Emphasis; SRLGE: Short-Run Low Gray-level Em-phasis; SRHGE: Short-Run High Gray-level Emphasis; LRLGE: Long-Run Low Gray-level Emphasis; LRHGE: Long-Run High Gray-level Emphasis; GLNU: Gray-Level Non-Uniformity; RLNU: Run Length Non-Uniformity; RP: Run Percentage; SZE: Short-zone emphasis; LZE: Long-zone emphasis; LGZE: Low Gray-level Zone Emphasis; HGZE: High Gray-level Zone Emphasis; SZLGE: Short-Zone Low Gray-level Emphasis; SZHGE: Short-Zone High Gray-level Em-phasis; LZLGE: Long-Zone Low Gray-level Emphasis; LZHGE: Long-Zone High Gray-level Emphasis; ZLNU: Zone Length Non-Uniformity. Extraction of RF by LIFEx is only possible for VOI of at least 64 voxels, therefore 16 patients were excluded from the study because the volume of the TIs uptake was below this limit. As a consequence, the final number of patients included in the study was 221.

2.4. Statistical Analysis

Statistical analysis was performed using MedCalc Software version 18.1 (8400, Ostend, Belgium) and R (http://www.R-project.org/) software version 4.1.1 (Statistics Department of the University of Auckland, Auckland, New Zealand). In the descriptive analysis, the categorical variables were represented as simple and relative frequencies, while the numeric variables with mean, standard deviation, and range values. For both scanners, the kernel density estimation built on the RF values were qualitatively compared and the presence of significant differences were evaluated with the Mann–Whitney test.

The general statistical analysis line of the study was structured of various steps. First of all, a univariate analysis (with a logistic regressor, in a 10-cross-fold validation) was performed for the group of patients evaluated on scanner 1, 1 for the group of patients of scanner 2 and 1 for the entire group of patients (scanner 1 and scanner 2 considered together). This first analysis had the purpose to evaluate the influence of the two scanners on the ability of RF to correlate with the final clinical outcome.

Furthermore, a bivariate analysis was performed with the purpose of developing 3 predictive models (1 for scanner 1, 1 for scanner 2 and 1 for both scanners considered together), by analyzing all of the possible couples of variables (the cartesian product of semiquantitative parameters, RF and the major clinical features such as age, gender and ultrasound dimension of the Tis). This bivariate analysis was performed with a bivariate logistic regression model was applied in order to classify them on the basis of the area under the curve (AUC) under the receiving operator curve (ROC) after a 10-cross fold validation training/testing test. This bivariate model had the purpose to clearly explore all the space of RF presented in the study. Similarly, for each couple of variables, the accuracy was extrapolated and to obtain a more complete statistic, the p-value were also extracted.

Lastly, a selection of the models with the best bivariate logistic regression was performed for scanner 1, scanner 2 and for both scanners considered together. In this setting an AUC higher than 0.8 was arbitrarily considered optimal to predict the final diagnosis of TIs, while an AUC between 0.6 and 0.8 was considered acceptable. Similarly, a p-value < 0.05 was arbitrarily considered as statistically significant.

3. Results
3.1. Patients Characteristics

A total of 221 patients were included in the study (Table 2), with a mean age of 66 years (range 16–88). The majority of the patients were female (n = 149, 67%) while 72 (33%) were male. No significant difference in terms of sex between the 2 groups of malignant TIs and benignant TIs was underlined (p value = 0.07).

Table 2. Characteristics of the 221 patients included in the study.

Characteristic	N. (%)
Age, mean ± SD (range)	66 ± 14 (16–88)
Sex	
Male	72 (33%)
Female	149 (67%)
Thyroid Lobe	
Right	123 (56%)
Left	87 (39%)
Isthmus	11 (5%)
Ultrasound diameter (mm), mean ± SD (range)	17 ± 12 (5–75)
Final Diagnosis	
Benign	150 (68%)
Malign	71 (32%)
Cytology (N. = 118)	
TIR2	35 (30%)
TIR3a	24 (20%)
TIR3b	30 (25%)
TIR4	13 (11%)
TIR5	16 (14%)
Histology (N. = 71)	
Anaplastic carcinoma	3 (4%)
Follicular carcinoma	7 (10%)
Papillary carcinoma	61 (86%)
PET/CT Scanner	
Scanner 1 (Discovery 690)	128 (58%)
Scanner 2 (Discovery STE)	93 (42%)

Table 2. *Cont.*

Characteristic	N. (%)
Semiquantitative PET/CT parameters	
SUVmax, mean ± SD (range)	7.9 ± 8 (1.3–56.7)
SUVmean, mean ± SD (range)	4.3 ± 4 (1.0–37.1)
SUVlbm, mean ± SD (range)	5.8 ± 6 (1.0–41.3)
SUVbsa, mean ± SD (range)	2.0 ± 2 (0.4–12.6)
MTV, mean ± SD (range)	9.2 ± 18 (0.4–198.0)
TLG, mean ± SD (range)	35.0 ± 75 (1.9–722.4)

N.: number, SD: standard deviation, mm: millimeters, SUVmax: standardized uptake value body weight max, SUVmean: standardized uptake value body mean, SUVlbm: standardized uptake value lean body mass, SUVbsa: standardized uptake value body surface area, MTV: metabolic tumor volume, TLG: total lesion glicolysis.

TIs were most frequent findings on the right thyroid lobe with 123 (56%) subjects, while in 87 (39%) the incidental uptake were discovered on the left lobe and only in 11 (5%) cases they were underlined at the isthmus. Again, the site of TIs was not significantly correlated with the final diagnosis (p value = 0.79).

The mean diameter of the TIs, evaluated on subsequent ultrasound evaluation, was of 17 mm (range 5–75).

Overall, the final diagnosis of TIs was malignant for 71 (32%) patients and benignant in 150 (68%) patients. In this setting, for the correct evaluation of their final diagnosis, 97 (44%) subjects were evaluated only with ultrasound exams, with a mean follow-up of 24 months (range 12–168). Five (2%) patients performed a ^{99m}Tc thyroid scintigraphy, that revealed the presence of an hyperfunctioning adenoma.

For 118 (53%) patients, a cytological examination for the correct diagnosis of incidental ^{18}F-FDG uptakes was performed, classifying the results according to the Italian Thyroid Cytology Classification System [27]. In particular, in 16 (14%) cases the result of the cytological examination was TIR5, in 13 (11%) it was TIR4, in 54 (45%) it was TIR3 while in 35 (30%) it was TIR2. Furthermore, of the 54 patients with a TIR3 classification, 24 (44%) had a TIR3a result while TIR3b was the final cytological result for 30 (56%) patients. A histological diagnosis of the TIs was performed in 71 (32%) cases and all of them revealed the presence of malignancy. In particular, in 3 (4%) cases the presence of anaplastic carcinoma was revealed, in 7 (10%) the presence of follicular carcinoma was underlined and in 61 (86%) there was a final diagnosis of papillary carcinoma. An evaluation of the predictive abilities of semiquantitative PET/CT parameters and of RF to predict the final cytological or histologic diagnosis was not performed because of the low sample of subjects beneath all the subgroups mentioned before.

A total of 128 (58%) scans were performed on the Discovery 690 tomograph (scanner 1), while 93 (42%) of them were acquired on the Discovery STE tomograph (scanner 2). The mean value of the SUVmax of the TIs was 7.9, it was 4.3 for SUVmean, 5.8 for SUVlbm, 2.0 for SUVbsa, 9.2 for MTV and 35.0 for TLG. (Figure 1).

Analyzing PET/CT acquisition depending on the tomograph used for their execution, in 92 (72%) scans performed on scanner 1 the incidental uptake resulted of benign nature while in 36 (28%) cases the final diagnosis was malignancy (1 anaplastic carcinoma, 4 follicular carcinomas and 31 papillary carcinomas). Regarding scanner 2, in 58 (62%) scans the final diagnosis of incidental uptake was benignancy while in 35 (38%) cases the presence of malignancy was underlined (2 anaplastic carcinomas, 3 follicular carcinomas and 30 papillary carcinomas). No significant difference in terms of final diagnosis was reported between the 2 scanners (p value = 0.1).

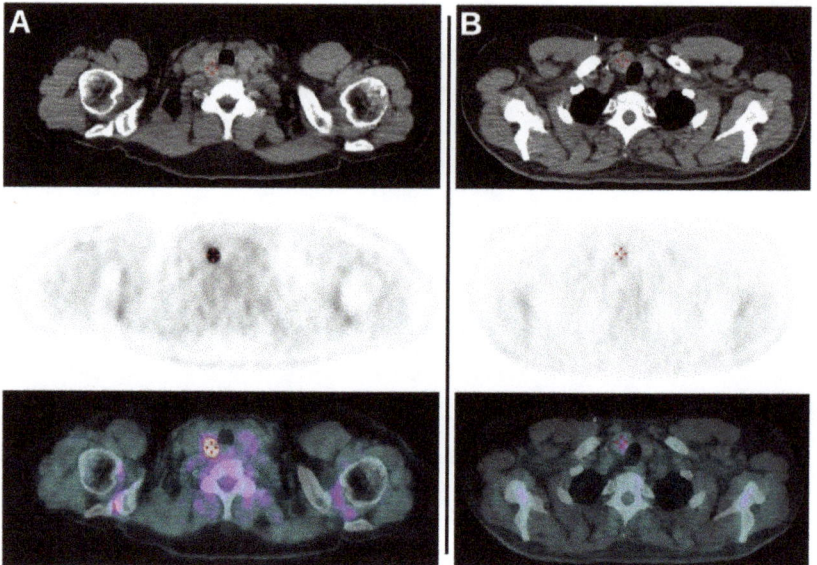

Figure 1. (**A**): Axial CT, axial PET and axial fused PET/CT images demonstrating the presence of TI revealed as intense focal uptake of ^{18}F-FDG on the right lobe of thyroid. The lesion had a SUVmax of 44.47, an MTV of 0.7 and a TLG of 18.1 and subsequent cytological exam revealed no malignancy (TIR2). (**B**): Axial CT, axial PET and axial fused PET/CT images of another scan demonstrating again the presence of TI as a faint uptake on the right lobe of thyroid. The values of SUVmax, MTV and TLG of the lesion were 2.64, 6.9 and 10.3, respectively. Cytological evaluation (TIR5) and subsequent total thyroidectomy revealed the presence of papillary carcinoma.

3.2. Comparison between the Two Scanners

The major clinical and epidemiological characteristics of the patients (age, sex, ultrasound dimension and final diagnosis of the TIs) were not significantly different between the two scanners.

Regarding semiquantitative parameters of PET/CT, only the values of SUVmax resulted significantly different between the 2 scanners (p value = 0.046), while the remaining parameters were not. In particular, the SUVmax values resulted higher on scanner 1 compared to scanner 2.

Focusing on RF, only 9 of 42 resulted in significant differences between the 2 scanners. In particular, RF with apparent correlation on the type of scanner used for the acquisition were Histo entropy_log10, Histo entropy_log2, Histo Energy, GLRLM LGRE, GLRLM SRLGE, NGLDM busyness, GLZLM SZE, GLZLM SZHGE and GLZLM ZLNU (Table 3). However, cross-correlation maps of RF between the two scanners were quite similar (Figure 2).

Table 3. Comparison of clinical parameters, semiquantitative PET/CT parameters and radiomics features between the two scanners.

Parameters		p-Value
Clinical		
	Age	0.787
	Sex	0.522
	Diameters at ultrasound	0.446

Table 3. *Cont.*

Parameters	*p*-Value
Semiquantitative PET/CT parameters	
SUVmax	0.046
SUVmean	0.118
SUVlbm	0.119
SUVbsa	0.076
MTV	0.595
TLG	0.869
Radiomics features	
Histo skewness	0.193
Histo kurtosis	0.924
Histo excess kurtosis	0.924
Histo entropy_log10	0.023
Histo entropy_log2	0.024
Histo energy	0.017
Shape volume_mL	0.211
Shape volume_vx	0.560
Shape sphericity	0.088
Shape compacity	0.518
GLCM homogeneity	0.104
GLCM energy	0.638
GLCM contrast	0.132
GLCM correlation	0.889
GLCM entropy_log10	0.319
GLCM entropy_log2	0.315
GLCM dissimilarity	0.145
GLRLM SRE	0.123
GLRLM LRE	0.113
GLRLM LGRE	0.026
GLRLM HGRE	0.069
GLRLM SRLGE	0.036
GLRLM SRHGE	0.069
GLRLM LRLGE	0.098
GLRLM LRHGE	0.135
GLRLM GLNU	0.260
GLRLM RLNU	0.962
GLRLM RP	0.126
NGLDM coarseness	0.471
NGLDM contrast	0.476
NGLDM busyness	0.006
GLZLM SZE	0.017

Table 3. Cont.

Parameters	p-Value
GLZLM LZE	0.168
GLZLM LGZE	0.053
GLZLM HGZE	0.086
GLZLM SZLGE	0.069
GLZLM SZHGE	0.041
GLZLM LZLGE	0.102
GLZLM LZHGE	0.561
GLZLM GLNU	0.366
GLZLM ZLNU	0.026
GLZLM ZP	0.093

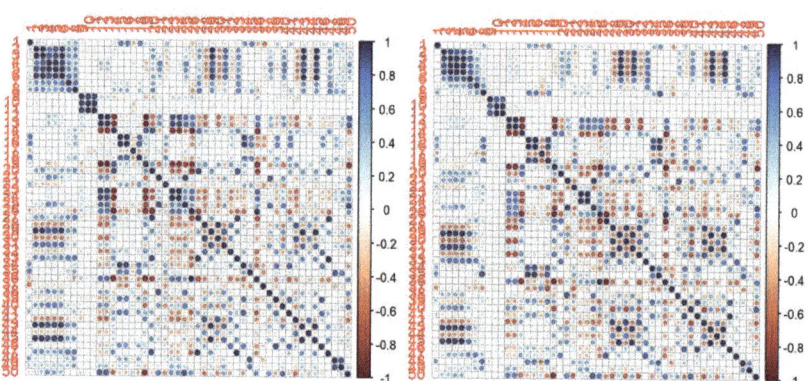

Figure 2. Correlation maps for first and second order RF between the two scanners. Scanner 1 (Discovery 690) is presented on the left, while scanner 2 (Discovery STE) is presented on the right. Blue means high positive correlation; red means high negative correlation; white means no correlation.

3.3. Predictive Accuracy

At univariate analysis (Table 4), for scanner 1 (Discovery 690) all PET/CT semiquantitative parameters and RF obtained an AUC value between 0.6 and 0.8. Regarding scanner 2 (Discovery STE), again all of the semiquantitative PET/CT parameters and RF reached a value of AUC between 0.6 and 0.8; in general, these values were lower than the those reported for scanner 1. Furthermore, the evaluation of *p*-value allowed the selection of some parameters with the best performances for the prediction of the final diagnosis of Tis, for both scanner 1 and scanner 2.

Considering the combined analysis of both the scanners together (scanner 1 + 2), in general PET/CT semiquantitative parameters revealed a higher AUC compared to RF, with significant *p*-value. Interestingly, the combined evaluation of both scanners revealed acceptable values of UAC with significant *p*-value for some RF, even if the same RF did not reach these values at the analysis for single scanner.

Table 4. Univariate analysis for semiquantitative PET/CT parameters and for radiomics features for the single scanner and for both scanners considered together. Only values with AUC > 0.6 and p-value < 0.05 are reported.

	Mean AUC			Mean p-Value		
Parameters	Scanner 1	Scanner 2	Scanner 1 + 2	Scanner 1	Scanner 2	Scanner 1 + 2
SUVmax	0.762	0.679	0.748	<0.01	0.02	<0.01
SUVmean	0.724	0.675	0.748	<0.01	<0.01	<0.01
SUVlbm	0.757	0.685	0.748	<0.01	0.01	<0.01
SUVbsa	0.756	0.689	0.742	<0.01	0.01	<0.01
Histo entropy_log10	0.709	0.674	0.724	<0.01	<0.01	<0.01
Histo entropy_log2	0.705	0.674	0.724	<0.01	<0.01	<0.01
GLCM entropy_log10	0.713	0.664	0.702	0.02	0.03	<0.01
GLCM entropy_log2	0.712	0.664	0.703	0.02	0.03	<0.01
GLCM dissimilarity	0.719	0.682	0.727	0.01	<0.01	<0.01
GLRLM HGRE	0.731	0.693	0.741	0.03	0.03	<0.01
GLRLM SRHGE	0.739	0.682	0.744	0.02	0.02	<0.01
GLRLM LRLGE	0.707	0.653	0.715	0.01	0.01	<0.01
GLZLM SZE	0.734	0.671	0.693	<0.01	<0.01	0.01
GLZLM HGZE	0.740	0.668	0.740	0.02	0.03	<0.01
GLZLM SZHGE	0.758	0.693	0.733	0.02	0.03	<0.01
GLZLM ZP	0.692	0.669	0.699	<0.01	0.01	<0.01
Variables with good performances only at Scanner 1 + 2 analysis						
GLCM contrast			0.733			0.01
GLZLM ZLNU			0.729			0.04
GLRLM LRLGE			0.715			<0.01
GLZLM LGZE			0.706			<0.01
GLRLM LGRE			0.703			<0.01
GLCM homogeneity			0.702			<0.01
GLRLM SRLGE			0.687			<0.01
NGLDM busyness			0.684			0.01
GLRLM RP			0.660			0.04
GLZLM SZLGE			0.651			<0.01

AUC: area under the curve.

After performing a bivariate analysis, for both the single scanners and for both of the scanners considered together, the best combinations between PET/CT semiquantitative parameters and RF are summarized in Table 5. Similarly to univariate analysis, none of the combinations reached an optimal AUC of 0.8 and the couples of parameters generally obtained higher AUC values on scanner 1 than on scanner 2. Furthermore, for this analysis, the p-values were statistically more significant on scanner 1 than on scanner 2. In this setting, even if a comparison between the couples of variables obtained before is complex given the heterogeneity between the two scanners, in general GLCM-related parameters variously combined resulted the ones with best performances. This is true for both scanner 1 and scanner 2 and these findings are confirmed by the good results at univariate analysis previously described. The GLRLM-related and GLZLM-related RF also revealed good performances in this setting. Interestingly, PET/CT semiquantitative parameters were confirmed as good predictors only for scanner 2 (Figure 3).

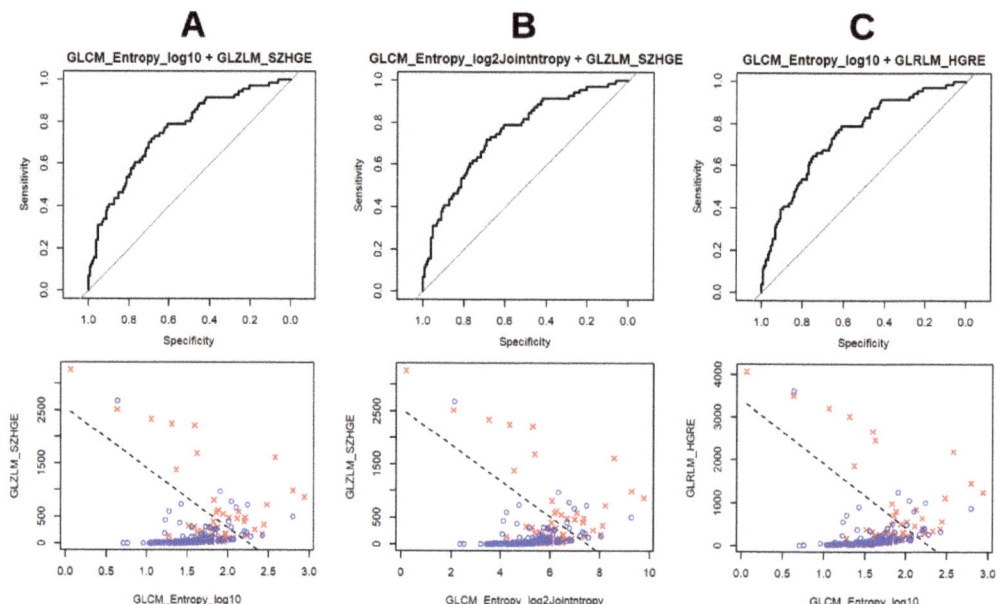

Figure 3. Visual representations of the three combinations ((**A**) GLCM Entropy_log10+GLZLM_SZHGE, (**B**) GLCM Entropy_log2+GLZLM:SZHGE; (**C**) GLCM Entropy_lo10+GLRLM_HGRE) with best performances at bivariate analysis for both scanners considered together.

Table 5. Bivariate analysis for clinical, semiquantitative PET/CT parameters and radiomics features for the single scanner and for both scanners considered together. For each analysis, only the couples with best performances are reported.

Covariate 1	Covariate 2	Mean *p*-Value 1	Mean *p*-Value 2	Mean AUC
		Scanner 1		
GLZLM GLNU	MTV	<0.01	0.01	0.779
GLRLM RLNU	MTV	0.02	0.03	0.776
GLCM energy	GLCM entropy_log2	0.04	<0.01	0.771
GLCM energy	GLCM entropy_log10	0.04	<0.01	0.771
GLCM entropy_log2	GLRLM HGRE	0.01	0.03	0.763
GLCM entropy_log10	GLZLM HGZE	0.02	0.02	0.762
GLCM entropy_log10	GLRLM HGRE	0.01	0.03	0.761
GLCM entropy_log2	GLZLM HGZE	0.02	0.02	0.760
GLCM entropy_log10	GLZLM SZHGE	0.01	0.02	0.760
GLCM entropy_log2	GLZLM SZHGE	0.01	0.02	0.759
GLRLM RP	GLZLM SZHGE	0.04	0.02	0.751
GLRLM HGRE	GLRLM RP	0.02	0.03	0.745
MTV	TLG	<0.01	0.01	0.741

Table 5. Cont.

Covariate 1	Covariate 2	Mean *p*-Value 1	Mean *p*-Value 2	Mean AUC
GLRLM SRE	GLZLM HGZE	0.03	0.01	0.740
NGLDM coarseness	NGLDM busyness	<0.01	0.01	0.738
Shape volume_mL	GLRLM GLNU	0.03	0.01	0.736
GLRLM GLNU	NGLDM coarseness	0.03	<0.01	0.734
GLRLM SRE	GLZLM SZHGE	0.03	0.02	0.732
GLRLM SRE	GLRLM HGRE	0.03	0.02	0.730
GLRLM LRLGE	NGLDM coarseness	<0.01	0.04	0.730
Shape volume_vx	GLRLM GLNU	0.02	0.02	0.723
GLCM entropy_log10	GLZLM SZHGE	0.04	<0.01	0.713
Shape compacity	GLZLM GLNU	0.01	<0.01	0.707
Shape volume_mL	MTV	0.02	0.02	0.693
Ultrasound dimension	MTV	0.01	0.02	0.691
GLCM correlation	NGLDM coarseness	<0.01	<0.01	0.690
Shape compacity	NGLDM coarseness	0.03	0.01	0.680
Ultrasound dimension	GLRLM GLNU	0.01	0.01	0.677
Scanner 2				
GLRLM SRE	SUVmean	0.04	0.01	0.712
GLCM entropy_log10	SUVbsa	0.05	0.01	0.697
GLCM entropy_log2	SUVbsa	0.05	0.02	0.696
GLCM entropy_log2	GLZLM SZHGE	0.03	0.02	0.689
GLCM entropy_log10	GLZLM SZHGE	0.03	0.02	0.689
GLRLM RP	SUVmean	0.05	0.02	0.686
GLCM entropy_log2	GLZLM HGZE	0.05	0.02	0.682
GLCM entropy_log10	GLZLM HGZE	0.05	0.02	0.680
GLCM entropy_log10	GLRLM HGRE	0.04	0.02	0.679
GLCM energy	GLRLM LRHGE	0.01	0.02	0.679
GLCM entropy_log2	GLRLM HGRE	0.04	0.02	0.679
NGLDM coarseness	GLZLM ZP	0.03	<0.01	0.677
Histo energy	GLRLM HGRE	0.04	0.03	0.676
GLCM homogeneity	NGLDM coarseness	<0.01	0.06	0.675
GLCM contrast	GLCM entropy_log10	0.04	0.04	0.673
GLCM contrast	GLCM entropy_log2	0.04	0.04	0.673
Histo energy	GLZLM SZHGE	0.04	0.03	0.669
GLRLM SRE	GLRLM HGRE	0.04	0.03	0.669
GLRLM SRE	NGLDM coarseness	0.01	0.05	0.668
GLRLM LRE	SUVmean	0.04	0.01	0.668
NGLDM coarseness	NGLDM busyness	0.02	0.02	0.666
GLZLM GLNU	MTV	0.02	0.02	0.663
GLCM energy	GLZLM SZHGE	0.06	<0.01	0.660
GLCM energy	GLRLM HGRE	0.06	<0.01	0.659

Table 5. *Cont.*

Covariate 1	Covariate 2	Mean *p*-Value 1	Mean *p*-Value 2	Mean AUC
GLRLM RP	NGLDM coarseness	0.01	0.05	0.657
GLRLM RLNU	MTV	0.01	0.01	0.650
NGLDM coarseness	MTV	0.04	0.03	0.627
Scanner 1 + 2				
GLCM entropy_log2	GLZLM SZHGE	<0.01	<0.01	0.769
GLCM entropy_log10	GLRLM HGRE	<0.01	<0.01	0.769
GLCM entropy_log10	GLZLM SZHGE	<0.01	<0.01	0.769
GLCM entropy_log10	GLZLM HGZE	<0.01	<0.01	0.769
GLCM entropy_log2	GLRLM HGRE	<0.01	<0.01	0.768
GLCM entropy_log2	GLZLM HGZE	<0.01	<0.01	0.768
GLRLM SRE	SUVmean	<0.01	<0.01	0.763
GLRLM GLNU	NGLDM Coarseness	<0.01	<0.01	0.756
GLCM homogeneity	GLRLM HGRE	<0.01	<0.01	0.749
GLCM homogeneity	GLZLM HGZE	<0.01	<0.01	0.749
Histo energy	GLRLM HGRE	<0.01	<0.01	0.749
Histo energyUniformity	GLZLM SZHGE	<0.01	<0.01	0.748
GLCM homogeneity	GLZLM SZHGE	<0.01	<0.01	0.748
NGLDM coarseness	NGLDM busyness	<0.01	<0.01	0.746
GLRLM SRE	GLRLM HGRE	<0.01	<0.01	0.742
GLRLM RP	GLZLM HGZE	<0.01	<0.01	0.742
GLRLM SRE	GLZLM HGZE	<0.01	<0.01	0.742
GLRLM HGRE	GLRLM RP	<0.01	<0.01	0.742
NGLDM coarseness	GLZLM ZP	<0.01	<0.01	0.741
GLZLM GLNU	MTV	<0.01	<0.01	0.738
GLRLM SRE	GLZLM SZHGE	<0.01	<0.01	0.738
GLRLM RP	GLZLM SZHGE	<0.01	<0.01	0.737
GLRLM LRE	GLRLM LRHGE	<0.01	<0.01	0.737
GLRLM RLNU	MTV	<0.01	<0.01	0.730
Histo energy	GLCM energy	<0.01	<0.01	0.717
Shape compacity	NGLDM coarseness	<0.01	<0.01	0.681
GLCM correlation	NGLDM coarseness	<0.01	<0.01	0.654
Shape compacity	GLZLM GLNU	<0.01	<0.01	0.640

AUC: area under the curve.

4. Discussion

The aim of this study was to verify the predictive abilities of semiquantitative PET/CT parameters and of RF to discriminate between benignant and malignant nature of TIs revealed at ^{18}F-FDG imaging.

On the basis of the resulting evidence we identified some remarkable points concerning the effect of different PET scanners on RF extraction and the predictive features and associated models.

In our experimental setting, we had to deal with images coming from different PET/CT tomographs and this fact required a preliminary investigation of the effect of different technologies in producing images and subsequent image features. The results showed that the scanner technology concretely affects some RF, as previously underlined in literature, and in clinical day practice the use of different tomographs in the same department is frequent [20,28–34]. In particular, the acquisition of the same phantoms on different tomographs with different scintillators and algorithm used for the reconstruction (number of iterations, number of subsets or on the presence of partial volume correction) demonstrated this evidence.

These findings suggest two relevant points: the former indicates that different scanners can potentially have different preferred features in terms of correlations with a clinical outcome; the second point suggests that we must critically consider radiomics models coming from centers adopting different technologies. In other words, on one hand a unique radiomic best model trained on many scanners is probably suboptimal for each of them and on the other hand, any radiomic model coming from different centers should be internally validated before considering its use in the daily practice. In particular, in the literature only one study which evaluated the predictive role of RF in TIs [23] used different scanners for the extraction of RF: this means that the reproducibility of the results (which is one of the biggest challenges in radiomics) still remain uninvestigated in this field. Furthermore, in our evaluation, only a small amount of RF demonstrated to be significantly different between the two scanners, together with SUVmax, but nevertheless the cross-correlation maps resulted quite similar, adding value to our results. In this setting, of the parameters that after bivariate analysis demonstrated the best performances, GLZLM SZHGE was the only one significantly different between the two scanners.

Regarding the predictive role of RF for the correct evaluation of TIs, at univariate and bivariate analysis a good percentage of the aforementioned parameters revealed an acceptable AUC between 0.6 and 0.8. However, none of them demonstrated an AUC above 0.8. Similarly, these AUC were coupled with a significant p-value in a high percentage of the cases. It is worth underlining the fact that at bivariate analysis performed for both the scanner considered together, the AUC values and the p-values were the best in the whole study. This fact underlines a good predictive ability of some RF such as GLCM-related (in particular GLCM entropy_log2 e GLCM entropy_log10), GLRLM-related and GLZLM-related.

Only a small amount of works that investigate the predictive role of radiomics in the evaluation of TIs at ^{18}F-FDG PET/CT are available in literature [21–24].

Even if not clearly characterized by the presence of a proper texture analysis, the first study to evaluate the distributive heterogeneity of ^{18}F-FDG in TIs was produced by Kim et al. [24]. In this work, the authors revealed that this heterogeneity was a promising parameter which was able to predict the final nature of these TIs.

Subsequently, Sollini et al. [23] were the first to evaluate the predictive abilities of texture analysis in this setting. Data of this study underlined the fact that SUVstd (the standard deviation of the distribution of SUV inside the considered VOI), SUVmax, MTV, TLG, Histo skewness, Histo kurtosis and GLCM correlation were the only parameters that were able to predict the final diagnosis of TIs, with a general positive predictive value of 54% and a general negative predictive value of 85%.

A similar analysis was also performed by Aksu et al. [22], who underlined how the semiquantitative PET/CT parameters and some shape-related, GLCM-related, GLRLM-related and GLZLM-related RF obtained AUC values superior to 0.7. These findings were partially confirmed in our study, where the same parameters confirmed these good results, with the exception of semiquantitative parameters and shape-related RF. Furthermore, the authors of the study developed a machine-learning algorithm using GLRLM RLNU e SUVmax with a good general AUC value (0.731).

Lastly, Ceriani et al. [21] demonstrated the ability to predict the final nature of TIs of some PET/CT semiquantitative parameters (SUVmax, SUVmean, SUVpeak, MTV e TLG) and some RF. In this case, the authors performed texture analysis with a different software from LIFEx and so RF resulted partly different in comparison to the ones used in our study. In general, some shape-related and GLCM-related features demonstrated good performances and multivariate analysis confirmed TLG, SUVmax and Shape sphericity as able to predict the final nature of TIs.

It is interesting to underline that PET/CT semiquantitative parameters resulted good predictors in all of the studies, while in our work only SUVmean obtained a certain predictive role at bivariate analysis. In this setting, we reported that AUC of semiquantitative parameters were quite similar to AUC of RF only at monovariate analysis. Given the fact that the bivariate predictive model did not confirm this evidence, we can assume that these parameters do not perform well when trying to build models with multiple variables as in our case. Furthermore, as previously described, data in literature about the role of these parameters for the assessment of TIs are really heterogeneous and our findings confirm these insights. Moreover, RF describe quality and parameters of images that cannot be visually assessed and this is why we focused our attention on the evaluation of these features, allowing us to better understand the role of ^{18}F-FDG PET/CT in the prediction of TIs nature.

Our study surely presents some limitations. First of all, this is a retrospective study with the use of tomography that are not the actual state. Furthermore, the relatively low sample of patients included in the work, even if higher than similar studies, appears sub-optimal to clearly evaluate the predictive abilities of texture analysis. Furthermore, RF extrapolation with a single software appears another limit of our analysis. Lastly, the aforementioned problem of the reproducibility of radiomics analysis in terms of multicentric evaluation is still an open issue and, in this setting, further research in this field are mandatory.

5. Conclusions

In conclusion, our study enabled the selection of some RF that are able to predict with a certain good accuracy, the final nature of TIs discovered at ^{18}F-FDG PET/CT imaging. Classic semiquantitative and volumetric PET/CT parameters did not reveal this ability. Furthermore, a good overlap in the extraction of RF between the two scanners was underlined.

Author Contributions: Conceptualization, F.D., R.G. (Roberto Gattaand) and D.A.; methodology, R.G. (Raffaele Giubbini) and N.P.; formal analysis, F.D. and R.G. (Roberto Gattaand); writing—original draft preparation, F.D., D.A. and R.G. (Raffaele Giubbini); writing—review and editing, N.P. and F.B. All authors have read and agreed to the published version of the manuscript.

Funding: This research received no external funding.

Institutional Review Board Statement: Ethical review and approval were waived for this study due to the retrospective design of the study according to the local laws.

Informed Consent Statement: Informed consent was obtained from all subjects involved in the study.

Data Availability Statement: Data are not public, but are present in our institution.

Conflicts of Interest: The authors declare no conflict of interest.

References

1. DeGroot, L.J.; Kaplan, E.L.; McCormick, M.; Straus, F.H. Natural history, treatment, and course of papillary thyroid carcinoma. *J. Clin. Endocrinol. Metab.* **1990**, *71*, 414–424. [CrossRef] [PubMed]
2. Schlumberger, M.J. Papillary and follicular thyroid carcinoma. *N. Engl. J. Med.* **1998**, *338*, 297–306. [CrossRef] [PubMed]
3. Stokkel, M.P.; Duchateau, C.S.; Dragoiescu, C. The value of FDG-PET in the follow-up of differentiated thyroid cancer: A review of the literature. *Q. J. Nucl. Med. Mol. Imaging* **2006**, *50*, 78–87. [PubMed]
4. Bertagna, F.; Treglia, G.; Piccardo, A.; Giubbini, R. Diagnostic and clinical significance of F-18-FDG-PET/CT thyroid incidentalomas. *J. Clin. Endocrinol. Metab.* **2012**, *97*, 3866–3875. [CrossRef] [PubMed]
5. Filetti, S.; Durante, C.; Hartl, D.; Leboulleux, S.; Locati, L.D.; Newbold, K.; Papotti, M.G.; Berruti, A.; ESMO Guidelines Committee. Thyroid cancer: ESMO Clinical Practice Guidelines for diagnosis, treatment and follow-up. *Ann. Oncol.* **2019**, *30*, 1856–1883. [CrossRef] [PubMed]

6. Vaccarella, S.; Franceschi, S.; Bray, F.; Wild, C.P.; Plummer, M.; Dal Maso, L. Worldwide Thyroid-Cancer Epidemic? The Increasing Impact of Overdiagnosis. *N. Engl. J. Med.* **2016**, *375*, 614–617. [CrossRef] [PubMed]
7. Haugen, B.R.; Alexander, E.K.; Bible, K.C.; Doherty, G.M.; Mandel, S.J.; Nikiforov, Y.E.; Pacini, F.; Randolph, G.W.; Sawka, A.M.; Schlumberger, M.; et al. 2015 American Thyroid Association Management Guidelines for Adult Patients with Thyroid Nodules and Differentiated Thyroid Cancer: The American Thyroid Association Guidelines Task Force on Thyroid Nodules and Differentiated Thyroid Cancer. *Thyroid* **2016**, *26*, 1–133. [CrossRef]
8. Luster, M.; Clarke, S.E.; Dietlein, M.; Lassmann, M.; Lind, P.; Oyen, W.J.; Tennvall, J.; Bombardieri, E. European Association of Nuclear Medicine (EANM). Guidelines for radioiodine therapy of differentiated thyroid cancer. *Eur. J. Nucl. Med. Mol. Imaging* **2008**, *35*, 1941–1959. [CrossRef]
9. Bertagna, F.; Bosio, G.; Biasiotto, G.; Rodella, C.; Puta, E.; Gabanelli, S.; Lucchini, S.; Merli, G.; Savelli, G.; Giubbini, R.; et al. F-18 FDG-PET/CT evaluation of patients with differentiated thyroid cancer with negative I-131 total body scan and high thyroglobulin level. *Clin. Nucl. Med.* **2009**, *34*, 756–761. [CrossRef]
10. Dong, M.J.; Liu, Z.F.; Zhao, K.; Ruan, L.X.; Wang, G.L.; Yang, S.Y.; Sun, F.; Luo, X.G. Value of ^{18}F-FDG-PET/PET-CT in differentiated thyroid carcinoma with radioiodine-negative whole-body scan: A meta-analysis. *Nucl. Med. Commun.* **2009**, *30*, 639–650. [CrossRef]
11. Elzein, S.; Ahmed, A.; Lorenz, E.; Balasubramanian, S.P. Thyroid incidentalomas on PET imaging—Evaluation of management and clinical outcomes. *Surgeon* **2015**, *13*, 116–120. [CrossRef] [PubMed]
12. Bomanji, J.B.; Costa, D.C.; Ell, P.J. Clinical role of positron emission tomography in oncology. *Lancet Oncol.* **2001**, *2*, 157–164. [CrossRef]
13. Chen, Y.K.; Ding, H.J.; Chen, K.T.; Chen, Y.L.; Liao, A.C.; Shen, Y.Y.; Su, C.T.; Kao, C.H. Prevalence and risk of cancer of focal thyroid incidentaloma identified by 18F-fluorodeoxyglucose positron emission tomography for cancer screening in healthy subjects. *Anticancer Res.* **2005**, *25*, 1421–1426. [PubMed]
14. Shi, H.; Yuan, Z.; Yuan, Z.; Yang, C.; Zhang, J.; Shou, Y.; Zhang, W.; Ping, Z.; Gao, X.; Liu, S. Diagnostic Value of Volume-Based Fluorine-18-Fluorodeoxyglucose PET/CT Parameters for Characterizing Thyroid Incidentaloma. *Korean J. Radiol.* **2018**, *19*, 342–351. [CrossRef] [PubMed]
15. Burguera, B.; Gharib, H. Thyroid incidentalomas. Prevalence, diagnosis, significance, and management. *Endocrinol. Metab. Clin. N. Am.* **2000**, *29*, 187–203. [CrossRef]
16. Are, C.; Hsu, J.F.; Schoder, H.; Shah, J.P.; Larson, S.M.; Shaha, A.R. FDG-PET detected thyroid incidentalomas: Need for further investigation? *Ann. Surg. Oncol.* **2007**, *14*, 239–247. [CrossRef]
17. Kim, T.Y.; Kim, W.B.; Ryu, J.S.; Gong, G.; Hong, S.J.; Shong, Y.K. ^{18}F-fluorodeoxyglucose uptake in thyroid from positron emission tomogram (PET) for evaluation in cancer patients: High prevalence of malignancy in thyroid PET incidentaloma. *Laryngoscope* **2005**, *115*, 1074–1078. [CrossRef]
18. Kim, B.H.; Na, M.A.; Kim, I.J.; Kim, S.J.; Kim, Y.K. Risk stratification and prediction of cancer of focal thyroid fluorodeoxyglucose uptake during cancer evaluation. *Ann. Nucl. Med.* **2010**, *24*, 721–728. [CrossRef]
19. Wilson, R.; Devaraj, A. Radiomics of pulmonary nodules and lung cancer. *Transl. Lung Cancer Res.* **2017**, *6*, 86–91. [CrossRef]
20. Albano, D.; Gatta, R.; Marini, M.; Rodella, C.; Camoni, L.; Dondi, F.; Giubbini, R.; Bertagna, F. Role of ^{18}F-FDG PET/CT Radiomics Features in the Differential Diagnosis of Solitary Pulmonary Nodules: Diagnostic Accuracy and Comparison between Two Different PET/CT Scanners. *J. Clin. Med.* **2021**, *10*, 5064. [CrossRef]
21. Ceriani, L.; Milan, L.; Virili, C.; Cascione, L.; Paone, G.; Trimboli, P.; Giovanella, L. Radiomics Analysis of [^{18}F]-Fluorodeoxyglucose-Avid Thyroid Incidentalomas Improves Risk Stratification and Selection for Clinical Assessment. *Thyroid* **2021**, *31*, 88–95. [CrossRef] [PubMed]
22. Aksu, A.; Şen, N.P.K.; Acar, E.; Kaya, G.Ç. Evaluating Focal ^{18}F-FDG Uptake in Thyroid Gland with Radiomics. *Nucl. Med. Mol. Imaging* **2020**, *54*, 241–248. [CrossRef] [PubMed]
23. Sollini, M.; Cozzi, L.; Pepe, G.; Antunovic, L.; Lania, A.; Di Tommaso, L.; Magnoni, P.; Erba, P.A.; Kirienko, M. [^{18}F]FDG-PET/CT texture analysis in thyroid incidentalomas: Preliminary results. *Eur. J. Hybrid Imaging* **2017**, *1*, 3. [CrossRef] [PubMed]
24. Kim, S.J.; Chang, S. Predictive value of intratumoral heterogeneity of F-18 FDG uptake for characterization of thyroid nodules according to Bethesda categories of fine needle aspiration biopsy results. *Endocrine* **2015**, *50*, 681–688. [CrossRef]
25. Boellaard, R.; Delgado-Bolton, R.; Oyen, W.J.; Giammarile, F.; Tatsch, K.; Eschner, W.; Verzijlbergen, F.J.; Barrington, S.F.; Pike, L.C.; Weber, W.A.; et al. FDG PET/CT: EANM procedure guidelines for tumour imaging: Version 2.0. *Eur. J. Nucl. Med. Mol. Imaging* **2014**, *42*, 328–354. [CrossRef]
26. Nioche, C.; Orlhac, F.; Boughdad, S.; Reuzè, S.; Goya-Outi, J.; Robert, C.; Pellot-Barakat, C.; Soussan, M.; Frouin, F.; Buvat, I. LIFEx: A Freeware for Radiomic Feature Calculation in Multimodality Imaging to Accelerate Advances in the Characterization of Tumor Heterogeneity. *Cancer Res.* **2018**, *78*, 4786–4789. [CrossRef]
27. Nardi, F.; Basolo, F.; Crescenzi, A.; Fadda, G.; Frasoldati, A.; Orlandi, F.; Palombini, L.; Papini, E.; Zini, M.; Pontecorvi, A.; et al. Italian consensus for the classification and reporting of thyroid cytology. *J. Endocrinol. Investig.* **2014**, *37*, 593–599. [CrossRef]
28. Reynes-Llompart, G.; Sabatè-Llobera, A.; Linares-Tello, E.; Martì-Climent, J.; Gamez-Cenzano, C. Image quality evaluation in a modern PET system: Impact of new reconstructions methods and a radiomics approach. *Sci. Rep.* **2019**, *9*, 10640. [CrossRef]
29. Ha, S.; Choi, H.; Paeng, J.C.; Cheon, G.J. Radiomics in Oncological PET/CT: A Methodological Overview. *Nucl. Med. Mol. Imaging* **2019**, *53*, 14–29. [CrossRef]

30. Lodge, M.A. Repeatability of SUV in Oncologic ^{18}F-FDG PET. *J. Nucl. Med.* **2017**, *58*, 523–532. [CrossRef]
31. Cook, G.J.R.; Azad, G.; Owczarczyk, K.; Siddique, M.; Goh, V. Challenges and Promises of PET Radiomics. *Int. J. Radiat. Oncol. Biol. Phys.* **2018**, *102*, 1083–1089. [CrossRef] [PubMed]
32. Zwanenburg, A. Radiomics in nuclear medicine: Robustness, reproducibility, standardization, and how to avoid data analysis traps and replication crisis. *Eur. J. Nucl. Med. Mol. Imaging* **2019**, *46*, 2638–2655. [CrossRef] [PubMed]
33. Lovinfosse, P.; Visvikis, D.; Hustinx, R.; Hatt, M. FDG PET radiomics: A review of the methodological aspects. *Clin. Transl. Imaging* **2018**, *6*, 379–391. [CrossRef]
34. Pfaehler, E.; van Sluis, J.; Merema, B.B.J.; van Ooijen, P.; Berendsen, R.C.M.; van Velden, F.H.P.; Boellaard, R. Experimental Multicenter and Multivendor Evaluation of the Performance of PET Radiomic Features Using 3-Dimensionally Printed Phantom Inserts. *J. Nucl. Med.* **2020**, *61*, 469–476. [CrossRef]

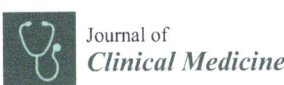

Article

A Prospective Investigation of Tumor Hypoxia Imaging with ^{68}Ga-Nitroimidazole PET/CT in Patients with Carcinoma of the Cervix Uteri and Comparison with ^{18}F-FDG PET/CT: Correlation with Immunohistochemistry

Kgomotso M. G. Mokoala [1], Ismaheel O. Lawal [1,2], Letjie C. Maserumule [1], Khanyisile N. Hlongwa [1], Honest Ndlovu [1], Janet Reed [1], Meshack Bida [3], Alex Maes [1,4], Christophe van de Wiele [1,5], Johncy Mahapane [1], Cindy Davis [1], Jae Min Jeong [6,7], Gbenga Popoola [8], Mariza Vorster [1,2] and Mike M. Sathekge [1,2,*]

1. Department of Nuclear Medicine, University of Pretoria, Pretoria 0001, South Africa; kgomotso.mokoala@up.ac.za (K.M.G.M.); ismaheellawal@gmail.com (I.O.L.); letjie.maserumule@gmail.com (L.C.M.); khanyi29@gmail.com (K.N.H.); ndlovuhonest@gmail.com (H.N.); drjanreed@gmail.com (J.R.); alex.maes@azgroeninge.be (A.M.); cvdwiele@hotmail.com (C.v.d.W.); jkmahapane@gmail.com (J.M.); sbahtherapy@gmail.com (C.D.); marizavorster@gmail.com (M.V.)
2. Nuclear Medicine Research Infrastructure (NuMeRI), Steve Biko Academic Hospital, Pretoria 0001, South Africa
3. Department of Anatomical Pathology, National Health Laboratory Services, Pretoria 0001, South Africa; meshack.bida@nhls.ac.za
4. Department of Nuclear Medicine, Katholieke University Leuven, 8500 Kortrijk, Belgium
5. Department of Radiology and Nuclear Medicine, University of Ghent, 9000 Ghent, Belgium
6. Radiation Applied Life Sciences, Department of Nuclear Medicine, Institute of Radiation Medicine, Seoul National University College of Medicine, Seoul 03080, Korea; jmjng@snu.ac.kr
7. Cancer Research Institute, Seoul National University College of Medicine, Seoul 03080, Korea
8. Department of Epidemiology and Community Health, University of Ilorin, Ilorin 240102, Nigeria; g.popoola45@gmail.com
* Correspondence: mike.sathekge@up.ac.za

Abstract: Hypoxia in cervical cancer has been associated with a poor prognosis. Over the years ^{68}Ga labelled nitroimidazoles have been studied and have shown improved kinetics. We present our initial experience of hypoxia Positron Emission Tomography (PET) imaging in cervical cancer with ^{68}Ga-Nitroimidazole derivative and the correlation with ^{18}F-FDG PET/CT and immunohistochemistry. Twenty women with cervical cancer underwent both ^{18}F-FDG and ^{68}Ga-Nitroimidazole PET/CT imaging. Dual-point imaging was performed for ^{68}Ga-Nitroimidazole PET. Immunohistochemical analysis was performed with hypoxia inducible factor-1α (HIF-1α). We documented SUVmax, SUVmean of the primary lesions as well as tumor to muscle ratio (TMR), tumor to blood (TBR), metabolic tumor volume (MTV) and hypoxic tumor volume (HTV). There was no significant difference in the uptake of ^{68}Ga-Nitroimidazole between early and delayed imaging. Twelve patients had uptake on ^{68}Ga-Nitroimidazole PET. Ten patients demonstrated varying intensities of HIF-1α expression and six of these also had uptake on ^{68}Ga-Nitroimidazole PET. We found a strong negative correlation between HTV and immunohistochemical staining (r = −0.660; p = 0.019). There was no correlation between uptake on PET imaging and immunohistochemical analysis with HIF-1α. Two-thirds of the patients demonstrated hypoxia on ^{68}Ga-Nitroimidazole PET imaging.

Keywords: cervical cancer; hypoxia; ^{68}Ga-Nitroimidazole; ^{18}F-FDG; HIF-1α; immunohistochemistry

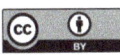

1. Introduction

Despite widespread awareness programs and improvements in screening, cervical cancer continues to be a major cause of morbidity and mortality amongst women in low- and middle-income states [1]. Some of the challenges related to the management include late presentation, access to treatment and poor response to therapy [2,3]. Hypoxia is a common phenomenon linked to resistance to most forms of therapy in various malignancies including cervical cancer [4–7]. Hypoxia refers to a state of sub-physiological levels of tissue oxygen that develops due to excessive tumor growth which outgrows its blood supply and the inability of the new impaired blood vessels to keep up with the demand [8,9]. The presence or absence of hypoxia has therapeutic and prognostic implications.

Strategies to overcome hypoxia have been the subject of investigations over the years as treatment becomes more personalized. Several methods have been implemented to try and overcome hypoxia including intensity modulated radiation therapy (IMRT) which is closely linked to dose-painting, and hypoxia sensitizing drugs [10,11]. Due to the high costs and side effects of some of these therapies, it is vital to select patients that will likely benefit from these additional therapies. Therefore, detection of hypoxia in cancer lesions may help aid treatment planning.

The Eppendorf probe is considered the gold standard for hypoxia detection, however there are many reasons that have seen it fall out of favor. The analysis of genes and molecular markers that are upregulated in hypoxic states is another strategy to assess for hypoxia. These markers include hypoxia inducible factor 1 alpha (HIF-1α), vascular endothelial growth factor (VEGF) and carbonic anhydrase IX (CAIX), to name a few [12]. Other non-invasive methods have been sought and by far positron emission tomography (PET) imaging has been the most widely investigated. Fluorinated nitroimidazole derivates, specifically ^{18}F-FMISO, were among the first tracers to be investigated for hypoxia imaging and are by far the most robust [13]. Due to its inherent limitations (slow tracer kinetics and non-specific washout) second and third generation nitroimidazole compounds such as ^{18}F-FAZA, ^{18}F-FETNIM and ^{18}F-HX4 were developed [14–16]. The $^{60/64}$Cu-ATSM radionuclides were also developed and investigated as hypoxia markers [17]. The feasibility of all these tracers for hypoxia imaging in cervical cancers has been demonstrated, however some of them are not widely available. While imaging with the ^{18}F-FDG plays a major role in oncology for staging and therapy planning, several studies have demonstrated that its role in imaging hypoxia is limited.

The chemistry of ^{68}Ga makes for easy labelling with several peptides and molecules. With the increase in availability of the ^{68}Ga generator this makes the ^{68}Ga-labelled nitroimidazole derivatives attractive because ^{68}Ga is available from a generator with a shelf life of almost a year [18]. The pre-clinical work on these tracers have demonstrated the feasibility of imaging hypoxia [19–23]. In these studies, ^{68}Ga-Nitroimidazole compounds were more hydrophilic than the ^{18}F-labelled radiotracers and were selectively taken up in hypoxic areas [24]. The aim of this paper was to investigate the feasibility of PET imaging of hypoxia with ^{68}Ga-Nitroimidazole in cervical cancer lesions and to correlate imaging findings to findings on ^{18}F-FDG PET/CT as well as immunohistochemical staining for HIF-1α.

2. Materials and Methods

2.1. Patients

Twenty women with histologically confirmed locally advanced cervical cancer were prospectively recruited into the study. The patients were enrolled consecutively from January 2020 to November 2021. The ^{18}F-FDG PET/CT was performed as part of their work-up for initial staging to plan therapy. These patients were recruited as part of an ongoing study on hypoxia imaging. Informed consent was obtained from the patients for the scan as well as to access their hospital records. In the patients that were recruited, the hemoglobin levels at the time of imaging were determined and recorded. The study was approved by the Human Research Ethics Committee of the University of Pretoria (protocol number: 691/2019). All procedures were performed in accordance with the ethical standards of the institutional research committee in alignment with the 1964 Helsinki declaration and its latter amendments.

2.2. Radiochemistry of ^{68}Ga-Nitroimidazole

The synthesis of ^{68}Ga-Nitroimidazole was performed as previously described [21]. Briefly, we obtained ^{68}Ga from our inhouse ^{68}Ge/^{68}Ga generator (iThemba LABS, Somerset West, South Africa). We received the Nitroimidazole peptide complexed with TRAP chelator from Korea (Radiation Applied Life Sciences, Department of Nuclear Medicine and Cancer Research Institute of Radiation Medicine, Seoul National University College of Medicine, Seoul, Korea). This nitroimidazole residue, 2-(2-nitroimidazolyl)ethylamine was conjugated with TRAP via an acid-amine coupling reaction in dimethylsulfoxide (DMSO) using 2-(1H-benzotriazol-1-yl)-1,1,3,3-tetramethyluronium hexafluorophosphate (HBTU) as a coupling agent in the presence of N,N-diisopropylethylamine (DIPEA) as a base. Radiolabeling was conducted at pH of 4.5 at 95 °C in a heating block for 10 min. Labelling efficiency was verified by instant thin layer chromatography (ITLC) using 0.1 M Na_2CO_3. Radiochemical yields of the prepared derivatives were found to be >96% for all the derivatives.

2.3. ^{68}Ga-Nitroimidazole PET/CT Imaging Procedure

There was no specific patient preparation applied for the ^{68}Ga-Nitroimidazole scan.

The injected activity of ^{68}Ga-Nitroimidazole was weight based (1.8–2.2 MBq) and ranged between 111–185 MBq. We obtained a pelvic image at 30 min. post tracer injection. This was followed by a whole body (vertex to mid-thigh) PET/CT image at 60 min post tracer injection. Lasix was administered at the time of tracer injection. Patients were catheterized prior to the 60-min image to reduce bladder activity. PET imaging was acquired in 3D mode at 3 min per bed position. We used CT data for attenuation correction and for anatomic delineation of lesions. We performed image reconstruction using ordered subset expectation maximization iterative reconstruction algorithm (four iterations, eight subsets) followed by post reconstruction filtering with a Gaussian filter applied at 5.0 mm FWHM.

2.4. ^{18}F-FDG PET/CT Imaging Procedure

Patient preparation for ^{18}F-FDG PET/CT included a minimum of 4 h of fasting which is in keeping with published guidelines [25,26]. Blood sugar before ^{18}F-FDG injections was less than 7.1 mmol/L in all cases. The injected activity of ^{18}F-FDG was between 3–5 MBq/kg. We imaged patients after an uptake period of 60 min. Thirteen of the patients were imaged on a Biograph 40 Truepoint PET/CT scanner (Siemens Medical Solutions, Lincolnshire, IL, USA), while the other seven were imaged on a Biograph Vision 450 PET/CT scanner (Siemens Medical Solutions, Lincolnshire, IL, USA). We performed a vertex to mid-thigh CT scan with parameters adjusted for patients' weight (120 KeV, 40–150 mAs) with a section width of 5 mm and pitch of 0.8.

2.5. Image Analysis

Two Nuclear Medicine Physicians with over two decades experience reporting PET/CT images reviewed the hypoxia ^{68}Ga-Nitroimidazole PET/CT images. Reconstructed images were displayed as maximum intensity projection image, PET, CT, and fused PET/CT in the axial, coronal and sagittal planes on a dedicated workstation equipped with syngo software (Siemens Medical Solutions, Lincolnshire, IL, USA).

2.6. Qualitative Analysis

The 60-min whole body images were analysed for bio-distribution as well as additional tumor related information. We performed qualitative assessment of the images and recorded our findings using a grading scale of 0–3 with 0 = no uptake/uptake less than normal background tissues, 1 = uptake similar to background activity, 2 = focal uptake above background activity and 3 = uptake markedly above background activity [27]. For this visual analysis, the background was considered as the blood pool.

2.7. Semi-Quantitative Analysis

Semi-quantitative analyses were also used with calculation of SUVmax, SUVmean, HTV and Tumor to muscle ratio (TMR) as well as Tumor to blood ratio (TBR). The muscle tissue for the calculation of the TMR was the gluteus muscle and the aorta and left ventricle were used for the tumor to blood ratio. The tumor to muscle or blood ratio was calculated as the tumor SUVmax uptake divided by the SUVmean uptake in the gluteus muscle or the blood (aorta). Hypoxic tumors were identified based on the semi-quantitative analysis as those with at least one voxel with a ^{68}Ga-Nitroimidazole signal greater than the calculated threshold. A semi-automatic spherical volume of interest (VOI) was drawn encircling the primary lesion in the cervix using an SUV threshold of 1.4 and a 3D isocontour of 41%. The VOI was manually adjusted to exclude areas of physiological uptake adjacent to the primary lesion. The maximum and mean standardized uptake values (SUVmax and SUVmean) and the hypoxic tumor volume (HTV) of the primary lesion in each patient were recorded. The hypoxic tumor volume (HTV) was defined as the volume in the ^{68}Ga-Nitroimidazole PET dataset with an intensity greater than the determined threshold. This analysis was based on similar principles as the MTV determination. We divided the HTV by the MTV of the primary tumor to calculate a fractional HTV.

^{18}F-FDG PET/CT images were analyzed for the presence of nodal and distant metastases. Nodal metastasis was differentiated from inflammation based on the experience of the interpreting nuclear physicians using the following criteria as indicative of metastatic nodes: the presence of asymmetry, size, architecture or consistency (absence of fatty hilum/center, necrosis), the degree of uptake and the location. Disagreements were resolved by consensus.

2.8. Immunohistochemical Assessment

The slides obtained from endocervical biopsies of the cervix for initial diagnosis were retrieved for immunohistochemical analysis. The slides were evaluated by an experienced pathologist from the department of Anatomical Pathology, National Health Laboratory Services (NHLS) at our institute. Hypoxia inducible factor 1 alpha (HIF-1α) monoclonal rabbit anti-human antibodies (clone EP118) were used to evaluate the HIF-1α expression. The tissue samples had all been fixed in 10% buffered formalin, processed and embedded in paraffin routinely. Sections were cut at 3 µm using a Leica TP1020 microtome and dried overnight at 60 °C. After deparaffinization in xylene, the sections were rehydrated in decreasing ethanol solutions and incubated in 0.3% hydrogen peroxide for 10 min, to block endogenous peroxidase. DAKO auto-stainer with PT link method of antigen retrieval was done. Citrate buffer solution (pH 6) for 20 min was done. Peroxidase was incubated for 5 min. Then, the slides were washed in PBS and put in the auto-stainer. Then the antibody was put in for 30 min and washed again in PBS. Envision fluid (polymer-peroxidase method, EnVision+/HRP, DAKO, Glostrup Kommune, Denmark) was added, followed by incubation for 30 min. Bound antibodies were visualized by using 0.05% 3,3′-diaminobenzidine solution (DAB solution, DAKO). Finally, sections were counterstained with Meyer's hematoxylin and mounted in Entellan (Merck, Darmstadt, Germany). The grade of staining was defined via a light microscope. HIF-1α protein expression, (nuclear unless otherwise specified), was graded in intensity form 0 (negative) to 3 (strong), with 1 for weak intensity, 2 for moderate intensity. The distribution of staining was assessed as 25%, 50%; 75% and 100% of the tumor cells and allocated scores 1, 2, 3 and 4. A value of the sum of intensity and distribution out of 6 was used to score the positivity of the staining. HIF score = [intensity (I) + distribution (D)].

2.9. Statistical Analysis

Baseline clinical and demographic information of the patients was analyzed with descriptive statistics. Categorical data are presented as frequencies while continuous variables are presented as mean ± standard deviation (SD) or as median (interquartile range, IQR). Statistical analysis was performed using the commercially available software package SPSS 28.0. Normalcy was assessed by means of the Kolmogorov–Smirnov test. For non-normal distributed data, the Mann–Whitney test, Kruskal–Wallis test and Spearman-rank test were used when appropriate. For normal distributed data, ANOVA with post-hoc Bonferroni correction, the student t-tests and the Pearson correlation test were used when appropriate.

Multivariate analysis was performed using Cox-regression including in sequential order of statistical significance those variables that were found to be significant in univariate analysis. Statistical significance was defined as a p-value ≤ 0.05

3. Results

All 20 women included in the study underwent both ^{68}Ga-Nitroimidazole PET/CT and ^{18}F-FDG PET/CT on different days with a median interval of 6 days (range: 1–32) between the two scans. The mean age of the study population was 44.65 ± 11.43 years (range: 26–72). The majority (n = 16/20; 80%) of the patients had squamous cell carcinoma while the rest had various other histological subtypes of cervical cancer. Most patients were referred for a scan with an initial clinical impression of locally advanced disease, however, some of the patients were upstaged by the ^{18}F-FDG PET/CT. Seventeen patients had a FIGO clinical stage of between IIB and IIIC2 while two patients had stage IVA and one stage IVB. Thirteen patients demonstrated pelvic lymph node metastases on ^{18}F-FDG PET/CT. The median hemoglobin level was 10 g/dL (IQR: 9–11.75 g/dL). Demographic characteristics of the patients are displayed in Table 1 below.

Table 1. Demographic characteristics of the patient cohort.

Variable	Frequency	Percent
Age (years)		
Mean ± SD	44.65 ± 11.43	
Range	26–72	
Histological subtype		
Mucinous endocervical carcinoma	1	5.0
Papillary squamourethelial carcinoma	1	5.0
Squamous cell carcinoma	16	80.0
Papillary surface serous carcinoma	1	5.0
Adenocarcinoma	1	5.0
FIGO stage		
IIB	3	15.0
IIIA	1	5.0
IIIB	9	45.0
IIIC	2	10.0
IIIC1	1	5.0
IIIC2	1	5.0
IVA	2	10.0
IVB	1	5.0

SD: Standard Deviation; FIGO: International Federation of Gynecology and Obstetrics.

3.1. Qualitative and Semiquantitative Analysis of the PET/CT Images

The biodistribution was as anticipated with minimal tracer seen in the blood pool with excretion through the urinary system. A few patients demonstrated liver and gallbladder uptake. There was minimal background activity noted in the fat and muscles. The mean SUVmax and SUVmean of the primary tumor on ^{18}F-FDG PET/CT imaging was 22.1 ± 21.4 and 8.9 ± 7.6, respectively; while the mean SUVmax and SUVmean of the primary lesion on ^{68}Ga-Nitroimidazole PET/CT imaging was 3.54 ± 1.5 and 1.8 ± 0.8 for the early time point and 3.43 ± 1.5 and 1.4 ± 0.4 for the delayed imaging. There was no statistical difference noted in the mean SUVmax and SUVmean of the primary lesion between the two time points on the ^{68}Ga-Nitroimidazole scan ($p = 0.461$; $p = 0.510$, respectively). Qualitatively, 12 patients had discernable focal uptake above background, three patients had uptake similar to background and the remaining five patients had no uptake on ^{68}Ga-Nitroimidazole scan. The mean TMR on ^{18}F-FDG PET/CT and at both time points on the ^{68}Ga-Nitroimidazole scans were 38.3, 10.1 and 11.7, respectively. The mean TBRs on ^{18}F-FDG PET/CT was 13.6 ± 11.3 and 13.5 ± 12.6 when using the aorta and ventricle as the blood pool surrogate. The median TBR on the delayed images on ^{68}Ga-Nitroimidazole when using the aorta and ventricle were 2, while the mean TBR was 2.5 ± 1.6 and 3.3 ± 3.2. Figure 1 below demonstrates the semi-quantitative parameters on both ^{18}F-FDG and ^{68}Ga-Nitroimidazole PET/CT imaging.

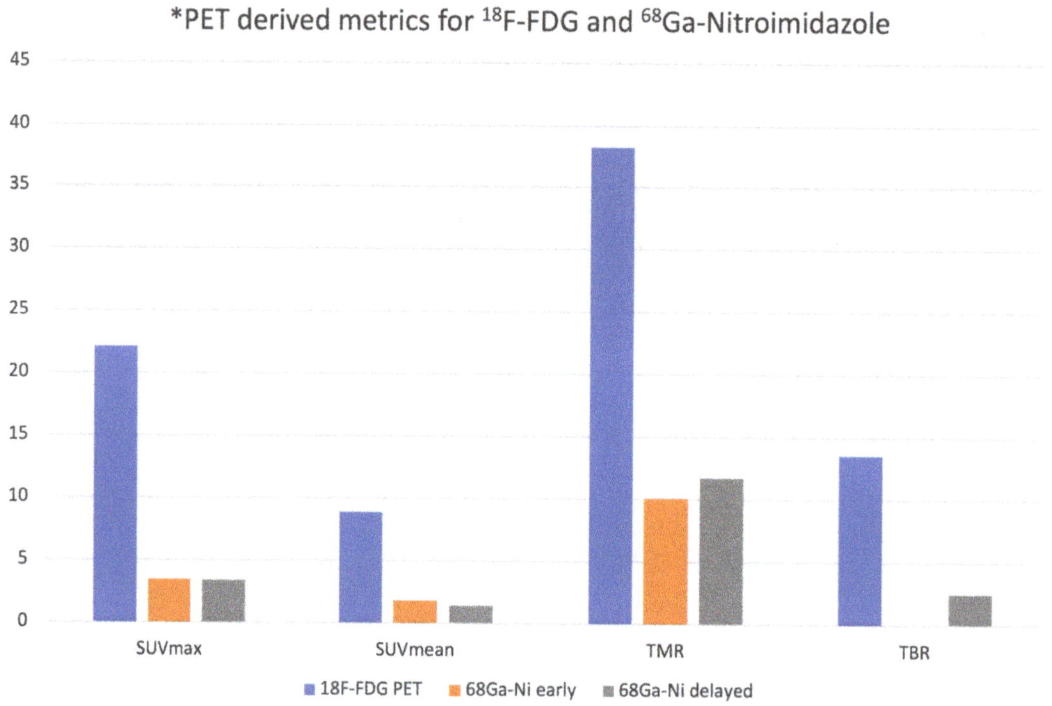

Figure 1. The mean SUVmax, SUVmean, tumor to muscle ratio (TMR) and tumor to blood ratio (TBR) for ^{18}F-FDG and ^{68}Ga-Nitroimidazole at 30 and 60 min. * PET: Positron Emission Tomography

The median MTV on the ^{18}F-FDG PET/CT was 150.5 (18.41–548.93). The median hypoxic tumor volumes on the early and delayed images were 50 and 60.85, respectively. The hypoxic subvolume as a percentage of the MTV ranged from 2 to 98% (median 37%).

3.2. Immunohistochemistry Findings

We successfully retrieved histological specimen for 15 patients. Five patients had negative staining for HIF-1α on immunohistochemistry. The remainder of the patients had varying intensities of staining for HIF-1α with three (3) patients having weak staining, two (2) had moderate intensity and five (5) patients had strong intensity. When considering the hypoxia score, seven patients were considered positive for hypoxia. Table 2 represents the intensity and percentage distribution of the HIF-1α expression within the tumor specimen. In 70% (n = 7) of the patients with any level of HIF-1α expression on immunohistochemistry, we demonstrated uptake on the ^{68}Ga-Nitroimidazole hypoxia PET scan (Figures 2 and 3). Statistically there was a very weak, almost negligible correlation between these findings (r = 0.058; p = 0.837).

Table 2. Immunohistochemical analysis and correlation to ^{68}Ga-Nitroimidazole imaging qualitative assessment.

Patient No.	Histological Subtype	Intensity of Staining of HIF-1α	Percentage Distribution of HIF-1α Expression	Sum of Intensity and Distribution (Out of 6)	Qualitative ^{68}Ga-Nitroimidazole PET Findings
1	Squamous cell carcinoma	3	25%	4	2
2	Squamous cell carcinoma	3	75 %	6	2
3	Squamous cell carcinoma	3	75%	6	2
4	Papillary surface serous carcinoma	2	75%	5	0
5	Squamous cell carcinoma	3	75%	6	0
6	Adenocarcinoma	3	75%	6	2
7	Squamous cell carcinoma	0	-	0	2
8	Squamous cell carcinoma	2	25%	3	2
9	Squamous cell carcinoma	0	-	0	2
10	Papillary squamo-urothelial carcinoma	1	25%	2	1
11	Squamous cell carcinoma	0	-	0	1
12	Squamous cell carcinoma	1	25%	2	2
13	Squamous cell carcinoma	0	-	0	2
14	Squamous cell carcinoma	0	-	0	0
15	Squamous cell carcinoma	1	25%	2	2

Intensity of staining: 0 = no staining, 1 = weak intensity, 2 = moderate intensity, 3 = strong intensity. Sum of intensity and percentage distribution out of a total of 6 (see methods section for detailed description). Values above 3 were considered positive for hypoxia. Qualitative ^{68}Ga-Nitroimidazole PET findings: 0 = no uptake, 1 = uptake similar to background, 2 = focal uptake above background, 3 = focal uptake markedly above background.

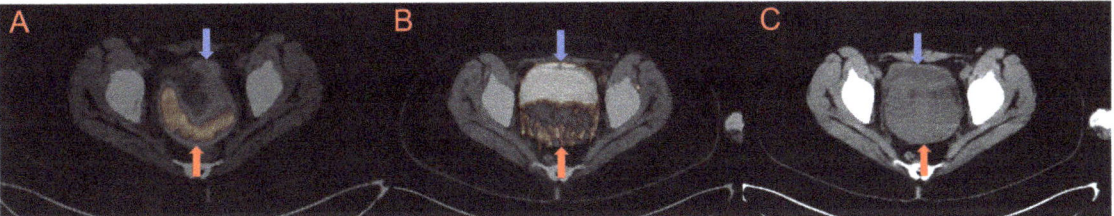

Figure 2. A 36-year-old female patient with FIGO stage II, squamous cell carcinoma of the cervix. (**A**). ^{18}F-FDG PET transaxial image through the pelvis demonstrating uptake in the primary tumor (red arrow) with minimal uptake in the urinary bladder (blue arrow) (**B**). ^{68}Ga-Nitroimidazole PET transaxial image through the same plane exhibiting spatially incongruent uptake with inhomogeneous uptake in parts of the tumor (red arrow) and intense activity in the urinary bladder (blue arrow). (**C**) is the corresponding CT only image in the same plane with target organs marked with arrows. The fractional hypoxic volume was 36%.

3.3. Correlation between ^{68}Ga-Nitroimidazole PET/CT, ^{18}F-FDG PET/CT Imaging and Immunohistochemistry

There was no statistically significant correlation between the hemoglobin levels, ^{18}F-FDG SUVmax, ^{68}Ga-Nitroimidazole imaging and immunohistochemical analysis. The median SUVmax and TMR on both ^{18}F-FDG and ^{68}Ga-Nitromimidazole at both time points did not demonstrate any statistical difference in hypoxic and non-hypoxic states as assessed by immunohistochemistry. When considering the hypoxia score, we found that five of the seven patients considered positive for hypoxia on immunohistochemistry, displayed uptake above background on the ^{68}Ga-Nitroimidazole scan. Table 3. Demonstrates the results of the Kruskal–Wallis test assessing the difference between quantitative parameters on both ^{18}F-FDG and ^{68}Ga-Nitroimidazole PET/CT imaging in hypoxic and non-hypoxic states. There was no significant association between the presence of metastasis on ^{18}F-FDG and the presence of hypoxia both on imaging and immunohistochemistry. None of the variables under study proved significantly different between those patients presenting with distant metastasis versus those who without ($p \geq 0.162$). When assessing the HTV, we found no significant difference in the HTV of patients with positive results on immunohistochemical staining and those with negative results. Importantly we found a strong negative correlation between HTV and immunohistochemical staining (r = −0.660; $p = 0.019$). Additionally, hypoxia positivity proved moderately and significantly correlated to SUVmean values of the primary tumor derived from the early and delayed ^{68}Ga-nitroimidazole PET examinations r = 0.531 ($p = 0.42$) and r = 0.580 ($p = 0.024$), see Figure 4. Additionally, upon dichotomization of the primary tumor hypoxia score (group 0, scores: 0, 1 and 2 and group 1, scores: 3, 4, 5 and 6) TMR derived from the early ^{68}Ga-nitroimidazole PET examination proved significantly higher in tumors with score 1 versus those with score 0 (13.2 ± 7.3 versus 8 ± 13.2, respectively).

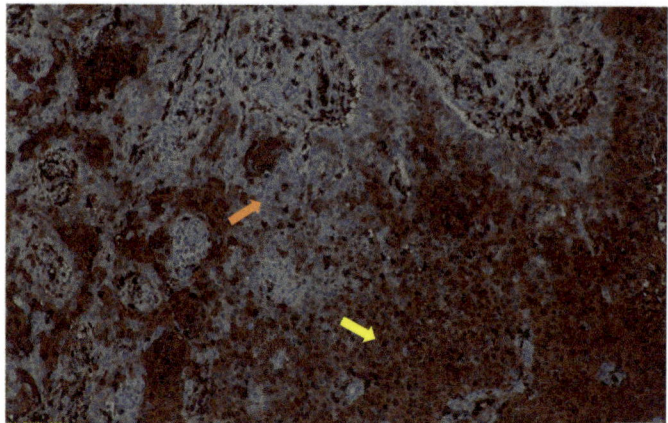

Figure 3. The immunohistochemical staining of HIF-1α expression in the endocervical biopsy specimen of the patient in Figure 2. Well differentiated squamous cell carcinoma ×20 magnification. The tumor areas with well differentiated cells (*yellow arrow*) with brown staining, demonstrate HIF-1α expression, while the areas with other cell types (*orange arrow*) demonstrate little to no HIF-1α expression.

Table 3. SUVmax and TMR from the ^{18}F-FDG and ^{68}Ga-Nitroimidazole PET/CT scans correlated with the HIF-1α expression.

	Hypoxia on Staining					
	Negative	Weak	Moderate	Strong		
	Median (Range)	Median (Range)	Median (Range)	Median (Range)	K	*p* Value
^{18}F-FDG SUVmax	17.32 (11.82–17.81)	21.21 (11.64–22.42)	13.70 (13.41–13.99)	17.50 (16.09–30.77)	2.927	0.403
^{18}F-FDG TMR	30.00 (21.00–43.00)	38.00 (22.00–46.00)	27.00 (27.00–27.00)	32.00 (18.00–50.00)	0.670	0.880
^{68}Ga-Ni SUVmax(1)	3.73 (1.00–4.00)	3.38 (3.00–4.00)	2.08 (2.00–2.00)	4.10 (2.00–5.00)	2.795	0.424
^{68}Ga-Ni SUVmax(2)	3.71 (1.60–4.19)	3.06 (3.04–3.15)	1.77 (1.62–1.91)	3.57 (2.78–4.32)	4.342	0.227
^{68}Ga-Ni TMR	8.00 (4.00–10.00)	9.50 (8.00–11.00)	10.00 (6.00–14.00)	15.00 (7.00–24.00)	2.669	0.446
^{68}Ga-Ni TMR 2	11.00 (6.00–16.00)	15.00 (7.00–17.00)	7.50 (7.00–8.00)	12.00 (7.00–26.00)	1.852	0.604

K: Kruskal–Wallis test, ^{68}Ga-Nitroimidazole maximum standardized uptake value (^{68}Ga-Ni SUVmax): ^{68}Ga-Ni SUVmax (1) and ^{68}Ga-Ni SUVmax (2): SUVmax at 30 and 60 min post tracer injection, respectively; ^{68}Ga-Nitroimidazole tumor to muscle ratio (^{68}Ga-Ni TMR): ^{68}Ga-Ni TMR and ^{68}Ga-Ni TMR 2 are the tumor to muscle ratio at 30 and 60 min post tracer injection, respectively.

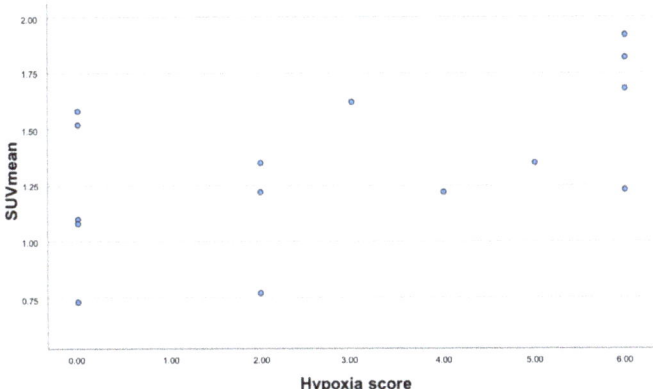

Figure 4. Scatterplot showing the relationship between the hypoxia score (data shown in the X-axis) and SUVmean of the primary tumor derived from the delayed ^{68}Ga-Nitroimidazole PET images.

4. Discussion

The presence of hypoxia in solid tumors has a bearing on treatment and outcomes; therefore, non-invasive modalities that can map it are essential for therapy planning. Several PET tracers have been utilized for this purpose in various cancer entities with variable results. Our study aimed to image hypoxia in cervical cancer lesions/tumors with ^{68}Ga-Nitroimidazole which is more hydrophilic and has demonstrated improved properties compared to 1st, 2nd and 3rd generation ^{18}F-labelled nitroimidazole tracers. The biodistribution was as expected with intense activity seen in the kidney and urinary bladder because of the hydrophilicity. The qualitative assessment revealed that two-thirds of the patients had uptake in the primary tumor above background. This is similar to the >50% rate of hypoxic tumors in studies using invasive needle electrode measurements [6,7,28]. In a study of 38 women, Dehdashti and colleagues found discernable ^{60}Cu-ATSM uptake in all but one patient [29]. Another study using ^{18}F-FMISO also detected focal areas of uptake in all 16 patients [30]. Although the patient population in both studies was similar to ours (locally advanced tumors), the differences seen in the numbers of patients with uptake may be related to the differences in the tracers and tracer kinetics as well as interpretation criteria. Most studies on hypoxia imaging (pre-clinical and clinical) report on the SUVmean or none at all and we found the SUVmean on the delayed ^{68}Ga-Nitroimidazole to be strongly correlated to the positivity on immunohistochemical staining. This finding is most likely related to the heterogeneity of hypoxic regions within a tumor and may explain why most papers on this subject have reported on the SUVmean as opposed to the SUVmax. The median SUVmax in our series was 3.63 and 3.27 at 30 and 60 min, respectively, which is comparable to that reported in the clinical work using ^{18}F-FMISO in cervical cancer patients [30]. The other parameter that has been more commonly reported on, in the context of hypoxia imaging using different tracers is the TMR or TBR. Preclinical studies using ^{68}Ga-labelled nitromidazoles have demonstrated that TMR and TBR were highest at 1 h post imaging. We confirmed this finding as we found a median TMR of 8 ± 4.8 and 10 ± 5.1 at 30- and 60-min post injection, respectively. Initial pre-clinical work on ^{68}Ga-Nitroimidazole revealed median TMRs as high as 7.41 ±1.12, 5.70 ± 2.5, 5.64 ± 0.8 [19–21]. The work on ^{64}Cu-ATSM also revealed TMR 7.3 ± 1.8 [31]. These high TMRs contrast with the TMRs when using ^{18}F-labelled tracers and this may be attributed physical properties of these tracers which result in faster clearance from background tissues. We found no significant difference in the TMR and TBR between the 30 min and 60 min time points, suggesting that images may be obtained as early as 30 min post tracer injection without significantly compromising the image quality. Interestingly we also found higher TMRs on the early ^{68}Ga-Nitroimidazole scan in patients with hypoxia on immunohistochemistry than those with no hypoxia. This may further support early imaging. This is in contrast to ^{18}F-FMISO which has prolonged imaging times up to 2 h post tracer injection.

There is an abundance of literature demonstrating hypoxia in cervical cancer lesions using ^{18}F-labelled tracers and $^{60/64}$Cu-ATSM, however very few of them correlated their findings to immunohistochemistry which may be considered the gold standard. There are various genes that are upregulated in hypoxic environments including vascular endothelial growth factor (VEGF), Carbonic anhydrase IX (CAIX) and osteopontin to name a few. In a study of 44 women with advanced cervical cancer, the authors found no correlation between the expression of HIF-1α and tumor oxygenation as detected by an Eppendorf device [32]. Vercellino and colleagues assessed the feasibility of imaging hypoxic lesions with ^{18}F-FETNIM and correlated their findings to osteopontin which is also upregulated in hypoxic environments. They found no correlation between levels of osteopontin and ^{18}F-FETNIM uptake. Similarly, we also failed to find a correlation between the HIF-1α expression on immunohistochemistry and ^{68}Ga-Nitroimidazole imaging. We found that almost half of the patients with any level of HIF-1α expression on immunohistochemistry had discernable hypoxia on PET imaging, while five of the seven patients with positive hypoxia scores had uptake on ^{68}Ga-Nitroimidazole PET. This is contrary to the study by Grigsby et al. who correlated VEGF, CAIX, cyclo-oxygenase-2 (COX-2), epidermal growth factor and apoptotic index with ^{60}Cu-ATSM PET imaging of tumor hypoxia. Immunohistochemical markers were expressed in most, if not all the tumors seen to be hypoxic on ^{60}Cu-ATSM PET imaging [33]. Immunohistochemical analyses are fraught with challenges including operator dependence and sampling issues etc., and this may be a reason for the lack of correlation of these findings with imaging as seen in our study.

We believe there are unique patient groups or outcomes that deserve a special mention because of their interesting or unexpected findings. Two patients, namely patient 4 and 5 (Table 2) demonstrated hypoxia on immunohistochemistry, however their ^{68}Ga-Nitroimidazole PET scans demonstrated no discernable areas of uptake. The reasons for the above may be related to size of the tumor which may render the lesion/s prone to partial volume effect or being missed because of the inherent resolution limits of the imaging unit. In three patients (7, 9 and 13), we note the reverse, wherein the despite lack of HIF-1α, the ^{68}Ga-Nitroimidazole PET scan demonstrated uptake above background tissues. This outcome may be related to sampling errors for the HIF-1α staining in view of the heterogeneous nature of hypoxia.

Most oncology guidelines recommend the use of ^{18}F-FDG PET/CT in the staging and restaging of most malignancies including cancer of the cervix [34]. Often, ^{18}F-FDG PET/CT images are used for the visual estimation of uptake of hypoxia tracers within tumor lesions. Furthermore, in-vitro studies have demonstrated that hypoxia results in increased FDG uptake [35–37]. There are several studies which have correlated the findings on hypoxia PET imaging with those from metabolic imaging. Grigsby et al. found no correlation between uptake parameters on ^{18}F-FDG and ^{60}Cu-ATSM PET scans, however they did note a significant correlation between the presence of ^{18}F-FDG positive lymph nodes and the findings on ^{60}Cu-ATSM PET [33]. The lack of correlation between the metabolic and hypoxia imaging has been also demonstrated in other tumor entities [38,39]. Similarly, we could not demonstrate any correlation between PET-derived parameters (SUVmax, SUVmean, TMR and TBR) on the metabolic and hypoxic imaging. We also found no correlation between the presence of any metastasis on ^{18}F-FDG PET and ^{68}Ga-Nitroimidazole. The hypoxic volume was always less than the metabolic tumor volume in our patient cohort. This is in support of the reports of heterogeneity of hypoxia, therefore further highlighting the importance of hypoxia mapping with imaging studies.

We found a significant strong negative correlation between HTV and immunohistochemistry ($r = -0.660$; $p = 0.019$). This finding was not anticipated. We postulate that this finding may be due to several factors including tumoral environmental issues and technical factors. We believe that other factors besides upregulation of HIF-1α are at play in the hypoxic environment. A possible theory is the presence of a feedback mechanism between markers/genes within the tumor and HIF-1α. Another plausible explanation may be related to the different isoforms of HIF-α, as it has been shown that there are at least three, namely HIF-1α, HIF-2α and HIF-3α [40]. These α-subunits are regulated at the protein level by oxygen dependent mechanisms. It has been shown that HIF-1α expression is higher in acute hypoxia whereas that of HIF-2α is higher in chronic hypoxia [41,42]. This finding calls for larger studies with modified and improved protocols to be conducted as to unravel the association we found.

To the best of our knowledge, this is the first study to assess this novel ^{68}Ga-Nitroimidazole tracer in patients with cervical cancer. This very fact may prove to be a limitation since there are no prior studies to compare our findings to, therefore most of our comparisons are with pre-clinical studies, other ^{18}F-labelled or the ^{64}Cu-labelled hypoxia tracers. We could not draw any strong conclusion because of the small sample size. The main excretory pathway of the more hydrophilic ^{68}Ga-Nitroimidazole is through the renal system. This resulted in intense bladder uptake that may pose as a challenge for pelvic malignancies. Despite urinary catheterization of the majority of our patients, the urinary bladder was often incompletely drained, and this may pose a challenge in the interpretation of the scan. Therefore, for pelvic malignancies, a tracer with minimal renal excretion or the employment of radiomics, may optimize the interpretation of the findings. The immunohistochemistry was performed on biopsy specimen that were collected at initial diagnosis and this may misrepresent the true status of hypoxia in the entire tumor lesion. Lastly, immunohistochemical analysis is highly operator dependent and this too may pose as a limitation in our study. Future studies with pre-operative patients that will undergo surgery and subsequent immunohistochemistry on more representative samples of the surgical specimen may yield improved results. While it was our desire to perform survival analysis, local factors e.g., lack of centralized health informatic systems, proved to be a challenge. This information may have added further insight in this area.

5. Conclusions

We found that there was no difference in the tumor uptake on ^{68}Ga-Nitroimidazole PET/CT between early (30 min) and delayed (60 min) imaging, which may suggest that imaging can be acquired early without compromising the tumor to background ratio. Although we detected hypoxia in two-thirds of the patients on ^{68}Ga-Nitroimidazole PET imaging, we found no significant relationship between HIF-1α and clinicopathological features or ^{18}F-FDG and ^{68}Ga-Nitrimidazole PET/CT parameters. However, we found higher TMRs and SUVmeans in patients with hypoxia as assessed on immunohistochemistry. Furthermore, there was a negative correlation between HTV as assessed by PET hypoxia imaging and HIF-1α staining. Further, larger studies are required to determine the prognostic value of using ^{68}Ga-Nitroimidazole PET imaging to predict the pathological and prognostic course of cervical cancer.

Author Contributions: Conceptualization, K.M.G.M. and M.M.S.; methodology, M.M.S., M.B., J.M.J., J.M., C.D., M.V. and K.M.G.M.; formal analysis, K.M.G.M., C.v.d.W., A.M. and G.P.; investigation, K.M.G.M., I.O.L., L.C.M., K.N.H., H.N. and J.R.; resources, M.M.S. and J.M.J.; data curation, K.M.G.M.; writing—original draft preparation, K.M.G.M.; writing—review and editing, K.M.G.M., I.O.L., M.M.S. and M.V.; visualization, K.M.G.M. and M.M.S.; supervision, M.M.S. and M.V.; project administration, K.M.G.M. and M.M.S. All authors have read and agreed to the published version of the manuscript.

Funding: This research received no external funding.

Institutional Review Board Statement: The study was conducted according to the guidelines of the Declaration of Helsinki and its later amendments, and approved by the Institutional Review Board (or Ethics Committee) of the University of Pretoria (691/2019)

Informed Consent Statement: Informed consent was obtained from all subjects involved in the study.

Data Availability Statement: The data presented in this study are available on request from the corresponding author.

Acknowledgments: We would like to acknowledge the support staff including but not limited to the Nuclear Medicine Technologists, Administration staff and the staff in the departments of radiation oncology and pathology.

Conflicts of Interest: The authors declare no conflict of interest.

References

1. Sung, H.; Ferlay, J.; Siegel, R.L.; Laversanne, M.; Soerjomataram, I.; Jemal, A.; Bray, F. Global Cancer Statistics 2020: Globocan Estimates of Incidence and Mortality Worldwide for 36 Cancers in 185 Countries. *CA Cancer J. Clin.* **2021**, *71*, 209–249. [CrossRef] [PubMed]
2. Denny, L.; Anorlu, R. Cervical cancer in Africa. *Cancer Epidemiol. Biomark. Prev.* **2012**, *21*, 1434–1438. [CrossRef] [PubMed]
3. Denny, L. Cervical cancer treatment in Africa. *Curr. Opin. Oncol.* **2011**, *23*, 469–474. [CrossRef]
4. McKeown, S.R. Defining normoxia, physoxia and hypoxia in tumours-implications for treatment response. *Br. J. Radiol.* **2014**, *87*, 20130676. [CrossRef] [PubMed]
5. Vaupel, P.; Thews, O.; Hoeckel, M. Treatment resistance of solid tumors: Role of hypoxia and anemia. *Med. Oncol.* **2001**, *18*, 243–259. [CrossRef]
6. Hockel, M.; Vorndran, B.; Schlenger, K.; Baussmann, E.; Knapstein, P.G. Tumor oxygenation: A new predictive parameter in locally advanced cancer of the uterine cervix. *Gynecol. Oncol.* **1993**, *51*, 141–149. [CrossRef]
7. Hockel, M.; Vaupel, P. Oxygenation of cervix cancers: Impact of clinical and pathological parameters. *Adv. Exp. Med. Biol.* **2003**, *510*, 31–35.
8. Hockel, M.; Vaupel, P. Tumor hypoxia: Definitions and current clinical, biologic, and molecular aspects. *J. Natl. Cancer Inst.* **2001**, *93*, 266–276. [CrossRef]
9. Challapalli, A.; Carroll, L.; Aboagye, E.O. Molecular mechanisms of hypoxia in cancer. *Clin. Transl. Imaging* **2017**, *5*, 225–253. [CrossRef]
10. Ling, C.C.; Humm, J.; Larson, S.; Amols, H.; Fuks, Z.; Leibel, S.; Koutcher, J.A. Towards multidimensional radiotherapy (MD-CRT): Biological imaging and biological conformality. *Int. J. Radiat. Oncol. Biol. Phys.* **2000**, *47*, 551–560. [CrossRef]
11. Supiot, S.; Lisbona, A.; Paris, F.; Azria, D.; Fenoglietto, P. ["Dose-painting": Myth or reality?]. *Cancer Radiother.* **2010**, *14*, 554–562. [CrossRef] [PubMed]
12. Semenza, G.L. Hypoxia-inducible factor 1 and cancer pathogenesis. *IUBMB Life* **2008**, *60*, 591–597. [CrossRef] [PubMed]
13. Xu, Z.; Li, X.F.; Zou, H.; Sun, X.; Shen, B. ^{18}F-Fluoromisonidazole in tumor hypoxia imaging. *Oncotarget* **2017**, *8*, 94969–94979. [CrossRef]
14. Busk, M.; Horsman, M.R.; Jakobsen, S.; Keiding, S.; van der Kogel, A.J.; Bussink, J.; Overgaard, J. Imaging hypoxia in xenografted and murine tumors with ^{18}F-fluoroazomycin arabinoside: A comparative study involving microPET, autoradiography, PO2-polarography, and fluorescence microscopy. *Int. J. Radiat. Oncol. Biol. Phys.* **2008**, *70*, 1202–1212. [CrossRef] [PubMed]
15. Yang, D.J.; Wallace, S.; Cherif, A.; Li, C.; Gretzer, M.B.; Kim, E.E.; Podoloff, D.A. Development of F-18-labeled fluoroerythronitroimidazole as a PET agent for imaging tumor hypoxia. *Radiology* **1995**, *194*, 795–800. [CrossRef] [PubMed]
16. Sanduleanu, S.; Wiel, A.; Lieverse, R.I.Y.; Marcus, D.; Ibrahim, A.; Primakov, S.; Wu, G.; Theys, J.; Yaromina, A.; Dubois, L.J.; et al. Hypoxia PET Imaging with [^{18}F]-HX4-A Promising Next-Generation Tracer. *Cancers* **2020**, *12*, 1322. [CrossRef] [PubMed]
17. Fujibayashi, Y.; Taniuchi, H.; Yonekura, Y.; Ohtani, H.; Konishi, J.; Yokoyama, A. Copper-62-ATSM: A new hypoxia imaging agent with high membrane permeability and low redox potential. *J. Nucl. Med.* **1997**, *38*, 1155–1160.
18. Roesch, F. Maturation of a key resource—The germanium-68/gallium-68 generator: Development and new insights. *Curr. Radiopharm.* **2012**, *5*, 202–211. [CrossRef]
19. Hoigebazar, L.; Jeong, J.M.; Hong, M.K.; Kim, Y.J.; Lee, J.Y.; Shetty, D.; Lee, Y.S.; Lee, D.S.; Chung, J.K.; Lee, M.C. Synthesis of ^{68}Ga-labeled DOTA-nitroimidazole derivatives and their feasibilities as hypoxia imaging PET tracers. *Bioorg. Med. Chem.* **2011**, *19*, 2176–2181. [CrossRef]
20. Hoigebazar, L.; Jeong, J.M.; Choi, S.Y.; Choi, J.Y.; Shetty, D.; Lee, Y.S.; Lee, D.S.; Chung, J.K.; Lee, M.C.; Chung, Y.K. Synthesis and characterization of nitroimidazole derivatives for ^{68}Ga-labeling and testing in tumor xenografted mice. *J. Med. Chem.* **2010**, *53*, 6378–6385. [CrossRef]
21. Seelam, S.R.; Lee, J.Y.; Lee, Y.S.; Hong, M.K.; Kim, Y.J.; Banka, V.K.; Lee, D.S.; Chung, J.K.; Jeong, J.M. Development of ^{68}Ga-labeled multivalent nitroimidazole derivatives for hypoxia imaging. *Bioorg. Med. Chem.* **2015**, *23*, 7743–7750. [CrossRef] [PubMed]
22. Fernandez, S.; Dematteis, S.; Giglio, J.; Cerecetto, H.; Rey, A. Synthesis, in vitro and in vivo characterization of two novel ^{68}Ga-labelled 5-nitroimidazole derivatives as potential agents for imaging hypoxia. *Nucl. Med. Biol.* **2013**, *40*, 273–279. [CrossRef] [PubMed]
23. Mittal, S.; Sharma, R.; Mallia, M.B.; Sarma, H.D. ^{68}Ga-labeled PET tracers for targeting tumor hypoxia: Role of bifunctional chelators on pharmacokinetics. *Nucl. Med. Biol.* **2021**, *96–97*, 61–67. [CrossRef] [PubMed]
24. Ramogida, C.F.; Pan, J.; Ferreira, C.L.; Patrick, B.O.; Rebullar, K.; Yapp, D.T.; Lin, K.S.; Adam, M.J.; Orvig, C. Nitroimidazole-Containing H$_2$dedpa and H$_2$CHXdedpa Derivatives as Potential PET Imaging Agents of Hypoxia with ^{68}Ga. *Inorg. Chem.* **2015**, *54*, 4953–4965. [CrossRef]

25. Boellaard, R.; O'Doherty, M.J.; Weber, W.A.; Mottaghy, F.M.; Lonsdale, M.N.; Stroobants, S.G.; Oyen, W.J.; Kotzerke, J.; Hoekstra, O.S.; Pruim, J.; et al. FDG PET and PET/CT: EANM procedure guidelines for tumour PET imaging: Version 1.0. *Eur. J. Nucl. Med. Mol. Imaging* **2010**, *37*, 181–200. [CrossRef]
26. Boellaard, R.; Delgado-Bolton, R.; Oyen, W.J.; Giammarile, F.; Tatsch, K.; Eschner, W.; Verzijlbergen, F.J.; Barrington, S.F.; Pike, L.C.; Weber, W.A.; et al. FDG PET/CT: EANM procedure guidelines for tumour imaging: Version 2.0. *Eur. J. Nucl. Med. Mol. Imaging* **2015**, *42*, 328–354. [CrossRef]
27. Souvatzoglou, M.; Grosu, A.L.; Roper, B.; Krause, B.J.; Beck, R.; Reischl, G.; Picchio, M.; Machulla, H.J.; Wester, H.J.; Piert, M. Tumour hypoxia imaging with [^{18}F]FAZA PET in head and neck cancer patients: A pilot study. *Eur. J. Nucl. Med. Mol. Imaging* **2007**, *34*, 1566–1575. [CrossRef]
28. Fyles, A.; Milosevic, M.; Hedley, D.; Pintilie, M.; Levin, W.; Manchul, L.; Hill, R.P. Tumor hypoxia has independent predictor impact only in patients with node-negative cervix cancer. *J. Clin. Oncol.* **2002**, *20*, 680–687. [CrossRef]
29. Dehdashti, F.; Grigsby, P.W.; Lewis, J.S.; Laforest, R.; Siegel, B.A.; Welch, M.J. Assessing tumor hypoxia in cervical cancer by PET with ^{60}Cu-labeled diacetyl-bis(N4-methylthiosemicarbazone). *J. Nucl. Med.* **2008**, *49*, 201–205. [CrossRef]
30. Pinker, K.; Andrzejewski, P.; Baltzer, P.; Polanec, S.H.; Sturdza, A.; Georg, D.; Helbich, T.H.; Karanikas, G.; Grimm, C.; Polterauer, S.; et al. Multiparametric [^{18}F]Fluorodeoxyglucose/[^{18}F]Fluoromisonidazole Positron Emission Tomography/Magnetic Resonance Imaging of Locally Advanced Cervical Cancer for the Non-Invasive Detection of Tumor Heterogeneity: A Pilot Study. *PLoS ONE* **2016**, *11*, e0155333. [CrossRef]
31. Lewis, J.S.; Laforest, R.; Dehdashti, F.; Grigsby, P.W.; Welch, M.J.; Siegel, B.A. An imaging comparison of ^{64}Cu-ATSM and ^{60}Cu-ATSM in cancer of the uterine cervix. *J. Nucl. Med.* **2008**, *49*, 1177–1182. [CrossRef] [PubMed]
32. Dellas, K.; Bache, M.; Pigorsch, S.U.; Taubert, H.; Kappler, M.; Holzapfel, D.; Zorn, E.; Holzhausen, H.J.; Haensgen, G. Prognostic impact of HIF-1alpha expression in patients with definitive radiotherapy for cervical cancer. *Strahlenther. Onkol.* **2008**, *184*, 169–174. [CrossRef] [PubMed]
33. Grigsby, P.W.; Malyapa, R.S.; Higashikubo, R.; Schwarz, J.K.; Welch, M.J.; Huettner, P.C.; Dehdashti, F. Comparison of molecular markers of hypoxia and imaging with (60)Cu-ATSM in cancer of the uterine cervix. *Mol. Imaging Biol.* **2007**, *9*, 278–283. [CrossRef] [PubMed]
34. Marth, C.; Landoni, F.; Mahner, S.; McCormack, M.; Gonzalez-Martin, A.; Colombo, N.; Committee, E.G. Cervical cancer: ESMO Clinical Practice Guidelines for diagnosis, treatment and follow-up. *Ann. Oncol.* **2017**, *28* (Suppl. 4), iv72–iv83. [CrossRef]
35. Clavo, A.C.; Brown, R.S.; Wahl, R.L. Fluorodeoxyglucose uptake in human cancer cell lines is increased by hypoxia. *J. Nucl. Med.* **1995**, *36*, 1625–1632.
36. Minn, H.; Clavo, A.C.; Wahl, R.L. Influence of hypoxia on tracer accumulation in squamous-cell carcinoma: In vitro evaluation for PET imaging. *Nucl. Med. Biol.* **1996**, *23*, 941–946. [CrossRef]
37. Dierckx, R.A.; Van de Wiele, C. FDG uptake, a surrogate of tumour hypoxia? *Eur. J. Nucl. Med. Mol. Imaging* **2008**, *35*, 1544–1549. [CrossRef]
38. Rajendran, J.G.; Wilson, D.C.; Conrad, E.U.; Peterson, L.M.; Bruckner, J.D.; Rasey, J.S.; Chin, L.K.; Hofstrand, P.D.; Grierson, J.R.; Eary, J.F.; et al. [^{18}F]FMISO and [^{18}F]FDG PET imaging in soft tissue sarcomas: Correlation of hypoxia, metabolism and VEGF expression. *Eur. J. Nucl. Med. Mol. Imaging* **2003**, *30*, 695–704. [CrossRef]
39. Zimny, M.; Gagel, B.; DiMartino, E.; Hamacher, K.; Coenen, H.H.; Westhofen, M.; Eble, M.; Buell, U.; Reinartz, P. FDG–a marker of tumour hypoxia? A comparison with [^{18}F]fluoromisonidazole and pO2-polarography in metastatic head and neck cancer. *Eur. J. Nucl. Med. Mol. Imaging* **2006**, *33*, 1426–1431. [CrossRef]
40. Kietzmann, T.; Mennerich, D.; Dimova, E.Y. Hypoxia-Inducible Factors (HIFs) and Phosphorylation: Impact on Stability, Localization, and Transactivity. *Front. Cell Dev. Biol.* **2016**, *4*, 11. [CrossRef]
41. Uchida, T.; Rossignol, F.; Matthay, M.A.; Mounier, R.; Couette, S.; Clottes, E.; Clerici, C. Prolonged hypoxia differentially regulates hypoxia-inducible factor (HIF)-1alpha and HIF-2alpha expression in lung epithelial cells: Implication of natural antisense HIF-1alpha. *J. Biol. Chem.* **2004**, *279*, 14871–14878. [CrossRef] [PubMed]
42. Koh, M.Y.; Powis, G. Passing the baton: The HIF switch. *Trends Biochem. Sci.* **2012**, *37*, 364–372. [CrossRef] [PubMed]

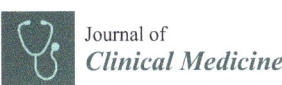

Article

Prognostic Role of Pre-Treatment Metabolic Parameters and Sarcopenia Derived by 2-[^{18}F]-FDG PET/CT in Elderly Mantle Cell Lymphoma

Domenico Albano [1,2,*,†], Nadia Pasinetti [3,†], Francesco Dondi [1,2], Raffaele Giubbini [2], Alessandra Tucci [4] and Francesco Bertagna [1,2]

1. Nuclear Medicine, ASST Spedali Civili Brescia, 25128 Brescia, Italy; f.dondi@outlook.com (F.D.); francesco.bertagna@unibs.it (F.B.)
2. Nuclear Medicine Department, University of Brescia, 25121 Brescia, Italy; raffaele.giubbini@unibs.it
3. Radiation Oncology Department, ASST Valcamonica Esine and University of Brescia, 25128 Brescia, Italy; nadia.pasinetti@unibs.it
4. Hematology, ASST Spedali Civili of Brescia, 25128 Brescia, Italy; alessandra.tucci@asst-spedalicivili.it
* Correspondence: domenico.albano@unibs.it
† These authors contributed equally to this work.

Abstract: The goal of this retrospective study was to analyze and compare the prognostic role of fluorine-18-fluorodeoxyglucose positron emission tomography/computed tomography (2-[^{18}F]-FDG PET/CT) features and sarcopenia, estimated by CT of PET in elderly (≥65 years) Mantle Cell Lymphoma (MCL). We recruited 53 patients, who underwent pre-treatment 2-[^{18}F]-FDG PET/CT and end-of-treatment PET/CT, and the main semiquantitative parameters were calculated. Sarcopenia was measured as skeletal muscle index (SMI, cm^2/m^2) and derived by low-dose PET/CT images at the L3 level. Specific cut-offs for SMI were calculated by receiver operator curve and divided by gender. Metabolic response was evaluated at end-of-treatment PET/CT, applying the Deauville score. Progression Free Survival (PFS) and Overall Survival (OS) were calculated for the whole population and for different subgroups, defined as per different sarcopenia cut-off levels. The specific cut-offs to define sarcopenia were 53 cm^2/m^2 for male and 45.6 cm^2/m^2 for female. Thirty-two (60%) patients were defined as sarcopenic. The 3-year and 5-year PFS rates were 29% and 23%, while the 3-year and 5-year OS rates were 43% and 33%. Metabolic response, total metabolic tumor volume (tMTV), total lesion glycolysis (tTLG) and sarcopenia were independent prognostic factors for PFS. Considering OS, no variable was significantly associated. Combination between PET features and sarcopenia may help to predict PFS.

Keywords: Mantle Cell Lymphoma; PET/CT; MTV; TLG; sarcopenia; ^{18}F-FDG

1. Introduction

Mantle Cell Lymphoma (MCL) is a non-Hodgkin's lymphoma (NHL), with aggressive behavior and poor prognosis representing less than 10% of all NHLs [1,2]. MCL is an NHL frequent in advanced age; the median age at diagnosis ranges from 60 to 70 [3]. The prognosis of elderly lymphoma patients is, of course, worse than that of younger patients; this is probably due to the presence of age-related conditions and comorbidities that could increase the risk of side effects after treatments and worsen the prognosis. Sometimes, the chemotherapy regimen needs to be changed during the course of therapy, with a de-escalation of doses or a reduction in the cycles [4]. The risk of relapse or progression is very high and, nowadays, no clear and shared prognostic factors are available. Furthermore, the MCL International Prognostic Index (MIPI), proposed as the prognostic index, found controversial evidence in the literature [5,6]. The potential prognostic role of fluorine-18-fluorodeoxyglucose positron emission tomography/computed tomography (2-[^{18}F]-FDG PET/CT) and its features is yet an open question [7]. Several recent papers [8–10] demonstrated that metabolic response after first-line therapy, metabolic tumor volume (MTV) and total lesion glycolysis (TLG) were significantly related with progression free survival (PFS), not with overall survival (OS). A detection of shared prognostic criteria could be fundamental with the aim to stratify patients and personalize the patient management and treatment. In this scenario, the potential prognostic role of sarcopenia and its indexes are not evaluated. Sarcopenia can be considered a multi-factorial syndrome, defined by a progressive and generalized loss of strength and skeletal muscle mass, which may increase the risk of adverse events (until death) and reduce the quality of life [11]. In HL and diffuse large B cell lymphoma (DLBCL), the sarcopenia estimated by CT (low-dose CT of PET or high-dose CT) has been shown to be an independent prognostic factor [12,13], while in MCL, these analyses are anecdotal with low numbers [14,15] of patients included and mixed with other lymphoma histotypes [16,17].

For these reasons, the aim of this retrospective study was to analyze and compare the prognostic value of PET/CT features and sarcopenia, estimated by CT of PET in elderly MCL.

2. Materials and Methods

2.1. Patients

We have retrospectively screened about 42.011 2-[^{18}F]-FDG PET/CT scans performed in our Nuclear Medicine Department from January 2010 until December 2020 for any reason. Among them, 140 had a histological diagnosis of MCL. The other patients had different oncological or not oncological diseases. These patients were further selected according to some inclusion criteria: (1) patients who performed a baseline PET/CT scan and an end-of-treatment (eot) PET/CT after first line chemotherapy; (2) patients without a previous history of other malignancies; (3) patients with an age at the time of MCL diagnosis ≥65 years; (4) patients with at least 12 months of follow-up from the baseline 2-[^{18}F]-FDG PET/CT. Finally, 53 patients were recruited (Figure 1). The medical records of these patients were analyzed with attention to the main epidemiological (gender, age at diagnosis, BMI), clinical (B symptoms, MIPI score, β2-microglobulin level and lactate-dehydrogenase (LDH) level), histopathological (blastoid variant), size (bulky disease, splenomegaly), PET/CT semiquantitative data and sarcopenia features. MIPI score, β2-microglobulin and LDH values were dichotomized using a cutoff value of 2, 2.8 mg/L and 245 U/L respectively.

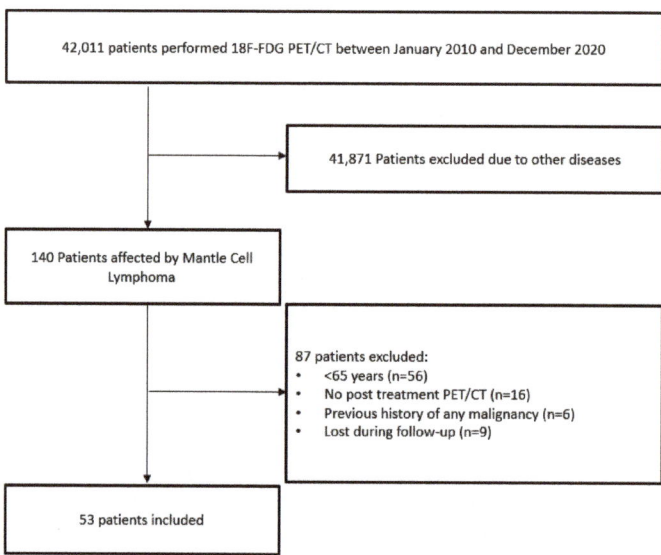

Figure 1. Flowchart of patients included.

All patients were treated according to the institution's standard protocol with chemotherapy regimen. In 22 cases R-BAC (Rituximab, Bendamustine and Cytarabine) regimen was performed up to six cycles of immuno-chemotherapy and in three cases, up to four cycles; in ten cases R-CHOP (Rituximab, Cyclophosphamide, Hydroxydoxorubicine, Oncovin and Prednisone) regimen was done up to six cycles and in five, up to three cycles; in three cases R-hyper-CVAD (rituximab, hyper-fractionated cyclophosphamide, vincristine, adriamycin, and dexamethasone alternating with rituximab, high-dose methotrexate, and high-dose cytarabine) regimen was chosen and in the remaining ten patients MCL 0208 trial which consisted of high-dose chemotherapy plus Rituximab, followed by Lenalidomide and autologous stem cell transplantation as maintenance therapy was used.

There was a minimal overlap (n 11 patients) with a previous paper already published [9].

2.2. 2-[^{18}F]-FDG PET/CT Imaging and Interpretation

All patients underwent a baseline 2-[^{18}F]-FDG PET/CT scan before any kind of therapy and, if available, an eotPET/CT. Then, 2-[^{18}F]-FDG PET/CT was acquired after at least 4 h fasting and with glucose blood level <150 mg/dL. An activity of 3.5–4.5 MBq/Kg of radiotracer was injected intravenously and scans began about 60 ± 10 min after the injection. The scan was performed from the skull base to the mid-thigh on two PET/CT scanners: Discovery ST and Discovery 690 PET/CT tomographs (General Electric Company—GE®—Milwaukee, WI, USA) with standard parameters (CT: 80 mA, 120 kV without contrast; 2.5–4 min per bed-PET-step of 15 cm). The matrix of reconstruction was 256 × 256 and the field of view was 60 cm. For both tomographs a standard non-contrast free-breathing helical low-dose CT was obtained for morphologic correlation and attenuation correction. The D-STE acquisition parameters were: 120 kV, fixed tube current ~73 mAs (40–160 mAs), 4 slices × 3.75 mm and 3.27 mm interval, pitch 1.5:1, tube rotation 0.8 s. The D690 acquisition parameters were: 120 kV, fixed tube current ~60 mAs (40–100 mAs), 64 slices × 3.75 mm and 3.27 mm interval, pitch 0.984:1, tube rotation 0.5 s. For D690, time-of-flight (TOF) and point spread function (PSF) were used as reconstruction algorithms; filter cutoff 5 mm, 18 subsets; three iterations. For D-STE, ordered subset expectation maximization (OSEM) was applied; filter cutoff 5 mm; 21 subsets, two iterations.

When available, eotPET/CT were performed at least three weeks after the last cycle of chemotherapy.

All PET images were analyzed visually and semi-quantitatively by a nuclear medicine physician with experience (DA) with the measurements of the maximum standardized uptake value body weight (SUVbw), the SUVmax corrected for the lean body mass (SUVlbm), the SUVmax corrected for body surface area (SUVbsa), lesion to liver SUVmax ratio (L-L SUV R), lesion to blood-pool SUVmax ratio (L-BP SUV R), MTV and TLG. Eot PET/CT was interpreted visually by the same nuclear medicine physician with more than 10 years of experience (DA) applying the Deauville scores. According to Deauville criteria [18], 2-[^{18}F]-FDG PET/CT was interpreted as follows: 1 = no uptake above background, 2 = uptake equal to or lower than mediastinum, 3 = uptake higher than mediastinum and lower than liver, 4 = uptake moderately increased compared to the liver and 5 = uptake markedly increased compared to the liver. After therapy, patients with a score of 1–3 were judged as having complete metabolic response, while patients with score 4–5 as not complete metabolic response. For the measurements of SUV, a region of interest (ROI) was drawn over the area of maximum activity of the lesion with highest uptake and the SUVmax was derived as the highest SUV of the pixels within the ROI. SUVmax of the liver was calculated at the VIII hepatic segment of axial PET images using a round-shape ROI of 10 mm; SUVmax of the blood-pool was calculated at the aortic arch by use not involving the vessel wall in a similar way. MTV was measured from attenuation-corrected PET images using an SUV-based automated contouring program (Advantage Workstation 4.6, GE HealthCare) with an isocounter threshold method based on 41% of the SUVmax, as previously recommended by European Association of Nuclear Medicine because of its high inter-observer reproducibility [19]. Total MTV (tMTV) was obtained by the sum of all nodal and extranodal lesions. Bone marrow involvement was included in volume measurement only if there was focal uptake; splenic involvement was considered if there was focal uptake in spleen or diffuse uptake higher than 150% in the liver background. Total TLG (tTLG) was calculated as the sum of the product of MTV of each lesion and its SUVmean. Semiquantitative analyses were performed by the same nuclear medicine physicians with long experience in lymphoma and in the use of Advantage Workstation 4.6, GE HealthCare for contouring.

2.3. Sarcopenia Analysis

Low-dose CT of 2-[^{18}F]-FDG PET/CT scans were analyzed by a researcher for the estimation of muscular and adipose tissues using Slice-O-Matic software V4.2 (Montreal, QC, Canada Tomovision). A transaxial slice with a multiplanar reconstruction at the third lumbar (L3) level was considered for the measurement of skeletal muscle area (SMA) considering psoas, paraspinal, abdominal transverse rectum, internal and external oblique, because the skeletal muscle in this area has been shown to represent the whole-body tissue quantities [11]. To measure the SMA (cm^2), CT Hounsfield unit thresholds were −29 to 150. If necessary, the tissue margins were manually corrected. Subsequently SMA was normalized for the height to obtain the skeletal muscle index (SMI) expressed in cm^2/m^2.

2.4. Statistical Analysis

MedCalc (Belgium) was used as software for statistical analysis. Categorical variables were expressed as simple and relative frequencies; the numeric variables were expressed as mean, standard deviation, minimum and maximum.

The receiver operating characteristic (ROC) curve analysis was carried out to find the best threshold point for each metabolic variable and SMI, which predict the risk of progression/relapse (Supplementary Table S1). Progression free survival (PFS) was calculated from the date of pre-treatment 2-[^{18}F]-FDG PET/CT to the date of first disease progression, relapse, death or the date of last follow-up. Overall survival (OS) was calculated from the date of pre-treatment 2-[^{18}F]-FDG PET/CT to the date of death from any cause or to the date of last follow-up. Survival curves were plotted according to the Kaplan–Meier method and differences between groups were analyzed by using a two-tailed log rank test. Cox regression was used to estimate the hazard ratio (HR) and its confidence interval (CI). A *p* value of < 0.05 was considered statistically significant.

3. Results

3.1. Patients Features

Among 53 patients included, there was a prevalence of male patients (74%); the average age was 72.7 years old. Most patients had advanced tumor stage disease, with stage IV in 45 patients. B-symptoms were present in 10 patients, while bulky disease in 6 cases. LDL and β2 microglobulin were higher than normal range values in 19 and 18 patients, respectively. Table 1 summarizes the clinical characteristics of the population. Pathological increased ^{18}F-FDG-uptake was present in all patients, showing the presence of at least one nodal or extranodal hypermetabolic lesion. The average SUVbw was 9.6 (range 3.3–27), average SUVlbm was 7.4 (range 2.4–22.3), average SUVbsa was 2.4 (range 0.9–7.3), average L-L SUV R 46.27 (1.7–54), average L-BP SUV R 5.3 (1–44), average tMTV was 358 cm^3 (3–1800 cm^3) and average TLG was 2023 (10–20088). The average SMI was 49.9 cm^2/m^2 (range 36.3–67) and was significantly higher in men, with a mean of 53.1 cm^2/m^2 (range 39–67), than women, with a mean value of 42 cm^2/m^2 (range 36.3–46.3) (Table 1). Based on Lugano classification metabolic response [18], 30 (57%) patients had a complete metabolic response at eotPET/CT. Fifteen (28%) patients had partial metabolic response and five (9%) patients had progression of disease. Three patients died before the execution of eotPET/CT.

Table 1. Main features of our sample (53 patients).

	Patients *n* (%)	Average ± SD (Range)
Age (years)		72.7 ± 5.6 (66–88)
Sex male	39 (74%)	
Sex female	14 (26%)	
BMI		26.15 ± 4.4 (16.8–34.8)
Tumor stage at diagnosis (Ann Arbor)		
I	0 (0%)	
II	4 (7.5%)	
III	4 (7.5%)	
IV	45 (85%)	
B symptoms	10 (19%)	
Blastoid variant	7 (13%)	
Bulky disease	6 (11%)	
LDH ≤ 245	34 (64%)	
>245	19 (36%)	
β 2 microglobulin ≤ 2.8	35 (66%)	
>2.8	18 (34%)	
Ki-67 score ≤ 15%	22 (44%)	
>15%	28 (56%)	
MIPI score ≤ 2	12 (23%)	
(>2)	41 (77%)	
SUVbw		9.6 ± 5.3 (3.3–27)
SUVlbm		7.4 ± 4.4 (2.4–22.3)
SUVbsa		2.4 ± 1.4 (0.9–7.3)
Lesion to BP SUVmax ratio		6.2 ± 8.8 (1.7–54)
Lesion to liver SUVmax ratio		5.3 ± 6.8 (1–44)
tMTV		358 ± 481 (3–1800)
tTLG		2023 ± 3147 (10–20,088)
SMI		49.9 ± 7.7 (36.3–67)
for male		53.1 ± 6.3 (39–67)
for female		42 ± 3.4 (36.3–46.3)

BMI: body mass index; LDH: lactate dehydrogenase; MIPI: Mantle international prognostic index; SUV: standardized uptake value; bw:body weight; lbm: lean body mass; bsa: body surface area; BP: blood pool; MTV: metabolic tumor volume; TLG: total lesion glycolysis; SMI: skeletal muscle index; SD: standard deviation.

3.2. Sarcopenic Analysis

For the definition of sarcopenia, in the absence of specific shared thresholds based on the MCL population, we derived our thresholds by applying ROC curve analysis. A separate analysis for male and female was performed (Supplemental Table S1). The gender-specific cut-offs were 53 cm^2/m^2 for male and 45.6 cm^2/m^2 for female. With these cut-offs, 32 (60%) of our patients were considered sarcopenic. There was a significantly higher prevalence of sarcopenia in females than males (93% vs. 47%, $p = 0.001$), with no significant differences found considering age, BMI, tumor stage, B symptoms, bulky disease, blood samples (LDH, β 2 microglobulin), MIPI score and complete metabolic response at eot PET (Table 2). Instead, the presence of the blastoid variant was significantly higher in patients with sarcopenia. Focusing on the relationship between semiquantitative PET/CT variables and sarcopenia, no significant differences among SUVbw, SUVlbm, SUVbsa, lesion to BP SUVmax ratio and lesion to liver SUVmax ratio were registered, comparing sarcopenic and not sarcopenic cases. Further, tMTV and tTLG were significantly higher in patients with low SMI.

Table 2. Comparison of baseline variables between sarcopenic and not sarcopenic patients applying cut-offs of 53 cm^2/m^2 for male and 45.6 cm^2/m^2 for female.

	Sarcopenia $n = 32$	Not Sarcopenia $n = 21$	p Value
Male:Female	21:13	18:1	0.001
Age (mean ± SD)	73.4 ± 5.7	71.4 ± 5.2	0.338
BMI	25.8	26.6	0.801
Tumor stage advanced	29 (91%)	19 (90%)	0.985
Bulky disease	4 (12.5%)	2 (10%)	0.745
Splenomegaly	14 (44%)	6 (29%)	0.093
Blastoid variant	7 (22%)	0 (0%)	0.021
LDH (mean ± SD)	276 ± 264	208 ± 83	0.257
β 2 microglobulin (mean ± SD)	4.5 ± 5.5	2.44 ± 2	0.526
MIPI score > 2	10 (31%)	5 (24%)	0.288
Complete metabolic response	17 (57%)	13 (62%)	0.537
SUVbw (mean ± SD)	8.7 ± 4.9	10.8 ± 5.7	0.139
SUVlbm (mean ± SD)	6.7 ± 4	8.35 ± 4.8	0.144
SUVbsa (mean ± SD)	2.2 ± 1.3	2.7 ± 1.6	0.160
Lesion to BP SUVmax ratio (mean ± SD)	4.7 ± 5.7	6.3 ± 10	0.411
Lesion to liver SUVmax ratio (mean ± SD)	5.4 ± 4.8	7.4 ± 9	0.402
tMTV (mean ± SD)	470 ± 57	192 ± 34	0.040
tTLG (mean ± SD)	2726 ± 378	985 ± 138	0.033

BMI: body mass index; LDH: lactate dehydrogenase; MIPI: mantle international prognostic index; SUV: standardized uptake value; bw: body weight; lbm: lean body mass; bsa: body surface area; BP: blood pool; MTV: metabolic tumor volume; TLG: total lesion glycolysis; SD: standard deviation.

3.3. Survival Analysis

At a median follow-up of 50 months, a progression of disease or relapse was registered in 37 patients (70%), with an average time of 17.2 months (range: 2–62 months), while death occurred in 26 patients (49%), with a mean time of 33.6 months (range: 2–120). Overall, the 3-year and 5-year PFS rates were 29% and 23%, while the 3-year and 5-year OS rates were 43% and 33%. In univariate analysis, blastoid variant, Deauville Score 4–5, tMTV, tTLG and SMI were significantly correlated with PFS ($p = 0.015$, $p = 0.032$, $p = 0.001$, $p < 0.001$, $p < 0.001$), while the other clinical and metabolic features were not (Figure 2, Table 3). In multivariate analysis, the Deauville Score 4–5, tMTV, tTLG and SMI were confirmed to be independent prognostic factors. Considering OS, only tMTV and tTLG were shown to be significantly related to outcome at univariate analysis, but not at multivariate analysis. SMI demonstrated no prognostic impact (Figure 3, Table 3). Combining tMTV and SMI thresholds, patients without sarcopenia and with low metabolic volume disease (<90 cm^3) had the best PFS, without any case of progression/relapse during the follow-up. The worst PFS was specific of patients with sarcopenia independent from the tMTV value (Figure 4).

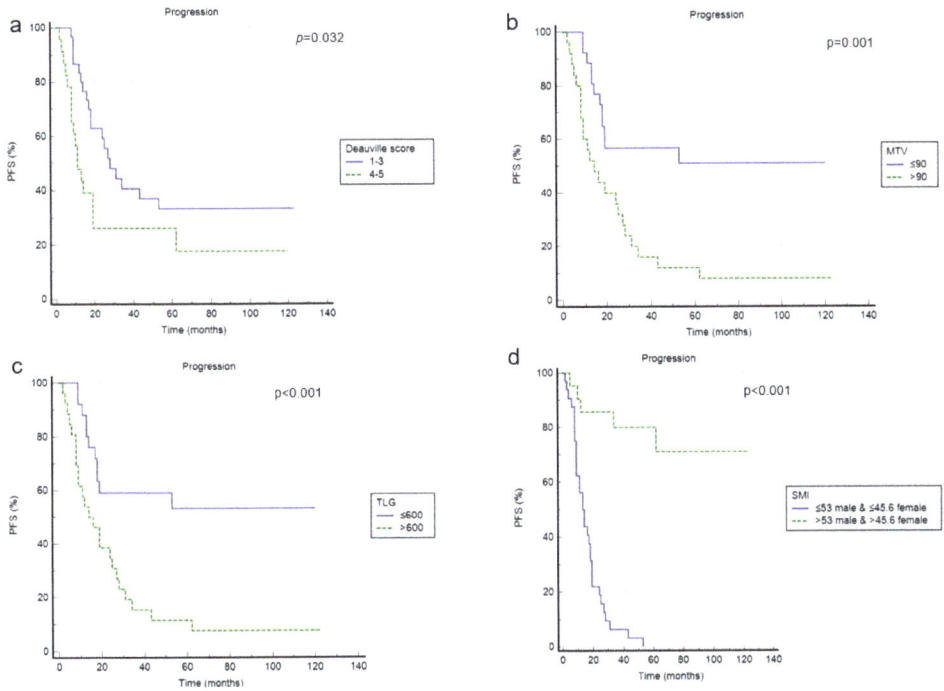

Figure 2. Progression free survival according to Deauville score (**a**), tMTV (**b**), tTLG (**c**) and SMI (**d**).

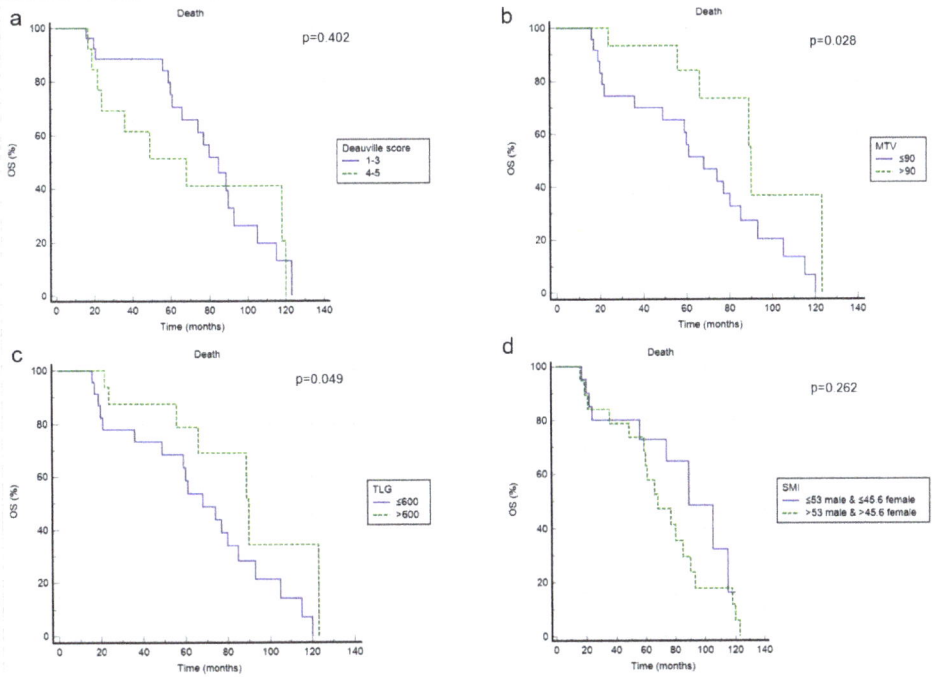

Figure 3. Overall survival according to Deauville score (**a**), tMTV (**b**), tTLG (**c**) and SMI (**d**).

Table 3. Univariate and multivariate analyses for PFS and OS.

	Univariate Analysis		Multivariate Analysis	
	p Value	HR (95% CI)	p Value	HR (95% CI)
PFS				
Sex	0.299	1.358 (0.500–2.333)		
Age	0.298	1.225 (0.284–2.585)		
MIPI score	0.582	1.989 (0.500–4.212)		
LDH level	0.121	0.610 (0.292–1.154)		
B2 microglobulin	0.895	1.053 (0.476–2.333)		
Bulky disease	0.458	0.124 (0.102–1.715)		
Splenomegaly	0.248	1.582 (0.123–3.002)		
Blastoid variant	0.015	1.292 (1.101–1.500)	0.102	1.250 (0.888–1.650)
Deauville score	0.032	2.155 (1.068–4.351)	0.042	2.255 (1.250–3.690)
SUVbw *	0.555	1.446 (0.759–3.042)		
SUVlbm *	0.434	1.111 (0.534–2.126)		
SUVbsa *	0.331	1.459 (0.339–2.856)		
L-L SUV R *	0.450	1.107 (0.756–2.122)		
L-BP SUV R *	0.324	1.222 (0.444–4.235)		
tMTV *	0.001	3.190 (1.568–6.374)	0.039	2.833 (1.053–7.619)
tTLG *	<0.001	3.258 (1.638–6.479)	0.022	2.075 (0.889–4.843)
SMI *	<0.001	0.125 (0.062–0.253)	<0.001	0.031 (0.007–0.132)
R-BAC vs other	0.401	0.852 (0.222–1.589)		
OS				
Sex	0.211	1.666 (0.389–5.026)		
Age	0.375	1.389 (0.445–3.005)		
MIPI score	0.690	0.987 (0.666–1.589)		
LDH level	0.480	0.825 (0.450–1.454)		
B2 microglobulin	0.333	0.858 (0.420–1.689)		
Bulky disease	0.387	1.258 (0.555–2.297)		
Splenomegaly	0.222	1.359 (0.801–1.987)		
Blastoid variant	0.342	0.659 (0.350–1.259)		
Deauville score	0.402	1.404 (0.596–3.310)		
SUVbw *	0.453	0.816 (0.464–1.408)		
SUVlbm *	0.160	0.698 (0.368–1.179)		
SUVbsa *	0.207	0.677 (0.363–1.245)		
L-L SUV R *	0.125	0.689 (0.376–1.127)		
L-BP SUV R *	0.307	0.631 (0.306–1.452)		
tMTV *	0.028	0.374 (0.172–0.811)	0.129	0.563 (0.105–1.009)
tTLG *	0.049	0.448 (0.207–0.970)	0.062	0.550 (0.102–1.120)
SMI *	0.262	1.574 (0.736–3.365)		
R-BAC vs. other	0.396	0.701 (0.386–1.499)		

PFS: progression free survival; OS: overall survival; HR: hazard ratio; CI: confidence interval; N°: number; SUV: standard uptake value; bw: body wheight; lbm: lean body mass; bsa: body surface area; L-L R: lesion to liver ratio; L-BP R: lesion to blood pool ratio; MTV: total metabolic tumor volume; TLG: total lesion glycolysis. * Variables dichotomized using cutoff values after ROC analysis reported in Supplemental Table S1.

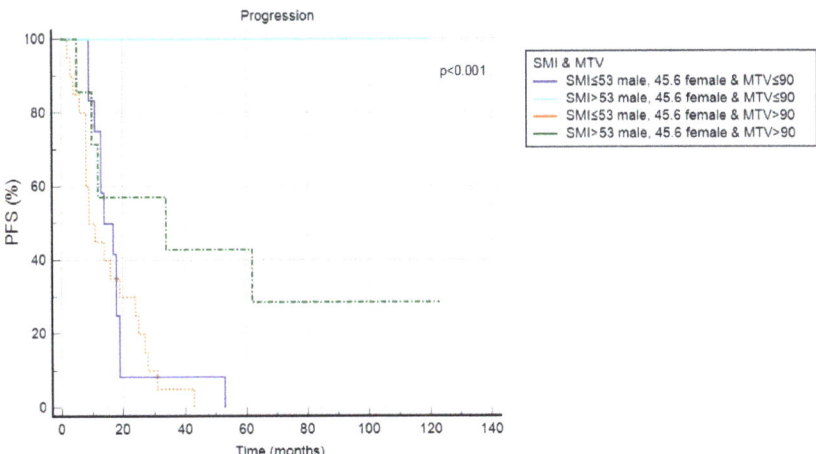

Figure 4. Kaplan–Meier curve considering the combination of tMTV and SMI.

4. Discussion

The clinical meaning of the sarcopenia has already been investigated and it is emerging as a promising tool for predicting the survival and treatment response [20–23]. However, in lymphoma patients, its usefulness is not yet clear because controversial evidence is available and the studies present are based specifically on HL and DLBCL [12,24], while for the other lymphoma histotyopes, specific studies are lacking. For this reason, we aimed to analyze patients affected by MCL, which is a lymphoma typical in advanced age. Just in this setting, the evaluation of the role of sarcopenia may be fundamental. For the measurements of sarcopenia, several techniques and imaging examinations have been proposed, such as hand-held dynamometer, CT and MRI [25,26]. These tools are very different for availability, cost, ease of execution and accuracy. CT seems to have the best compromise and it is often applied for the evaluation of the muscular area, due to its ability to distinguish adipose and muscular tissue from other soft tissues of the body. A recent paper demonstrated a good agreement and reproducibility between low-dose CT of PET and high-dose CT in the measurements of the adipose and muscular area [27]. These results underlined the possibility to use 2-[^{18}F]-FDG PET/CT, both for the measurements of "classical" PET/CT parameters (like SUV, MTV, TLG) and sarcopenia.

To the best of our knowledge, no studies about the rate and the role of sarcopenia in MCL are available, particularly in advanced age patients. We decided to select elderly MCL patients, because they are, by definition, frail patients with a high risk of toxicities and poor prognosis.

Due to the lack of consensus for optimal cut-off levels to define sarcopenia in lymphoma patients, and especially in MCL, we derived specific values for our population using ROC curve analysis. Many different thresholds have been proposed [12], specific for gender, BMI, ethnicity and geographic regions. Thus, it is hazardous to consider a unique threshold validated in other lymphoma variants. The cut-off values obtained in our analysis were 53 cm^2/m^2 for males and 45.6 cm^2/m^2 for females. Further studies with larger samples are essential to confirm or change these results, especially for women, where our cases are relatively low (n 14). However, these values may be considered a starting point to investigate. With these cut-offs, we found a prevalence of sarcopenia in 60% of our sample and it was more diffused in women than men. Besides gender, only the blastoid variant is significantly related to sarcopenia status, assuming a more aggressive disease in blastoid CML [28].

The second goal of our study was to analyze the prognostic role of several variables, including 2-[^{18}F]-FDG PET/CT features and sarcopenia, in terms of PFS and OS.

Besides quantitative parameters, visual analysis, applying the Deauville score, remains a valid prognostic variable for PFS in MCL, as demonstrated by several papers and confirmed in our analysis [9,29].

Among 2-[^{18}F]-FDG PET/CT parameters, MTV and TLG were shown to be superior than SUV-related factors, but also in this case, the significant correlation from the multivariate analysis was confirmed only for PFS. The same evidence was revealed considering sarcopenia. However, the combination of tMTV and sarcopenia better predicts the PFS. The absence of prognostic factors to predict OS may be explained by the advanced age of patients, which probably significantly influenced the outcome; moreover, it could be other variables not evaluated in this study with a prognostic impact. The open question, not yet resolute, is the choice of the cut-off values to apply to define sarcopenia with CT.

Several limitations affect the quality of this work, such as the retrospective study design, the heterogeneous management received by patients (for example primary treatment) and the relatively low number of patients included due to the inclusion criteria chosen. This is the first attempt to investigate the prognostic role of sarcopenia, detected by CT in combination with PET/CT features, in elderly MCL. Prospective studies are warranted to better define, in real-life settings, whether these easy and patient-level approaches retain their significance and utility and could be used to improve treatment tailoring in the setting of elderly MCL.

5. Conclusions

Baseline evaluation CT of PET may help to define sarcopenia, with a specific cutoff for gender in elderly MCL. Sarcopenia, together with Deauville score, tMTV and tTLG, may help to predict PFS. Instead, they had no role in predicting OS.

Supplementary Materials: The following supporting information can be downloaded at: https://www.mdpi.com/article/10.3390/jcm11051210/s1, Supplemental Table S1: Receiver operating characteristic (ROC) curve analysis of metabolic and sarcopenic PET/CT parameters.

Author Contributions: Conceptualization, D.A., F.B., R.G.; methodology, N.P., F.D., A.T.; formal analysis, N.P., D.A., R.G.; investigation, A.T.; F.B., F.D.; writing—original draft preparation, D.A., N.P.; writing—review and editing, D.A., R.G., F.B., F.D., N.P.; supervision, R.G. All authors have read and agreed to the published version of the manuscript.

Funding: This research received no external funding.

Institutional Review Board Statement: Ethical review and approval were waived for this study due to the retrospective design of the study, according to local laws.

Informed Consent Statement: Informed consent was obtained from all subjects involved in the study.

Data Availability Statement: Data are not public, but are present in our institution.

Conflicts of Interest: The authors declare no conflict of interest.

References

1. Swerdlow, S.H.; Campo, E.; Harris, N.L.; Jaffe, E.S.; Pileri, S.A.; Stein, H.; Thiele, J. *World Health Organization Classification of Tumours of Haematopoietic and Lymphoid Tissues*; IARC Press: Lyon, France, 2008.
2. Maddocks, K. Update on Mantle cell lymphoma. *Blood* **2018**, *132*, 1647–1656. [CrossRef] [PubMed]
3. Lynch, D.T.; Koya, S.; Acharya, U. Mantle Cell Lymphoma. 9 August 2021. In *StatPearls [Internet]*; StatPearls Publishing: Treasure Island, FL, USA, 2021.
4. Doordujin, J.K.; Kluin-Nelemans, H. Mangement of mantle cell lymphoma in the elderly patient. *Clin. Interv. Aging* **2013**, *8*, 1229–1236.
5. Hoster, E.; Dreyling, M.; Klapper, W.; Gisselbrecht, C.; van Hoof, A.; Kluin-Nelemans, H.C.; Pfreundschuh, M.; Reiser, M.; Metzner, B.; Einsele, H.; et al. A new prognostic index (MIPI) for patients with advanced-stage mantle cell lymphoma. *Blood* **2008**, *111*, 558–565. [CrossRef] [PubMed]
6. Shah, J.J.; Fayad, L.; Romaguera, J. Mantle Cell International Prognostic Index (MIPI) not prognostic after R-hyper-CVAD. *Blood* **2008**, *112*, 2583–2584. [CrossRef]
7. Albano, D.; Treglia, G.; Gazzilli, M.; Cerudelli, E.; Giubbini, R.; Bertagna, F. 18F-FDG PET or PET/CT in Mantle Cell Lymphoma. *Clin. Lymphoma Myeloma Leuk.* **2020**, *20*, 422–430. [CrossRef]

8. Mato, A.R.; Svodoba, J.; Feldman, T.; Zielonka, T.; Agress, H.; Panush, D.; Miller, M.; Toth, P.; Lizotte, P.M.; Nasta, S.; et al. Post-treatment (not interim) positron emission tomography-computed tomography scan status is highly predictive of outcome in mantle cell lymphoma patients treated with R-HyperCVAD. *Cancer* **2012**, *118*, 3565–3570. [CrossRef] [PubMed]

9. Albano, D.; Bosio, G.; Bianchetti, N.; Pagani, C.; Re, A.; Tucci, A.; Giubbini, R.; Bertagna, F. Prognostic role of baseline 18F-FDG PET/CT metabolic parameters in mantle cell lymphoma. *Ann. Nucl. Med.* **2019**, *33*, 449–458. [CrossRef]

10. Mayerhoefer, M.E.; Riedl, C.C.; Kumar, A.; Gibbs, P.; Weber, M.; Tal, I.; Schilksy, J.; Schoder, H. Radiomic features of glucose metabolism enable prediction of outcome in mantle cell lymphoma. *Eur. J. Nucl. Med. Mol. Imaging* **2019**, *46*, 2760–2769. [CrossRef]

11. Cruz-Jentoft, A.J.; Bahat, G.; Bauer, J.; Boirie, Y.; Bruyère, O.; Cederholm, T.; Cooper, C.; Landi, F.; Rolland, Y.; Sayer, A.A.; et al. Sarcopenia: Revised European consensus on definition and diagnosis. *Age Ageing* **2019**, *48*, 601. [CrossRef]

12. Albano, D.; Dondi, F.; Ravanelli, M.; Tucci, A.; Farina, D.; Giubbini, R.; Treglia, G.; Bertagna, F. Prognostic Role of "Radiological" Sarcopenia in Lymphoma: A Systematic Review. *Clin. Lymphoma Myeloma Leuk.* **2021**. [CrossRef] [PubMed]

13. Zilioli, V.R.; Albano, D.; Arcari, A.; Merli, F.; Coppola, A.; Besutti, G.; Marcheselli, L.; Gramegna, D.; Muzi, C.; Manicone, M.; et al. Clinical and prognostic role of sarcopenia in elderly patients with classical Hodgkin lymphoma: A multicentre experience. *J. Cachexia Sarcopenia Muscle* **2021**, *12*, 1042–1055. [CrossRef]

14. Burkart, M.; Schieber, M.; Basu, S.; Shah, P.; Venugopal, P.; Borgia, J.A.; Gordon, L.; Karmali, R. Evaluation of the impact of cachexia on clinical outcomes in aggressive lymphoma. *Br. J. Haematol.* **2019**, *186*, 45–53. [CrossRef]

15. Karmali, R.; Alrifai, T.; Fughhi, I.A.M.; Shah, P.; Venugopal, P.; Borgia, J.A.; Gordon, L.; Karmali, R. Impact of cachexia on outcomes in aggressive lymphomas. *Ann. Hematol.* **2017**, *96*, 951–956. [CrossRef] [PubMed]

16. Armenian, S.H.; Iukuridze, A.; The, J.B.; Mascarenhas, K.; Herrera, A.; McCune, J.S.; Zain, J.M.; Mostoufi-Moab, S.; McCormack, S.; Slavin, T.P.; et al. Abnormal body composition is a predic- tor of adverse outcomes after autologous haematopoietic cell transplantation. *J. Cachexia Sarcopenia Muscle* **2020**, *11*, 962–972. [CrossRef] [PubMed]

17. Caram, M.V.; Bellile, E.L.; Englesbe, M.J.; Terjimanian, M.; Wang, S.C.; Griggs, J.J.; Couriel, D. Sarcopenia is associated with autologous transplant-related outcomes in patients with lymphoma. *Leuk. Lymphoma* **2015**, *56*, 2855–2862. [CrossRef]

18. Barrington, S.F.; Mikhaeel, N.G.; Kostakoglu, L.; Meignan, M.; Hutchings, M.; Müeller, S.P.; Schwartz, L.H.; Zucca, E.; Fisher, R.I.; Trotman, J.; et al. Role of imaging in the staging and response assessment of lymphoma: Consensus of the International Conference on Malignant Lymphomas Imaging Working Group. *J. Clin. Oncol.* **2014**, *32*, 3048–3058. [CrossRef]

19. Boellaard, R.; Delgado-Bolton, R.; Oyen, W.J.; Giammarile, F.; Tatsch, K.; Eschner, W.; Verzijlbergen, F.J.; Barrington, S.F.; Pike, L.C.; Weber, W.A.; et al. FDG PET/CT: EANM procedure guidelines for tumour imaging: Version 2.0. *Eur. J. Nucl. Med. Mol. Imaging* **2015**, *42*, 328–354. [CrossRef] [PubMed]

20. Kamarajah, S.K.; Bundred, J.; Tan, B.H.L. Body composition assessment and sarcopenia in patients with gastric cancer: A systematic review and meta-analysis. *Gastric Cancer* **2019**, *22*, 10–22. [CrossRef]

21. Deng, H.Y.; Zha, P.; Peng, L.; Hou, L.; Huang, K.L.; Li, X.Y. Preoperative sarcopenia is a predictor of poor prognosis of esophageal cancer after esophagectomy: A comprehensive systematic review and meta-analysis. *Dis. Esophagus* **2019**, *32*, doy115. [CrossRef] [PubMed]

22. Mintziras, I.; Miligkos, M.; Wachter, S.; Manoharan, J.; Maurer, E.; Bartsch, D.K. Sarcopenia and sarcopenic obesity are significantly associated with poorer overall survival in patients with pancreatic cancer: Systematic review and meta-analysis. *Int. J. Surg.* **2018**, *59*, 19–26. [CrossRef]

23. Sun, G.; Li, Y.; Peng, Y.; Lu, D.; Zhang, F.; Cui, X.; Zhang, Q.; Li, Z. Can sarcopenia be a predictor of prognosis for patients with non-metastatic colorectal cancer? A systematic review and meta-analysis. *Int. J. Colorectal. Dis.* **2018**, *33*, 1419–1427. [CrossRef] [PubMed]

24. Surov, A.; Wienke, A. Sarcopenia predicts overall survival in patients with malignant hematological diseases: A meta-analysis. *Clin. Nutr.* **2021**, *40*, 1155–1160. [CrossRef] [PubMed]

25. Cooper, C.; Fielding, R.; Visser, M.; van Loon, L.J.; Rolland, Y.; Orwoll, E.; Reid, K.; Boonen, S.; Dere, W.; Epstein, S.; et al. Tools in the assessment of sarcopenia. *Calcif. Tissue Int.* **2013**, *93*, 201–210. [CrossRef] [PubMed]

26. Sinelnikov, A.; Qu, C.; Fetzer, D.T.; Pelletier, J.S.; Dunn, M.A.; Tsung, A.; Furlan, A. Measurement of skeletal muscle area: Comparison of CT and MR imaging. *Eur. J. Radiol.* **2016**, *85*, 1716–1721. [CrossRef] [PubMed]

27. Albano, D.; Camoni, L.; Rinaldi, R.; Tucci, A.; Zilioli, V.R.; Muzi, C.; Ravanelli, M.; Farina, D.; Coppola, A.; Camalori, M.; et al. Comparison between skeletal muscle and adipose tissue measurements with high-dose CT and low-dose attenuation correction CT of 18F-FDG PET/CT in elderly Hodgkin lymphoma patients: A two-centre validation. *Br. J. Radiol.* **2021**, *94*, 20200672. [CrossRef] [PubMed]

28. Jain, P.; Wang, M. Blastoid Mantle Cell Lymphoma. *Hematol. Oncol. Clin. N. Am.* **2020**, *34*, 941–956. [CrossRef] [PubMed]

29. Albano, D.; Laudicella, R.; Ferro, P.; Allocca, M.; Abenavoli, E.; Buschiazzo, A.; Castellino, A.; Chiaravalloti, A.; Cuccaro, A.; Cuppari, L.; et al. The Role of 18F-FDG PET/CT in Staging and Prognostication of Mantle Cell Lymphoma: An Italian Multicentric Study. *Cancers* **2019**, *11*, 1831. [CrossRef] [PubMed]

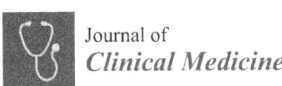

Article

Value of CT-Textural Features and Volume-Based PET Parameters in Comparison to Serologic Markers for Response Prediction in Patients with Diffuse Large B-Cell Lymphoma Undergoing CD19-CAR-T Cell Therapy

Christian Philipp Reinert [1,*], Regine Mariette Perl [1], Christoph Faul [2], Claudia Lengerke [2], Konstantin Nikolaou [1,3], Helmut Dittmann [4], Wolfgang A. Bethge [2,†] and Marius Horger [1,†]

1 Department of Radiology, Diagnostic and Interventional Radiology, University Hospital Tuebingen, Hoppe-Seyler-Str. 3, 72076 Tuebingen, Germany; regine.perl@med.uni-tuebingen.de (R.M.P.); konstantin.nikolaou@med.uni-tuebingen.de (K.N.); marius.horger@med.uni-tuebingen.de (M.H.)
2 Department of Hematology, Oncology, Clinical Immunology and Rheumatology, University Hospital Tuebingen, Hoppe-Seyler-Str. 3, 72076 Tuebingen, Germany; christoph.faul@med.uni-tuebingen.de (C.F.); claudia.lengerke@med.uni-tuebingen.de (C.L.); wolfgang.bethge@med.uni-tuebingen.de (W.A.B.)
3 Cluster of Excellence iFIT (EXC 2180) Image Guided and Functionally Instructed Tumor Therapies, University of Tuebingen, 72074 Tuebingen, Germany
4 Department of Radiology, Nuclear Medicine, University Hospital Tuebingen, Hoppe-Seyler-Str. 3, 72076 Tuebingen, Germany; helmut.dittmann@med.uni-tuebingen.de
* Correspondence: christian.reinert@med.uni-tuebingen.de; Tel.: +49-7071-298-7212; Fax: +49-7071-295-845
† These authors contributed equally to this work.

Abstract: The goal of this study was to investigate the value of CT-textural features and volume-based PET parameters in comparison to serologic markers for response prediction in patients with diffuse large B-cell lymphoma (DLBCL) undergoing cluster of differentiation (CD19)-chimeric antigen receptor (CAR)-T cell therapy. We retrospectively analyzed the whole-body (WB)-metabolic tumor volume (MTV), the WB-total lesion glycolysis (TLG) and first order textural features derived from ^{18}F-FDG-PET/CT, as well as serologic parameters (C-reactive protein [CRP] and lactate dehydrogenase [LDH], leucocytes) prior and after CAR-T cell therapy in 21 patients with DLBCL (57.7 ± 14.7 year; 7 female). Interleukin 6 (IL-6) and IL-2 receptor peaks were monitored after treatment onset and compared with patient outcome judged by follow-up ^{18}F-FDG-PET/CT. In 12/21 patients (57%), complete remission (CR) was observed, whereas 9/21 patients (43%) showed partial remission (PR). At baseline, WB-MTV and WB-TLG were lower in patients achieving CR (35 ± 38 mL and 319 ± 362) compared to patients achieving PR (88 ± 110 mL and 1487 ± 2254; $p < 0.05$). The "entropy" proved lower (1.81 ± 0.09) and "uniformity" higher (0.33 ± 0.02) in patients with CR compared to PR (2.08 ± 0.22 and 0.28 ± 0.47; $p < 0.05$). Patients achieving CR had lower levels of CRP, LDH and leucocytes at baseline compared to patients achieving PR ($p < 0.05$). In the entire cohort, WB-MTV and WB-TLG decreased after therapy onset ($p < 0.01$) becoming not measurable in the CR-group. Leucocytes and CRP significantly dropped after therapy ($p < 0.01$). The IL-6 and IL-2R peaks after therapy were lower in patients with CR compared to PR ($p > 0.05$). In conclusion, volume-based PET parameters derived from PET/CT and CT-textural features have the potential to predict therapy response in patients with DLBCL undergoing CAR-T cell therapy.

Keywords: diffuse-large B cell lymphoma; chimeric antigen receptor T cells; response assessment; positron emission tomography; computed tomography; texture analysis

1. Introduction

Diffuse large B-cell lymphoma (DLBCL) is the most common subtype of non-Hodgkin's lymphoma in adults with a prevalence of almost 40% [1]. Standard treatment regimens are efficacious, but up to 15% of patients will exhibit primary refractory disease and another 30–35% will experience relapse after initial response [2,3]. In the refractory/relapsed DLBCL patients, incidence of disease recurrence is high, even after salvage therapy combined with autologous stem cell support, leading to a dismal long-term survival rate [4]. In this setting, novel treatment strategies are explored. A promising, emerging therapy option are CD19 CAR (chimeric antigen receptor)-T cells, which consist of genetically modified autologous T cells by retroviral or lentiviral vectors containing DNA encoding a CAR [1]. It has been shown that CD19 CAR-T cells provide high and durable response rates even in refractory and relapsed DLBCL [5–7].

Imaging is playing a major role for diagnosis and treatment monitoring in patients with DLBCL, and the most frequently recommended technique is the positron emission tomography (PET) using ^{18}F-Fluorodeoxyglucose (FDG) as a tracer targeting glucose metabolism mostly in combination with computed tomography (CT) [8]. Hence, morphologic and glucometabolic changes in tumor herald either lymphoma response or relapse. The latter has been further refined by calculating the entire metabolic tumor volume (MTV) and the total lesion glycolysis (TLG). Both PET and CT image data can be additionally analyzed by using texture analysis with potential for tumor characterization either in the primary setting (baseline) for prognosis evaluation, or during therapy as an adjunct to morphologic and metabolic changes for more accurate response assessment [9,10]. Finally, some laboratory biomarkers like lactate dehydrogenase (LDH) in serum have been used for a long time as prognostic factors in lymphoma patients.

CD19-CAR T cell therapy as immunotherapy leads to a strong immunological response with T cell activation and cytokine release as illustrated by the most commonly observed adverse effect: cytokine release syndrome (CRS) and immune effector cell-associated neurotoxicity syndrome (ICANS). Manifestation of CRS goes along with hypersecretion of IL6, IL2-R, ferritin and CRP from activated macrophages following CAR-T cell activation [11].

Hence, the intention of this study was to investigate the value of CT-textural features and volume-based PET parameters in comparison to serologic markers for response prediction in patients with DLBCL undergoing CD19-CAR-T cell therapy.

2. Material and Methods

This retrospective image and laboratory data analysis was approved by the local ethics committee and the patients waived written consent (project number 277/2020BO2).

2.1. Patient Characteristics

Twenty-one consecutive patients with DLBCL (mean age 57.7 ± 14.7 year; seven female) undergoing CAR-T cell therapy from 06/2018 to 02/2021 were retrospectively evaluated. All patients had pathologically confirmed DLBCL. According to Ann-Arbor classification, 2/21 patients had a stage I, 3/21 patients had stage II, 5/21 patients had stage III and 11/21 patients were classified stage IV. According to the International Prognostic Index (IPI) scoring system, 3/21 patients were rated score 1, 9/21 patients were rated score 3 and 9/21 patients were rated score 4. Patient characteristics are summarized in Table 1.

Table 1. Patient characteristics.

	I	II	III	IV
Ann-Arbor stage	2	3	5	11
International Prognostic Index Score	3	0	9	9
Cytokine Release Syndrome Grade	10	7	2	1

At baseline staging, before CAR-T cell therapy, 17/21 patients underwent ^{18}F-FDG-PET/CT and 4/21 patients underwent CT using standardized protocols. All patients were additionally monitored by serologic parameters. At first follow-up after CAR-T cell therapy, 18/21 patients underwent ^{18}F-FDG-PET/CT and 3/21 patients underwent CT.

Therapy response was classified according to the Lugano classification system including CT-based response criteria and the Deauville five-point scale (Deauville 5PS) scoring system [12]. Each FDG-avid (or previously FDG-avid) lesion was rated independently by two readers. Response to CAR-T cell therapy was defined as PR in case of metabolically active disease (Deauville score 4), which is defined as lymphoma manifestations with ^{18}F-FDG-uptake slightly to moderately higher than the liver background ^{18}F-FDG-uptake without metric progression on CT. In case of no measurable ^{18}F-FDG-uptake and ^{18}F-FDG-uptake below or equal to uptake in the liver (Deauville score 1–3), CR was assigned.

2.2. Imaging Protocols

All PET/CT examinations were performed on a state-of-the art clinical scanner (Biograph mCT®, Siemens Healthineers, Erlangen, Germany). All patients fasted overnight before examination. Approximately 300 MBq ^{18}F-FDG were injected intravenously 60 min prior to image acquisition. Standardized CT examination protocols included weight-adapted 90–120 mL intravenous CT contrast agent (Ultravist 370®, Bayer Vital, Leverkusen, Germany). Portal-venous phase acquisitions were obtained with 70 s delay time using a tube voltage of 120 kV and a reference dose of 200 mAs. Image reconstruction was performed using iterative CT reconstruction (Siemens SAFIRE®, Forchheim, Germany). PET was acquired from the skull to the mid-thigh level over six to eight bed positions and reconstructed using a 3D ordered subset expectation maximization algorithm (two iterations, 21 subsets, Gaussian filter 2.0 mm, matrix size 400 × 400, and slice thickness 2.0 mm). PET acquisition time was 2–3 min per bed position.

CT was performed with patients in the supine position using a 128-slice MDCT scanner (SOMATOM Definition Flash, Siemens Healthcare, Erlangen, Germany). Contrast-enhanced portal-venous phases were obtained using 120-kV photon energy, 200-mAs tube current, a soft tissue image reconstruction kernel, and 1-mm slice thickness for image reconstruction. A weight-adapted iodine contrast agent (Ultravist [Iopromide] 370, Bayer Vital, Leverkusen, Germany) was given intravenously at a rate of 2 mL/s followed by a 30-mL saline chaser. Image acquisition began 70 s after the start of contrast agent injection. Image reconstruction was performed in all patients using filtered back projection.

2.3. Quantitative Image Analysis

The segmentation of lymphoma manifestations was performed by one reader using approved software for quantification of PET parameters on Syngo.via VB 30A (Siemens Healthineers, Erlangen, Germany). Evaluation included all lesions which were characterized by increased ^{18}F-FDG uptake above liver background activity (Deauville score 4). Segmentation of each lesion was performed manually using 50%-isocontour volumes of interests (VOIs) for quantification. Whole-body MTV and whole-body TLG were calculated as the sum of all quantified lymphoma manifestations per patient.

CT-texture analysis (CTTA) was performed in contrast-enhanced CT images derived from whole-body CT or whole-body ^{18}F-FDG-PET/CT obtained in the portal-venous enhancement phase using a standardized protocol and dedicated radiomics software (Siemens Healthcare, Erlangen, Germany) that is based on the pyradiomics package, a python package for the extraction of radiomics features from medical imaging [13]. A slice thickness of 1 mm was used. Regions of interests (ROIs) were drawn manually in lymphatic tissue carefully excluding neighboring tissues like blood vessels. This standardized procedure of ROI setting was performed by a radiologist with five years of experience in CTTA. Standardized measurements were performed to provide comparability for all data sets. All set ROIs were used to generate specific VOIs. The first step consisted of image filtration for selectively extracting features of different sizes and intensity variation. In the 2nd step, quantification of tissue texture followed. The computation of each texture type for an input VOI involved assigning a new value ("texture value") to all voxel of that VOI and thus creating a "texture image". This involved the creation of a three-dimensional VOI within the largest lymph node, the features of which were used to calculate texture values on a fine spatial scale.

Computation was performed on the current voxel and its neighborhood, and the results of that were stored as the current voxel's texture value. To ensure reliable statistics for this patient cohort, we limited analysis of textural parameters to the following 1st order features which describe the distribution of voxel intensities within the mask through commonly used and basic metrics: mean, uniformity, entropy, skewness. The definitions of these textural parameters are provided in Table 2.

Table 2. Definitions of measured 1st order textural features *.

1st Order Feature	Definition
Entropy	• Specifies the uncertainty/randomness in the image values. • Measures the average amount of information required to encode the image values.
Mean	• Mean of voxel intensities within the region
Skewness	• Measures the asymmetry of the distribution of values about the mean value. • Depends on where the tail is elongated and where the mass of the distribution is concentrated • Can be positive or negative.
Uniformity	• Sum of the squares of each intensity value. • Measure of the homogeneity of the image array, where a greater uniformity implies a greater homogeneity or a smaller range of discrete intensity values.

* Describe the distribution of voxel intensities within the image region defined by the mask through commonly used and basic metrics.

2.4. Laboratory Parameters

Laboratory parameters were extracted from the clinical data base on the same day as imaging. The upper limits of the reference ranges were: 250 U/L for serum LDH, 0.5 µg/dL for CRP, 130 U/L for AP, 4100–11,800 1/µL for leucocyte count, 158–613 U/mL for soluble IL-2R and 0–4 ng/L for IL-6.

2.5. Statistical Analysis

Statistical analysis was performed using SPSS Version 22 (IBM Corporation, Armonk, NY, USA). We tested all parameters for the normality with a Kolmogorov-Smirnov test. A Mann-Whitney-U test was used to test the differences in tumor volumetric parameters, 1st order textural features and laboratory parameters between the patient groups achieving CR or PR. To address the multiple comparisons, a Benjamin Hochberg correction was applied. The adjusted p-values were considered significant at a level of 0.05.

3. Results

In 12/21 DLBCL patients (57%), CR was observed after CAR-T cell therapy, whereas 9/21 patients (43%) showed PR. No patient had a progression at first follow-up after CAR-T cell therapy.

3.1. Quantitative Analysis of Tumor Volumetric Parameters

The whole-body MTV and whole-body TLG differed significantly ($p < 0.01$ and $p < 0.05$, respectively) between the subgroups assigned to CR or PR showing lower levels in the CR group at baseline (MTV: 35 ± 38 mL vs. 88 ± 110 mL; TLG: 319 ± 362 vs. 1488 ± 2254) (Figure 1).

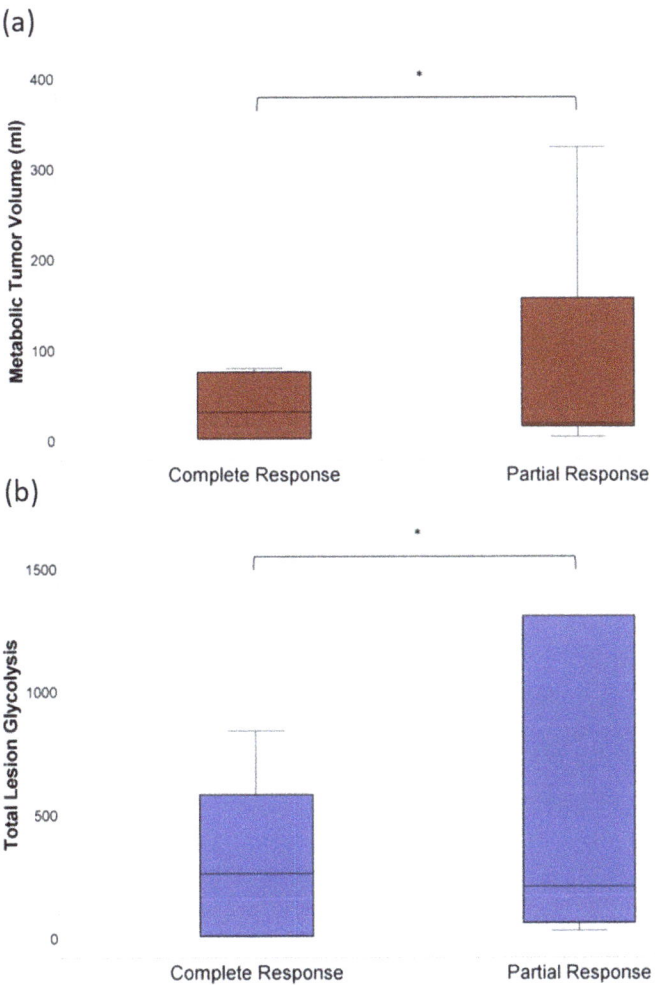

Figure 1. (a) At baseline ^{18}F-FDG PET/CT before CAR-T cell therapy, both the whole-body MTV (35 ± 38 mL vs. 88 ± 110 mL) and (b) the whole-body TLG (319 ± 362 vs. 1488 ± 2254) were lower in patients achieving CR compared to patients achieving PR ($p < 0.01$ and $p < 0.05$). The asterisk (*) indicates clinical significance ($p < 0.05$).

In the entire patient cohort, a significant ($p < 0.01$) decrease was observed for whole-body MTV (62 ± 86 mL vs. 4 ± 5 mL) and whole-body-TLG (925 ± 1722 vs. 33 ± 59) (Figure 2). After CAR-T cell therapy, MTV and TLG were not measurable in the subgroup achieving CR, whereas in the subgroup with PR, MTV (88 ± 110 mL vs. 7 ± 4 mL) and TLG (1488 ± 2254 vs. 41 ± 39) significantly decreased ($p < 0.01$).

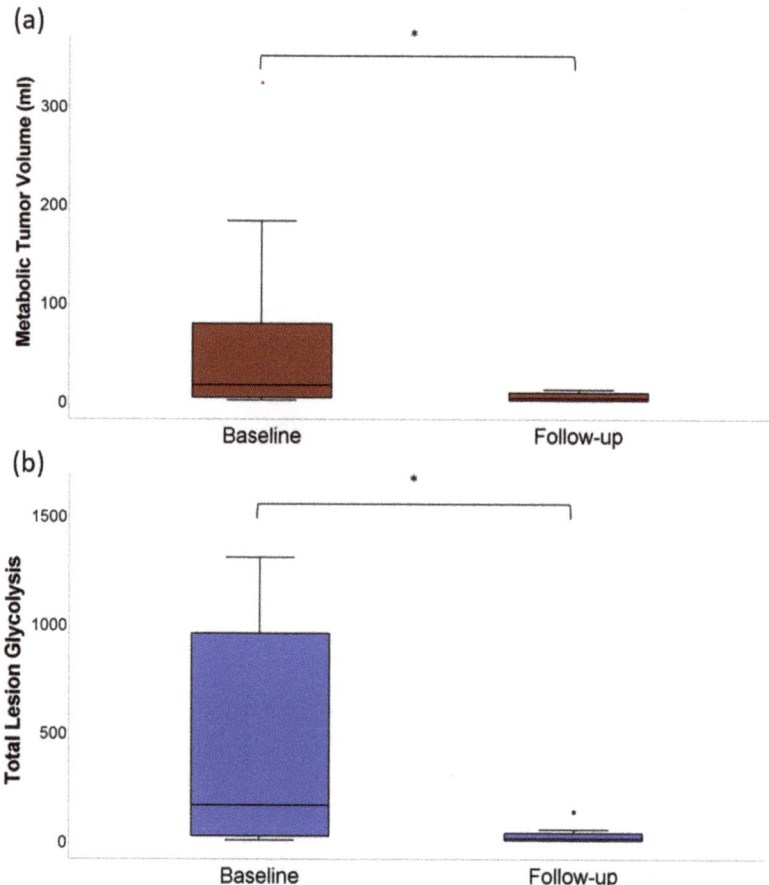

Figure 2. (**a**) Whole-body MTV at baseline ^{18}F-FDG-PET/CT before CAR T cell therapy (62 ± 86 mL) and at first follow-up ^{18}F-FDG-PET/CT (4 ± 5 mL) after CAR T cell therapy in the entire patient cohort ($p < 0.01$). (**b**) Whole-body TLG at baseline ^{18}F-FDG-PET/CT before CAR-T cell therapy (925 ± 1722) and at first follow-up ^{18}F-FDG-PET/CT (33 ± 59) after CAR-T cell therapy in the entire patient cohort ($p < 0.01$). The asterisk (*) indicates clinical significance ($p < 0.05$).

3.2. CT-Texture Analysis

At baseline, the "entropy" proved lower (1.81 ± 0.1) in patients achieving CR compared to patients achieving PR (2.08 ± 0.2; $p < 0.05$) (Figure 3a). In contrast, the "uniformity" was higher in patients with CR (0.33 ± 0.02) compared to patients with PR (0.28 ± 0.47; $p < 0.05$) (Figure 3b). No significant differences were found for "skewness" (0.11 ± 0.21 [CR] vs. −0.32 ± 1.23 [PR]; $p > 0.05$) and "mean" (66.1 ± 18.89 [CR] vs. 49.3 ± 23.9 [PR]; $p > 0.05$) with a trend in "mean" for higher values in patients with CR.

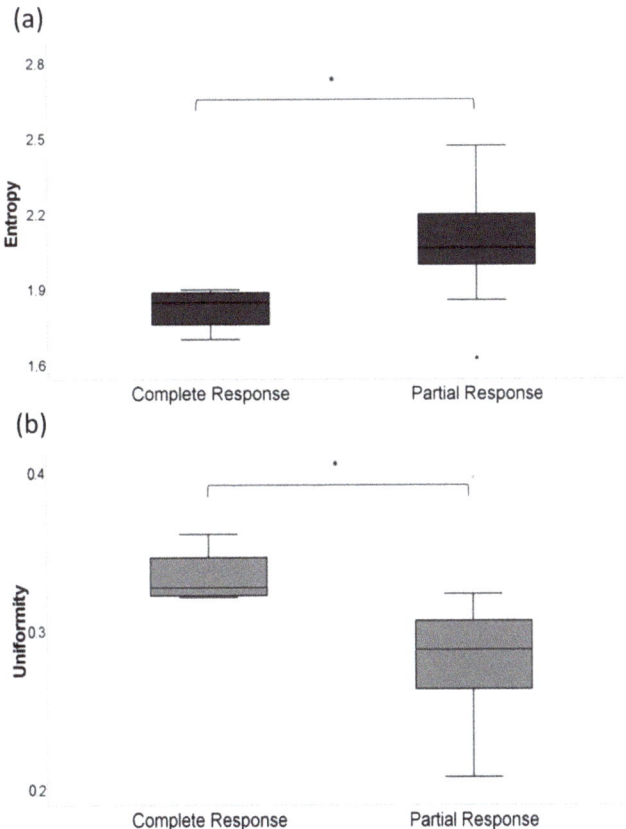

Figure 3. (a) Entropy at baseline imaging before CAR-T cell therapy in patients achieving CR (1.81 ± 0.1) vs. PR (2.08 ± 0.2; $p < 0.05$). (b) Uniformity at baseline imaging before CAR-T cell therapy in patients achieving CR (0.33 ± 0.02) vs. PR (0.28 ± 0.47; $p < 0.05$). The asterisk (*) indicates clinical significance ($p < 0.05$).

3.3. Laboratory Parameters

In the group of patients achieving CR after CAR-T cell therapy, the mean serum LDH proved significantly lower compared to the PR group at baseline (240 ± 28 U/L [CR] vs. 443 ± 262 U/L [PR]; $p < 0.05$) (Figure 4a). The CRP levels in serum at baseline also proved significantly lower in the CR group compared to the PR group (2.6 ± 4.6 µg/dL [CR] vs. 4.2 ± 6.6 µg/dL [PR]; $p < 0.05$) (Figure 4b). At baseline, no differences were found for the leucocyte count between patients achieving CR (5127 ± 766 1/µL) and PR (5290 ± 3142 1/µL; $p > 0.05$).

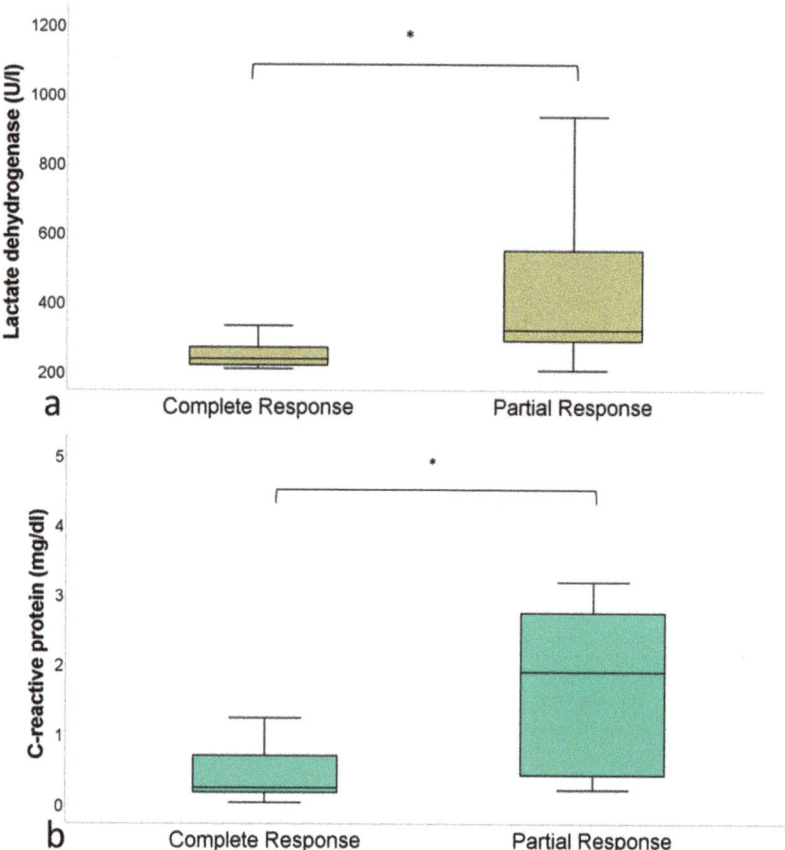

Figure 4. (**a**) Serum LDH at baseline before CAR-T cell therapy in patients achieving CR (240 ± 28 U/L) vs. patients achieving PR (443 ± 262 U/L; $p < 0.05$). (**b**) CRP at baseline before CAR-T cell therapy in patients achieving CR (2.6 ± 4.6 µg/dL) vs. patients achieving PR (4.2 ± 6.6 µg/dL; $p < 0.05$). The asterisk (*) indicates clinical significance ($p < 0.05$).

In the whole patient cohort, we observed a significant decrease of CRP (2.8 ± 5.6 µg/dL vs. 0.1 ± 0.2 µg/dL; $p < 0.01$) and leucocyte count (5348 ± 2514 1/µL vs. 2954 ± 2024 1/µL; $p < 0.01$) and trend towards lower serum LDH (366 ± 235 U/L vs. 242 ± 69 U/L; $p > 0.05$) after CAR-T cell therapy.

The mean time interval between re-infusion of CAR-T cells and IL-6 peak was 6.5 ± 4.3 days and between re-infusion of CAR-T cells and Il-2R peak the time was 7.4 ± 4.1 days. The IL-6 peak (867 ± 951 ng/L vs. 9121 ± 11,266 ng/L) and IL-2R peak (2483 ± 1164 U/mL vs. 5548 ± 3949 U/mL) were lower in patients with CR compared to PR, without statistical significance ($p > 0.05$) (Figure 5).

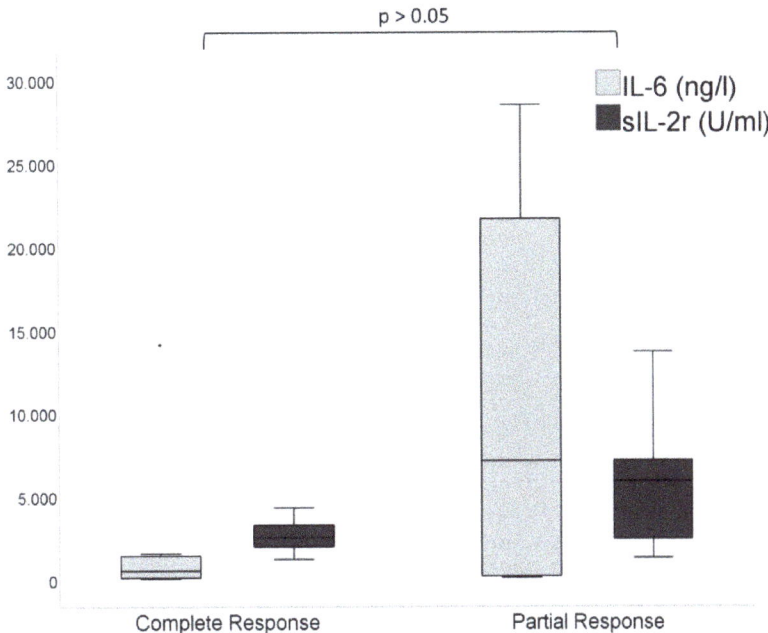

Figure 5. IL-6 peak (867 ± 951 ng/L vs. 9121 ± 11,266 ng/L) and IL-2R peak (2483 ± 1164 U/mL vs. 5548 ± 3949 U/mL) in patients with CR vs. PR ($p > 0.05$).

After CAR-T cell therapy, 20/21 patients developed a cytokine release syndrome (CRS). Of these, 10/21 patients had a CRS grade I, 7/21 patients had a CRS grade II, 2/21 patients had a CRS grade III and 1/21 patient had a CRS grade IV. In the group of patients with CR after CAR-T cell therapy, two patients had a manifest CRS (grade > 1), whereas eight patients with PR developed a manifest CRS.

4. Discussion

In this study, we investigated the predictive value of textural features derived from CT and volume-based parameters derived from ^{18}F-FDG-PET/CT in comparison to serologic markers in patients with DLBCL undergoing CD19-CAR-T cell therapy.

Patients achieving PR had a considerably higher MTV and TLG in the baseline setting compared to patients achieving morphological and metabolic CR. This is not surprising, as the MTV was already found to have predictive value in lymphoma [14–16]. Xie et al. reported a negative progression-free survival (PFS) in patients with DLBCL presenting high MTV and SUV_{max} values in the pre-treatment setting, irrespective of the applied treatment regimen [14]. Similarly, Zhou et al. described MTV as the only independent predictor of progression-free survival and overall survival in their patient cohort with DLBCL undergoing R-CHOP therapy [15]. In a subsequent analysis, the same authors found baseline TLG to be a significant predictor of PFS [16]. Quantification of the volumetric parameters MTV and TLG and calculation of cut-off values for response prediction were also performed by Xie and Sasanelli [16,17]. Furthermore, response prediction based on MTV was performed in patients with follicular lymphoma undergoing immuno-chemotherapy [18].

Expectedly, quantitative ^{18}F-FDG-PET proved also to be a good therapy monitoring tool with significant reduction in glucose metabolism in patients achieving PR and no residual uptake in patients achieving metabolic CR.

Other quantitative predicting and response monitoring metric features are those derived from texture analysis of either PET-metabolic or CT-morphologic image data, which are then post-processed by using radiomics parameters [13]. At this point, our results obtained from CT-radiomics analysis indicate that with increasing tumor tissue homogeneity and correspondingly decreasing heterogeneity in the baseline setting, the chances of achieving CR significantly increase. Similar results were reported in DLBCL patients undergoing immunochemotherapy [10]. Aide et al. demonstrated that ^{18}F-FDG-PET heterogeneity of the largest lymphoma lesion was an independent predictor of two years-event-free survival [10]. In this study, the only independent predictor when analyzed together with IPI and MTV was the long-zone high-grade level emphasis.

Texture analysis was further demonstrated to have potential in improving the value of pretreatment PET/CT for prediction of the interim response of primary gastrointestinal-DLBCL [9]. In this report, the SUV_{max}, MTV, as well as the entropy were significantly higher in the non-CR group. In the report by Aide et al., texture analysis of the skeleton in patients with DLBCL proved beneficial for diagnosis of infiltration with skewness being the only independent predictor of PFS [19].

The assumption that images contain information of disease-specific processes is the basis for the use of radiomics, which aims at enhancing the existing data by means of advanced mathematical analysis. Various studies from different fields in imaging highlight the potential of radiomics to support clinical decision-making [20,21]. However, various technical factors may influence the extracted radiomic features, which is a limitation of this approach that needs to be considered [22].

Although radiomics applications have yet to arrive in routine clinical practice, image interpretation using radiomics has potential in terms of a more personalized medicine in the future.

Another discipline in which radiomics is now increasingly being applied is pathology [23]. The idea to genetically classify tumors without biopsy using non-invasive extraction of image information promises support in diagnostics, individualized prognosis and therapy planning.

LDH is a non-specific marker for lymphoma whose prognostic significance is well established for both indolent and aggressive lymphomas at the time of diagnosis, which indirectly reflects the tumor burden. As expected, we found lower serum levels of LDH at baseline in DLBCL patients, which reached CR after CAR-T cell therapy. LDH significantly decreased after therapy accompanied also by decreasing serum levels of CRP and leucocyte count.

Of interest, the IL-6 and IL-2R serum peaks measured in the first week after CAR-T cell therapy onset proved lower in patients classified CR compared to patients classified PR. Almost half of our patient cohort developed a manifest CRS (grade 2 or higher) after CAR-T cell therapy, which was mainly observed in patients with PR after treatment.

Our results are in line with already existing data with respect to response prediction in DLBCL showing similar results of studies exploring the role of PET/CT and CT in immunotherapy.

Our study has some limitations. First, not all patients received the same CD19-CAR-T cells compound. Second, due to the retrospective study design, a selection bias or other confounding factors cannot be excluded. Third, the histologic subtype of DLBCL was not considered because of the small size of the entire cohort hampering an otherwise statistical analysis. Our observations have to be confirmed by larger prospective studies using multivariate analyses which include tumor volumetric and serologic markers.

In conclusion, volume-based PET parameters derived from PET/CT and CT-textural features have the potential to predict therapy response in patients with DLBCL undergoing CAR-T cell therapy.

Author Contributions: Conceptualization, C.P.R. and M.H.; Data curation, C.P.R.; Formal analysis, C.P.R.; Investigation, M.H.; Methodology, C.P.R., C.F., H.D. and W.A.B.; Project administration, M.H.; Resources, C.L., K.N. and W.A.B.; Supervision, C.L., K.N., W.A.B. and M.H.; Validation, R.M.P. and H.D.; Writing—original draft, C.P.R. and M.H.; Writing—review & editing, R.M.P., C.F., C.L., K.N., H.D. and W.A.B. All authors have read and agreed to the published version of the manuscript.

Funding: This research received no external funding.

Institutional Review Board Statement: Our study protocol was approved for retrospective evaluation of patient data by our institutional ethics committee with a waiver of the informed consent requirement (Project number 277/2020BO2).

Informed Consent Statement: Not applicable.

Data Availability Statement: The data presented in this study are available on request from the corresponding author. The data are not publicly available due to privacy and ethical restrictions.

Conflicts of Interest: Marius Horger received institutional research funds and speaker's honorarium from Siemens Healthineers and is a scientific advisor of Siemens Healthcare Germany. The other authors have declared that no competing interests exist.

Abbreviations

CAR	chimeric antigen receptor
CD19	cluster of differentiation 19
CR	complete remission
CRS	cytokine release syndrome
CTTA	CT texture analysis
Deauville 5PS	Deauville five-point scale
DLBCL	diffuse large B-cell lymphoma
FDG	^{18}F- Fluorodeoxyglucose
ICANS	immune effector cell-associated neurotoxicity
IL	interleukin
IPI	international prognostic index
LDH	lactate dehydrogenase
MBq	megabecquerel
MTV	metabolic tumor volume
PFS	progression-free survival
PR	partial remission
R-CHOP	Rituximab in combination with cyclophosphamide, doxorubicin, vincristine, and prednisone
ROI	region of interest
SUV	uptake value
TLG	total lesion glycolysis
VOI	volume of interest

References

1. Hosen, N. CAR T cell therapy. *Immunol. Med.* **2020**, *44*, 69–73. [CrossRef] [PubMed]
2. Rovira, J.; Valera, A.; Colomo, L.; Setoain, X.; Rodríguez, S.; Martínez-Trillos, A.; Giné, E.; Dlouhy, I.; Magnano, L.; Gaya, A.; et al. Prognosis of patients with diffuse large B cell lymphoma not reaching complete response or relapsing after frontline chemotherapy or immunochemotherapy. *Ann. Hematol.* **2014**, *94*, 803–812. [CrossRef] [PubMed]
3. Bishton, M.; Hughes, S.M.; Richardson, F.; James, E.; Bessell, E.; Sovani, V.; Ganatra, R.; Haynes, A.P.; McMillan, A.K.; Fox, C.P. Delineating outcomes of patients with diffuse large b cell lymphoma using the national comprehensive cancer network-international prognostic index and positron emission tomography-defined remission status; a population-based analysis. *Br. J. Haematol.* **2015**, *172*, 246–254. [CrossRef] [PubMed]
4. Gisselbrecht, C.; Glass, B.; Mounier, N.; Gill, D.S.; Linch, D.C.; Trneny, M.; Bosly, A.; Ketterer, N.; Shpilberg, O.; Hagberg, H.; et al. Salvage Regimens With Autologous Transplantation for Relapsed Large B-Cell Lymphoma in the Rituximab Era. *J. Clin. Oncol.* **2010**, *28*, 4184–4190. [CrossRef] [PubMed]
5. Neelapu, S.S.; Locke, F.L.; Bartlett, N.L.; Lekakis, L.J.; Miklos, D.B.; Jacobson, C.A.; Braunschweig, I.; Oluwole, O.O.; Siddiqi, T.; Lin, Y.; et al. Axicabtagene Ciloleucel CAR T-Cell Therapy in Refractory Large B-Cell Lymphoma. *N. Engl. J. Med.* **2017**, *377*, 2531–2544. [CrossRef] [PubMed]
6. Locke, F.L.; Ghobadi, A.; Jacobson, C.A.; Miklos, D.B.; Lekakis, L.J.; Oluwole, O.O.; Lin, Y.; Braunschweig, I.; Hill, B.T.; Timmerman, J.M.; et al. Long-term safety and activity of axicabtagene ciloleucel in refractory large B-cell lymphoma (ZUMA-1): A single-arm, multicentre, phase 1–2 trial. *Lancet Oncol.* **2019**, *20*, 31–42. [CrossRef]

7. Schuster, S.J.; Bishop, M.R.; Tam, C.S.; Waller, E.K.; Borchmann, P.; McGuirk, J.P.; Jäger, U.; Jaglowski, S.; Andreadis, C.; Westin, J.R.; et al. Tisagenlecleucel in Adult Relapsed or Refractory Diffuse Large B-Cell Lymphoma. *N. Engl. J. Med.* **2019**, *380*, 45–56. [CrossRef]
8. Baratto, L.; Wu, F.; Minamimoto, R.; Hatami, N.; Liang, T.; Sabile, J.; Advani, R.H.; Mittra, E. Correlation of 18-fluorodeoxyglucose PET/computed tomography parameters and clinical features to predict outcome for diffuse large B-cell lymphoma. *Nucl. Med. Commun.* **2021**, *42*, 792–799. [CrossRef] [PubMed]
9. Sun, Y.; Qiao, X.; Jiang, C.; Liu, S.; Zhou, Z. Texture Analysis Improves the Value of Pretreatment 18F-FDG PET/CT in Predicting Interim Response of Primary Gastrointestinal Diffuse Large B-Cell Lymphoma. *Contrast Media Mol. Imaging* **2020**, *2020*, 2981585. [CrossRef] [PubMed]
10. Aide, N.; Fruchart, C.; Nganoa, C.; Gac, A.-C.; Lasnon, C. Baseline 18F-FDG PET radiomic features as predictors of 2-year event-free survival in diffuse large B cell lymphomas treated with immunochemotherapy. *Eur. Radiol.* **2020**, *30*, 4623–4632. [CrossRef]
11. Shagera, Q.A.; Cheon, G.J.; Koh, Y.; Yoo, M.Y.; Kang, K.W.; Lee, D.S.; Kim, E.E.; Yoon, S.-S.; Chung, J.-K. Prognostic value of metabolic tumour volume on baseline 18F-FDG PET/CT in addition to NCCN-IPI in patients with diffuse large B-cell lymphoma: Further stratification of the group with a high-risk NCCN-IPI. *Eur. J. Pediatr.* **2019**, *46*, 1417–1427. [CrossRef] [PubMed]
12. Cheson, B.D.; Fisher, R.I.; Barrington, S.F.; Cavalli, F.; Schwartz, L.H.; Zucca, E.; Lister, T.A. Recommendations for initial evaluation, stag-ing, and response assessment of Hodgkin and non-Hodgkin lymphoma: The Lugano classification. *J. Clin. Oncol.* **2014**, *32*, 3059–3068. [CrossRef] [PubMed]
13. Van Griethuysen, J.; Fedorov, A.; Parmar, C.; Hosny, A.; Aucoin, N.; Narayan, V.; Beets-Tan, R.; Fillion-Robin, J.C.; Pieper, S.; Aerts, H. Computational Radiomics System to Decode the Radiographic Phenotype. *Cancer Res.* **2017**, *77*, e104–e107. [CrossRef] [PubMed]
14. Xie, M.; Zhai, W.; Cheng, S.; Zhang, H.; Xie, Y.; He, W. Predictive value of F-18 FDG PET/CT quantization parameters for progression-free survival in patients with diffuse large B-cell lymphoma. *Hematology* **2015**, *21*, 99–105. [CrossRef] [PubMed]
15. Zhou, M.; Chen, Y.; Huang, H.; Zhou, X.; Liu, J.; Huang, G. Prognostic value of total lesion glycolysis of baseline 18F-fluorodeoxyglucose positron emission tomography/computed tomography in diffuse large B-cell lymphoma. *Oncotarget* **2016**, *7*, 83544–83553. [CrossRef] [PubMed]
16. Xie, M.; Wu, K.; Liu, Y.; Jiang, Q.; Xie, Y. Predictive value of F-18 FDG PET/CT quantization parameters in diffuse large B cell lymphoma: A meta-analysis with 702 participants. *Med. Oncol.* **2014**, *32*, 1–10. [CrossRef] [PubMed]
17. Sasanelli, M.; Meignan, M.; Haioun, C.; Berriolo-Riedinger, A.; Casasnovas, R.-O.; Biggi, A.; Gallamini, A.; Siegel, B.A.; Cashen, A.F.; Véra, P.; et al. Pretherapy metabolic tumour volume is an independent predictor of outcome in patients with diffuse large B-cell lymphoma. *Eur. J. Pediatr.* **2014**, *41*, 2017–2022. [CrossRef] [PubMed]
18. Meignan, M.; Cottereau, A.-S.; Versari, A.; Chartier, L.; Dupuis, J.; Boussetta, S.; Grassi, I.; Casasnovas, R.-O.; Haioun, C.; Tilly, H.; et al. Baseline Metabolic Tumor Volume Predicts Outcome in High–Tumor-Burden Follicular Lymphoma: A Pooled Analysis of Three Multicenter Studies. *J. Clin. Oncol.* **2016**, *34*, 3618–3626. [CrossRef] [PubMed]
19. Aide, N.; Talbot, M.; Fruchart, C.; Damaj, G.; Lasnon, C. Diagnostic and prognostic value of baseline FDG PET/CT skeletal textural features in diffuse large B cell lymphoma. *Eur. J. Pediatr.* **2017**, *45*, 699–711. [CrossRef]
20. Mannil, M.; von Spiczak, J.; Manka, R.; Alkadhi, H. Texture Analysis and Machine Learning for Detecting Myocardial Infarction in Noncontrast Low-Dose Computed Tomography: Unveiling the Invisible. *Investig. Radiol.* **2018**, *53*, 338–343. [CrossRef] [PubMed]
21. Neisius, U.; El-Rewaidy, H.; Nakamori, S.; Rodriguez, J.; Manning, W.J.; Nezafat, R. Radiomic Analysis of Myocardial Native T1 Imaging Discriminates Between Hypertensive Heart Disease and Hypertrophic Cardiomyopathy. *JACC Cardiovasc. Imaging* **2019**, *12*, 1946–1954. [CrossRef] [PubMed]
22. Chalkidou, A.; O'Doherty, M.J.; Marsden, P.K. False Discovery Rates in PET and CT Studies with Texture Features: A Systematic Review. *PLoS ONE* **2015**, *10*, e0124165. [CrossRef] [PubMed]
23. Lu, C.; Shiradkar, R.; Liu, Z. Integrating pathomics with radiomics and genomics for cancer prognosis: A brief review. *Chin. J. Cancer Res. (Chung-Kuo Yen Cheng Yen Chiu)* **2021**, *33*, 563–573. [CrossRef] [PubMed]

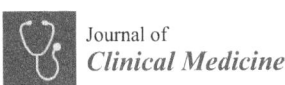

Article

Additional Value of [18F]FDG PET/CT in Detection of Suspected Malignancy in Patients with Paraneoplastic Neurological Syndromes Having Negative Results of Conventional Radiological Imaging

Marta Opalińska [1], Anna Sowa-Staszczak [2,*], Kamil Wężyk [3], Jeremiasz Jagiełła [4], Agnieszka Słowik [4] and Alicja Hubalewska-Dydejczyk [2]

1. Nuclear Medicine Unit, Department of Endocrinology, Oncological Endocrinology and Nuclear Medicine, University Hospital, 30-688 Kraków, Poland; mopalinska@su.krakow.pl
2. Chair and Department of Endocrinology, Jagiellonian University Medical College, 31-008 Kraków, Poland; alahub@cm-uj.krakow.pl
3. Department of Neurology, University Hospital, 30-688 Kraków, Poland; kwezyk@su.krakow.pl
4. Chair and Department of Neurology, Jagiellonian University Medical College, 31-008 Kraków, Poland; jeremiasz.jagiella@uj.edu.pl (J.J.); agnieszka.slowik@uj.edu.pl (A.S.)
* Correspondence: anna.sowa-staszczak@uj.edu.pl

Abstract: Background: Paraneoplastic neurological syndromes (PNS) affecting the CNS (central nervous system) are rare, presenting in less than 1% of all those with cancer. The pathogenesis of paraneoplastic neurological syndromes is not fully understood, but it is presumed to result from an immune attack on the underlying malignancy. The presence of different types of onconeural antibodies may occur in different tumors and can lead to different clinical manifestations, making the early detection of cancers challenging. Aim: An evaluation of [18F]FDG PET/CT in neoplastic tumor detection in patients with paraneoplastic neurological syndromes having negative or unremarkable results of conventional radiological imaging. Methods: Among all patients diagnosed with paraneoplastic neurological syndromes in the Neurology Department in 2016–2020, 15 patients with unremarkable conventional radiological findings who underwent [18F]FDG PET/CT were included in the study. Results: [18F]FDG PET/CT enabled localization of suspected malignancy in 53% (8 of 15) of PNS cases with previous unremarkable conventional radiological findings. Conclusion: [18F]FDG PET/CT may be considered as a useful tool for neoplastic tumor detection in patients with paraneoplastic neurological syndromes, accelerating the diagnostic process and enabling faster initiation of appropriate treatment.

Keywords: paraneoplastic syndromes; neurooncology; [18F]FDG PET/CT; PNS

1. Introduction

Paraneoplastic syndromes represent a wide range of symptoms associated with malignancy. They are usually systemic dysfunctions which are not a direct result of neoplastic tumor invasion or metastasis. They may manifest with symptoms from various systems and organs, causing endocrine, neurological, dermatological, rheumatological and hematological syndromes, usually, in areas and organs that are not directly affected by the neoplasm. The most common malignancies associated with paraneoplastic syndromes include breast, lung, pancreas, kidney as well as gynecological and hematological tumors. The incidence and prevalence of paraneoplastic disorders is estimated to be 0.89/100,000 person-years and 4.4 per 100,000, respectively [1]. In many cases, the etiology of the syndrome is unknown. Most often, they are autoimmune reactions to circulating tumor antigens or an effect of biologically active substances, such as hormones, growth factors or cytokines secreted by tumor cells.

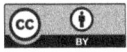

Paraneoplastic neurologic syndromes (PNS) in the large majority respond well to the symptomatic therapy; however, not in all cases is such treatment effective. The population-based study estimated an incidence of PNS at about 1/100,000 person-years and a prevalence of 4/100,000, with the incidence ratio increasing over time [2]. The clinical presentation of PNS is excessively variable (Table 1); hence, the proper diagnosis requires extensive workup and clinical experience. In 2004, an international panel of experts recommended diagnostic criteria defining a neurological syndrome as a paraneoplastic syndrome based on the coexistence of onconeural antibodies and the presence of clinical symptoms. Further, they categorized those presentation as "classical" and "non-classical" syndromes. "Classical" syndromes (e.g., Lambert–Eaton myaesthenic syndrome, limbic encephalitis, encephalomyelitis, subacute cerebellar degeneration, sensory neuronopathy, dermatomyositis, or opsoclonus-myoclonus) are more likely to be associated with an underlying malignancy [3].

According to the current knowledge, PNS occur in two main mechanisms of immune response. The first is the direct immune response against neuronal receptors or other cell membrane antigens. The most common types of abovementioned antibodies and their clinical significance are summarized in Table 2. Those syndromes usually present clinically by rapidly developing neurological dysfunction, which might not be related to tumor size or growth and frequently respond well to anti-inflammatory treatment. In the second type, the immunoreactivity is triggered by intra-cellular neuronal proteins, which are more often associated with the development of malignancy. In that mechanism, the immune response targets originate from intracellular antigens/proteins revealed by neuronal death. In those conditions, neurological damage is usually more severe and very often irreversible. The most common types of antibodies against intra-cellular neuronal proteins, associated with underlying malignancy, and their clinical symptoms are summarized in Table 3.

However, tumor removal itself is very seldom linked with good prognosis (e.g., teratoma removal in patients with NMDA (Anti-N-methyl-d-aspartate-mediated encephalitis) [4]), prompt identification and treatment are strongly recommended in order to eliminate proteins triggering the immune response (e.g., small cell carcinoma with anti Hu [5]). Within the pursuit of identifying the origin of malignancy, early imaging using radiological procedures (CT or MRI) often fails to establish the diagnosis. Among the widely available methods of advanced diagnostic procedures, a whole-body [18F]FDG PET/CT might be indispensable in the search for underlying pathology.

In the current state of knowledge, the value of [18F]FDG PET/CT as a pivotal imaging in doubtful cases is recommended but not fully elucidated. The rarity and complexity of neurological PNS leads to a paucity of information necessary to formulate strong diagnostic recommendations.

Table 1. Paraneoplastic syndromes of the nervous system classified by location. Adapted from Dalmau J, Rosenfeld MR. Paraneoplastic syndromes of the CNS. *Lancet Neurol.* 2008; 7(4): 327–340. [6].

	Brain, Cranial Nerves and Retina	Spinal Cord	Peripheral Nerves or Muscle	Neuromuscular Junction
Non-Classic PNS	Brainstem encephalitis	Stiff-person syndrome	Sensorimotor neuropathy	Myasthenia gravis
	Optic neuritis	Myelitis	Neuropathy and paraproteinaemia	
	Cancer-associated retinopathy	Necrotising myelopathy	Neuropathy with vasculitis	
	Melanoma-associated retinopathy	Motor-neuron syndromes	Polymyositis	
			Acute necrotising myopathy	
			Acquired neuromyotonia	
			Autonomic neuropathies	
Classic PNS	Cerebellar degeneration		Sensory neuronopathy	Lambert-Eaton myasthenic syndrome
	Limbic encephalitis		Intestinal pseudo-obstruction	
	Encephalomyelitis		Dermatomyositis	
	Opsoclonus-myoclonus			

Table 2. Major paraneoplastic onconeuronal antibodies reactive with neuronal membrane antigens. Adapted from Galli, J.; Greenlee, J. Paraneoplastic Diseases of the Central Nervous System [7].

Antibody	Common Neurological Phenotypes	Common Associated Malignancies
Anti-AMPAR	Limbic encephalitis	Breast Lung Thymus
Anti-LGI1/Anti-CASPR2	Limbic encephalitis Faciobrachial dystonic seizures Morvan's syndrome	Thymoma (especially in patients positive for both antibodies) Other neoplasms (rare)
Anti-GABAbR	Limbic encephalitis, status epilepticus	Small-cell lung cancer
Anti-mGluR1	Cerebellar degeneration	Hodgkin's disease
Anti-mGlur2	Cerebellar degeneration	Small-cell cancer; alveolar rhabdomyosarcoma
Anti-mGluR5	Limbic encephalitis	Hodgkin's disease
Anti-VGKC	Cerebellar degeneration (Lambert–Eaton myasthenic syndrome)	Small-cell lung cancer

Table 3. Major paraneoplastic onconeuronal antibodies reactive with intracellular neuronal antigens. Adapted from Galli, J.; Greenlee, J. Paraneoplastic Diseases of the Central Nervous System [7].

Antibody	Common Neurological Phenotypes	Common Associated Malignancies
Anti-CRMP5	Optic neuritis Cerebellar degeneration Encephalomyelitis	Small-cell lung cancer Breast carcinoma
Anti-GAD65	Stiff person syndrome Limbic encephalitis Cerebellar ataxia	Thymoma Renal cell carcinoma
Anti-Hu (ANNA-1)	Limbic encephalitis, encephalomyelitis, dorsal sensory neuropathy	Small-cell lung cancer Neuroendocrine tumors Retinoblastoma (infants)
Anti-Ma1	Limbic or brain-stem encephalitis	Non-small-cell lung cancer; other
Anti-Ma2	Limbic or brain-stem encephalitis	Testicular or other germ cell tumors Non-small-cell lung cancer
Anti-Ri (ANNA-2)	Cerebellar degeneration, opsoclonus myoclonus, brain-stem encephalitis	Breast Small-cell lung cancer
Anti-Tr	Cerebellar degeneration	Hodgkin's disease
Anti-Yo (PCA-1)	Cerebellar degeneration	Ovary, uterus, adnexa Breast

The aim of the study was to assess the usefulness of [18F]FDG PET/CT in patients with high risk of PNS and negative or unremarkable results of conventional radiological imaging.

2. Methods

Among the patients diagnosed with neurological syndromes between 2016–2020 in the Neurology Department of University Hospital in Krakow, we selected cases with a clinical picture strongly suggesting an underlying neoplastic background (rapid course of PNS and resistance to conventional first-line treatment).

In 15 of them, with positive or unremarkable results of onconeuronal antibodies, due to negative or unambiguous results of conventional screening (including radiological and endoscopy workup), the [18F]FGD PET/CT was applied.

Among these patients, seven were diagnosed with classical neurological PNS (cerebellar degeneration—3 cases, sensory polyneuropathy—1 case, autoimmune encephalitis—3 cases), and 7 with non-classic PNS (myasthenia gravis (MG)—1, myelitis—1, motor neuron disease—1, sensorimotor polyneuropathy—4). Additionally, a patient with Primary Angiitis of Central Nervous System (PACNS) (1) was included in the analysis, since several cases of sporadic presentation of that disease as a paraneoplastic syndrome are available in the literature.

All patients' demographic data, clinical presentation, cerebrospinal fluid (CSF) evaluation, previous imaging results and onconeuronal antibodies screening were recorded from the available patient database. The distribution of PNS types diagnosed among the analyzed group is presented in Table 4.

Table 4. The distribution of PNS types diagnosed among the analyzed group and the results of [18F]FDG examination.

Classic PNS	No of Patients with PNS Included to Analysis	No of Patients with Positive [18F]F-FDG PET/CT Findings	Percentage of PET/CT Positive Examination
Cerebellar degeneration	3	3	100
Sensory polyneuropathy	1	0	0
Autoimmune encephalitis	3	1	33
Non-classic PNS			
Myasthenia gravis	1	1	100
Myelitis	1	1	100
Sensorimotor polyneuropathy	4	2	50
Motor neuron disease	1	0	0
Others			
Primary Angiitis of Central Nervous System (PACS)	1	0	0
Sum	15	8	53

2.1. Image Acquisitions and Analysis

[18F]FDG PET/CT examinations were conducted in accordance with the standard protocol on GE DISCOVERY 690 VCT scanner (Krakow, Poland). All patients fasted at least 6 h before the procedure. Bedside fasting blood glucose of more than 11.0 mmol/L was not accepted. Imaging was performed 60 min after intravenous administration of the radiotracer. An initial low-dose CT without contrast enhancement (Smart mA with range: 50–180 mA) was performed, in order to correct for photon attenuation and to co-localize FDG uptake and anatomical structures. The FDG PET/CT was performed from the mid-thigh to the top of the head. Patients received 4 MBq [18F]FDG per 1 kg body mass (2 min per bed position in three-dimensional mode). The PET data were reconstructed with the use of the GE (matrix size 128×128, Vue Point FX reconstruction method: 16 subsets, 3 iterations reconstruction algorithm). Corrections were applied for attenuation, dead time, scatter and random coincidences. All image analyses were performed on fused PET/CT data sets. Slice thickness of the PET short-axis images was 3.3 mm. The estimated dose of radiation per patient was about 9.5 mSv.

All images were reviewed using first attenuation-corrected images. In all cases, a senior nuclear medicine consultant made an initial assessment of [18F]FDG-PET scans, which was then re-assessed by the consultant radiologist.

The PET/CT was binary classified, so a positive result was defined as the presence of a metabolically active tumor of any region of body, suspicion of metabolically active dissemination of neoplastic disease or increased focal uptake, being highly suspected to correspond with malignancy.

The negative results were considered as scans with no FDG uptake, and with any focal increased uptake with intensity higher than the surrounding tissues, but in localization not highly suspicious as a malignancy.

2.2. Statistical Analysis

Demographic and clinical characteristics were analyzed by producing tables of frequency for categorical variables and by calculation of the median and range for continuous variables. IBM SPSS Statistics for Windows, version 27 (IBM Corp., Armonk, NY, USA) was employed for the statistical analysis.

3. Results

A group of 15 patients (9 females and 6 males) were eligible for the study. The median age was 70 years (range: 32–88 years). All patients underwent anatomical neuroimaging of the brain—in 5 cases, head CT and in the remaining cases, MRI. A total of 14 patients also underwent lumbar puncture; in one patient, due to lack of consent, only blood tests were performed. The whole group was evaluated for the presence of onconeuronal antibodies [Table 5]. Positive results of [18F]FDG PET/CT were found in 8 out 15 cases, which were associated with 4 types of neurological PNS.

The following percentages of positive results were found: in patients with myelitis 100% (1 case), cerebral degeneration 75% (3 of 4 cases) and among patients with polyneuropathies 50% (2 of 4 cases).

Among patients with myasthenia gravis, primary angiitis of the central nervous system and motor neuron disease there were no positive results of PET/CT (total number of observations: 4). The increased FDG uptake was found in 4 cases in lungs, in 1 case in colon, in 2 cases in lymph nodes of neck and chest and in 1 case in stomach (Figure 1).

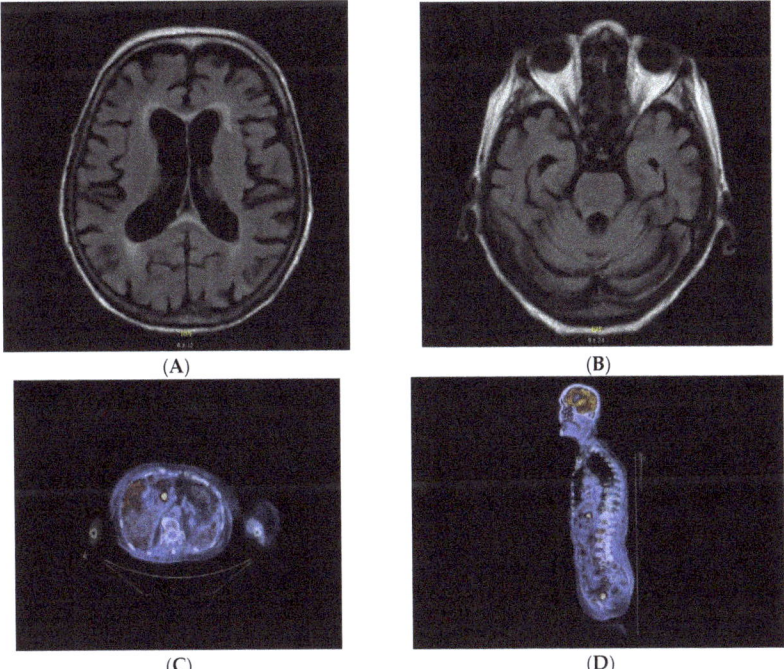

Figure 1. MRI and PET/CT results of a patient with cerebellar degeneration. (**A**,**B**) nonspecific vascular demyelination detected on MRI. (**C**,**D**) metabolically active area in the pylorus and in the locoregional lymph nodes detected on [18F]FDG PET/CT.

Table 5. Clinical. biochemical. and imaging data of patients included in the study.

Patient No	Sex, Age	Neuroimaging (CT, MR)	CSF Results	Antibodies	Metabolic Abnormalities of CNS	PET/CT Abnormalities
			Cerebellar Degeneration			
1.	F. 88	Brain MRI: nonspecific vascular demyelination; no clinical relevance	Cytosis 0.005×10^3/uL $(0$–0.005×10^3/uL) Protein 48.5 mg/dL (20.00–40.00) oligoclonal bands: positive	anti-Yo	none	metabolically active area in the pylorus and metabolically active lymph node next to the pylorus SUV max 7.8
2.	F. 83	Brain MRI: leukoaraiosis around lateral ventricles. nonspecific vascular demyelination. moderate cortical artrophy—mainly posterior. bilateral hyperintense changes in the thalami and caudate nuclei on diffusion weighted imaging (DWI).	Cytosis 0.004×10^3/uL $(0$–0.005×10^3/uL) Protein 34.8 mg/dL (20.00–40.00) oligoclonal bands: negative	anti-NMDA. anti-Yo	Generalized cortico-subcortical atrophy of the brain.	metabolically active lymph nodes in the mediastinum and chest—suspection of lymphoma SUV max 10.5
3.	M. 66	Brain MRI: not performed (due to contraindications) Brain CT: normal	Cytosis 0.006×10^3/uL $(0$–0.005×10^3/uL) Protein 40.6 mg/dL (20.00–40.00) oligoclonal bands: positive	not detected	not detected	metabolically active tumor in the transverse colon SUV max 5.0
			Autoimmune Encephalitis			
4.	F. 32	Brain MRI: normal	Cytosis 0.018×10^3/uL $(0$–0.005×10^3/uL) Protein 26.3 mg/dL (20.00–40.00) oligoclonal bands: negative	anti-NMDA	none	increased metabolism of FDG in the topography of numerous lesions in both lungs SUV max up to 7.5
5.	M. 30	Brain MRI: demyelinating lesions located bilaterally in the white matter of the frontal and parietal lobe, in the periventricular and subcortical areas.	Cytosis 0.002×10^3/uL $(0$–0.005×10^3/uL) Protein 47.2 mg/dL (20.00–40.00) oligoclonal bands: negative	anti-NMDA	none	not significant
6.	F. 74	Brain MRI: epidermal cysts located anteriorly from the medulla oblongata, on the left side; numerous demyelinating lesions located in the white matter of the centrum semiovale, periventricular and paraventricular areas; numerous, small signalless zones on Susceptibility-Weighted Imaging (SWI) which correspond to the presence of haemosiderin deposits—after microchemorrhages	Cytosis 0.002×10^3/uL $(0$–0.005×10^3/uL) Protein 37.3 mg/dL (20.00–40.00) oligoclonal bands: positive	anti-NMDA	cortical-subcortical atrophy of the brain	not significant
			Myasthenia Gravis			
7.	F. 79	Brain MRI: nonspecific vascular demyelination; no clinical relevance	not performed	anti-AChR	areas of porencephaly with decreased FDG metabolism	not significant
			Myelitis			
8.	F. 70	Brain MRI: leukoaraiosis around lateral ventricles; few. small changes with increased signal in T2 in the radial corona radiata in the frontal lobes; moderate cortical atrophy of the brain and cerebellum. Cervical Spine MRI: The zone of increased signal in the T2 sequences dependent on the central part of the spinal cord. extending from the C2 / C3 to C6 / C7 level	Cytosis 0.008×10^3/uL $(0$–0.005×10^3/uL) Protein 74 mg/dL (20.00–40.00) oligoclonal bands: negative	anti-AQP4	none	moderately metabolic active tumour in segment 4/5 of the right lung. SUV max 3.5
			Polyneuropathy			
9.	M. 59	Brain MRI: not performed. Brain CT: normal	not performed	not detected	none	metabolically active tumor in the apex of the left lung with the involvement of homonymous mediastinal lymph nodes—SUV max 9.4
10.	F. 56	MRI: not performed. Brain CT: normal	not performed	not detected	none	not significant
11.	F. 73	Brain MRI: not performed. Brain CT: normal	Cytosis 0.003×10^3/uL $(0$–0.005×10^3/uL) Protein 144.1 mg/dL (20.00–40.00) oligoclonal bands: negative	anti-PNMA2 (Ma2/Ta) anti-CV2.1	None	metabolically active cervical lymph node and a metabolically active soft tissue mass in the lower part of the neck and in the upper mediastinum SUV max 5.7
12.	M. 69	Brain MRI: nonspecific vascular demyelination; no clinical relevance.	not performed	anti-PNMA2 (Ma2/Ta)	none	not significant
13.	M. 65	Brain MRI: nonspecific vascular demyelination; no clinical relevance.	Cytosis 0.002×10^3/uL $(0$–0.005×10^3/uL) Protein 187 mg/dL (20.00–40.00) oligoclonal bands: negative	not detected	none	lesion in the 1 + 2 segment of left lung SUV max 2.2
			Primary Angiitis of Central Nervous System			
14.	M. 38	Brain MRI: disseminated demyelinating lesions located in the cortico-subcortical area of the right insula. bilaterally in the corona radiata. and single irregular lesions with cortico-subcortical distribution.	Cytosis 0.004×10^3/uL $(0$–0.005×10^3/uL) Protein 38.2 mg/dL (20.00–40.00) oligoclonal bands: negative	anti-Yo	none	nonspecific segmental metabolic stimulation in the loops of the small intestine SUV max 7.7
			Motor Neuron Disease			
15.	F. 67	Cervival Spine MRI: multi-level discopathy without pressure on the surrounding nerve roots.	Cytosis 0.001×10^3/uL $(0$–0.005×10^3/uL) Protein 67.96 mg/dL (20.00–40.00) oligoclonal bands: negative	anti-Yo	none	not significant

The mean value of SUV max in pathological findings were 6.59 (range 2.2–10.5).

The [18F]FDG PET/CT findings along with patients' demographic information, clinical presentation, results of brain/spinal cord imaging, presence and type of onconeural antibodies, and CSF analysis results are summarized in Table 5.

4. Discussion

PNS are rare (less than 1%) manifestation of malignancy. However, its significance is greater, because of diagnostic difficulties and demanding therapeutic process. Due to the increased availability of onconeural antibody tests, there is a progress in both early diagnosis and the implementation of effective targeted therapy.

According to published guidelines for PNS diagnosis [8] in all cases tumor removing is indicated, increasing chance for proper control of PNS symptoms. In patient (No. 4), the neurological symptoms including involuntary movements and psychotic symptoms, were refractory to therapy with steroids, intravenous immunoglobulins and monoclonal anti-CD20 antibody. Only identification and resection of the papillary thyroid cancer led to remission, however PET/CT examination revealed dissemination.

Other risk factors of neurological autoimmune disorders such as coexisting autoimmune disease or a family history of autoimmunity may mislead the initial diagnosis, but in all cases, exclusion of malignancy is mandatory. The evaluation of serum cancer markers such as CA-125, CA-15.3, prostate-specific antigen, and carcinoembryonic antigen with subsequent CSF assessment are usually the first steps in diagnostic workup. In our cohort, only one patient (No. 10) had an elevated carcinoma antigen 15-3 (Ca 15-3), suggesting an underlying paraneoplastic syndrome; however, the [18F]FDG PET/CT result was negative.

In many patients, CSF analysis demonstrates abnormalities such as elevated protein, pleocytosis, the presence of oligoclonal bands or mixed abnormalities, but normal CSF analysis results do not exclude the possibility of PNS [9]. Patients No. 2, 4 and 14 had normal CSF findings, although other elements of the clinical picture indicated the possibility of PNS. Finally, only in the patient with cerebellar syndrome (No. 2) did the PET/CT scan show metabolically active lymph nodes in the mediastinum and chest, suggesting myeloproliferative syndrome.

Onconeuronal antibodies may act as markers for the specific tumors, e.g., anti-Yo for breast or reproductive system tumors, anti-Hu for small-cell lung cancer, anti-Ri for breast or lung or anti-Ma2 for testicle malignancy. In these cases, targeted tumor seeking by CT, mammography, pelvic or testicular ultrasound is essential. However, in cases with high risk of malignancy established by the presence of antibodies directed against intracellular neuronal proteins and adequate clinical presentation, PET/CT with [18F]FDG may bring additional benefits due to the high sensitivity of PET/CT in the detection of small, aggressive tumors. Furthermore, many types of PNS and onconeuronal antibodies can appear in several types of tumors, such as Anti-Yo antibodies which were found in patients with cerebellar syndrome (No. 1, 2), primary CNS vasculitis (No. 14) and motor neuron disease (No. 15). In this context, in cases with positive, unspecific for particular malignancy, antibodies, PET/CT may have additional value, enabling whole-body screening during a single examination.

The meta-analysis evaluating the suitability of [18F]FDG PET/CT in PNS demonstrated a pooled sensitivity of 0.81 and specificity of 0.88 in patients with suspicion of paraneoplastic syndrome [10]. However, that high pooled sensitivity results from data analysis of all patients with PNS having both positive and inconclusive/negative results of prior conventional imaging. In our study, the efficacy of [18F]FDG PET/CT was 53%, but only patients with negative previous radiological and endoscopic exams were evaluated in whom PET/CT had a real clinical benefit.

In the clinical context, it is worth considering if and when PET/CT should be repeated in case of a negative initial study. The guidelines recommend regular oncological surveillance every 6 months for up to 4 years [11] for initially negative imaging results;

however, prolonged time of observation may be connected with unfavorable outcomes in some patients.

The worsening of a known autoimmune syndrome or the occurrence of a new one may suggest dissemination or recurrence of the malignancy. In two patients (No. 3 and 8), the PET/CT exam was repeated (after 12 and 3 months, respectively) due to progressing clinical symptoms. In patient 8 the second exam revealed lung malignancy.

Several studies have shown that whole-body [18F]FDG-PET and [18F]FDG PET/CT are very useful in the screening of patients with suspected paraneoplastic syndrome and positive paraneoplastic antibodies [12]. However, a recent study conducted by another group suggested that the presence of paraneoplastic antibody should not be an indispensable factor for performing [18F]FDG PET/CT [13,14]. In our study, the effectiveness of [18F]FDG PET/CT in the detection of pathology in patients with the presence and absence of onconeuronal antibodies was confirmed. In three PNS patients with negative onconeural antibodies and clinical presentation highly suggesting malignancy, PET/CT scans were positive. Furthermore, in total, there were 53% of positive [18F]FDG PET/CT results (50% and 57% of patients with non-classical and classical PNS, respectively).

The results of our study indicate the potential benefits of [18F]FDG PET/CT in a routine neurological practice in selected patients with PNS, regardless of their onconeural antibody status and type of PNS.

5. Highlights

[18F]FDG PET/CT may be effective in malignancy detection in a large group of PNS patients with negative results of prior diagnostic procedures.

In a routine neurological practice, selected patients with PNS may benefit from [18F]FDG PET/CT regardless of their onconeural antibody status and type of PNS.

Repeating [18F]FDG PET/CT may have additional value, but the optimal timing for the second examination remains uncertain.

Author Contributions: M.O.: Data collection, imaging review, data analysis, manuscript drafting, manuscript editing and approval, study coordination. A.S.-S.: Data collection, imaging review, data analysis, manuscript drafting, manuscript editing and approval. K.W.: Data collection, imaging review, manuscript drafting, manuscript editing and approval. A.S.: Analysis and interpretation of data, manuscript editing and approval. J.J.: Analysis and interpretation of data, manuscript editing and approval. A.H.-D.: Imaging review, data analysis, analysis and interpretation of data manuscript, editing and approval. All authors have read and agreed to the published version of the manuscript.

Funding: This research received no external funding.

Institutional Review Board Statement: Research was conducted ethically in accordance with the World Medical Association Declaration of Helsinki. The study protocol was approved by the Local Ethics Committee of the Jagiellonian University in Krakow (approval no 1072.6120.162.2021).

Informed Consent Statement: Written informed consent for participation was not required for this study in accordance with the national legislation and the institutional requirements.

Data Availability Statement: All data generated or analyzed during this study are included in this article. Further enquiries can be directed to the corresponding author.

Conflicts of Interest: The authors declare no conflict of interest.

References

1. Devine, M.F.; Kothapalli, N.; Elkhooly, M.; Dubey, D. Paraneoplastic neurological syndromes: Clinical presentations and management. *Ther. Adv. Neurol. Disord.* **2021**, *14*, 1756286420985323. [CrossRef] [PubMed]
2. Vogrig, A.; Gigli, G.L.; Segatti, S.; Corazza, E.; Marini, A.; Bernardini, A.; Valent, F.; Fabris, M.; Curcio, F.; Brigo, F.; et al. Epidemiology of paraneoplastic neurological syndromes: A population-based study. *J. Neurol.* **2020**, *267*, 26–35. [CrossRef] [PubMed]
3. Graus, F.; Delattre, J.Y.; Antoine, J.C.; Dalmau, J.; Giometto, B.; Grisold, W.; Honnorat, J.; Smitt, P.S.; Vedeler, C.; Verschuuren, J.J.; et al. Recommended diagnostic criteria for paraneoplastic neurological syndromes. *J. Neurol. Neurosurg. Psychiatry* **2004**, *75*, 1135–1140. [CrossRef] [PubMed]

4. Dai, Y.; Zhang, J.; Ren, H.; Zhou, X.; Chen, J.; Cui, L.; Lang, J.; Guan, H.; Sun, D. Surgical outcomes in patients with anti-N-methyl D-aspartate receptor encephalitis with ovarian teratoma. *Am. J. Obstet. Gynecol.* **2019**, *221*, 485.e1–485.e10. [CrossRef] [PubMed]
5. Baizabal-Carvallo, J.F.; Jankovic, J. Autoimmune and paraneoplastic movement disorders: An update. *J. Neurol. Sci.* **2018**, *385*, 175–184. [CrossRef] [PubMed]
6. Dalmau, J.; Rosenfeld, M.R. Paraneoplastic syndromes of the CNS. *Lancet Neurol.* **2008**, *7*, 327–340. [CrossRef]
7. Galli, J.; Greenlee, J. Paraneoplastic Diseases of the Central Nervous System. *F1000Research* **2020**, *9*, F1000. [CrossRef] [PubMed]
8. Titulaer, M.J.; Soffietti, R.; Dalmau, J.; Gilhus, N.E.; Giometto, B.; Graus, F.; Grisold, W.; Honnorat, J.; Sillevis Smitt, P.A.; Tanasescu, R.; et al. Screening for tumours in paraneoplastic syndromes: Report of an EFNS task force. European Federation of Neurological Societies. *Eur. J. Neurol.* **2011**, *18*, 19-e3. [CrossRef] [PubMed]
9. Dubey, D.; Pittock, S.J.; Kelly, C.R.; McKeon, A.; Lopez-Chiriboga, A.S.; Lennon, V.A.; Gadoth, A.; Smith, C.Y.; Bryant, S.C.; Klein, C.J.; et al. Autoimmune encephalitis epidemiology and a comparison to infectious encephalitis. *Ann. Neurol.* **2018**, *83*, 166–177. [CrossRef] [PubMed]
10. Sheikhbahaei, S.; Marcus, C.V.; Fragomeni, R.S.; Rowe, S.P.; Javadi, M.S.; Solnes, L.B. Whole-Body 18F-FDG PET and 18F-FDG PET/CT in Patients with Suspected Paraneoplastic Syndrome: A Systematic Review and Meta-Analysis of Diagnostic Accuracy. *J. Nucl. Med.* **2017**, *58*, 1031–1036. [CrossRef] [PubMed]
11. Vedeler, C.A.; Antoine, J.C.; Giometto, B.; Graus, F.; Grisold, W.; Hart, I.K.; Honnorat, J.; Sillevis Smitt, P.A.; Verschuuren, J.J.; Voltz, R. Management of paraneoplastic neurological syndromes: Report of an EFNS Task Force. Paraneoplastic Neurological Syndrome Euronetwork. *Eur. J. Neurol.* **2006**, *13*, 682–690. [CrossRef] [PubMed]
12. Harlos, C.; Metser, U.; Poon, R.; MacCrostie, P.; Mason, W. 18 F-Fluorodeoxyglucose positron-emission tomography for the investigation of malignancy in patients with suspected paraneoplastic neurologic syndromes and negative or indeterminate conventional imaging: A retrospective analysis of the Ontario PET Access Program. with systematic review and meta-analysis. *Curr. Oncol.* **2019**, *26*, e458–e465. [CrossRef] [PubMed]
13. Vatankulu, B.; Aksoy, S.Y.; Asa, S.; Sager, S.; Sayman, H.B.; Halac, M.; Sonmezoglu, K. Vccuracy of FDG-PET/CT and paraneoplastic antibodies in diagnosing cancer in paraneoplastic neurological syndromes. *Rev. Esp. Med. Nucl. Imagen Mol.* **2016**, *35*, 17–21. [CrossRef] [PubMed]
14. García Vicente, A.M.; Delgado-Bolton, R.C.; Amo-Salas, M.; López-Fidalgo, J.; Caresia Aróztegui, A.P.; García Garzón, J.R.; Orcajo Rincón, J.; García Velloso, M.J.; de Arcocha Torres, M.; Alvárez Ruíz, S. 18F-fluorodeoxyglucose positron emission tomography in the diagnosis of malignancy in patients with paraneoplastic neurological syndrome: A systematic review and meta-analysis. Oncology Task Force of Spanish Society of Nuclear Medicine and Molecular Imaging. *Eur. J. Nucl. Med. Mol. Imaging* **2017**, *44*, 1575–1587. [CrossRef] [PubMed]

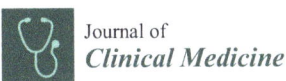

Review

Head-to-Head Comparison between ^{18}F-FES PET/CT and ^{18}F-FDG PET/CT in Oestrogen Receptor-Positive Breast Cancer: A Systematic Review and Meta-Analysis

Arnoldo Piccardo [1,*], Francesco Fiz [1], Giorgio Treglia [2,3,4], Gianluca Bottoni [1,†] and Pierpaolo Trimboli [2,5,†]

1. Nuclear Medicine Department, Ente Ospedaliero "Ospedali Galliera", 16128 Genoa, Italy; francesco.fiz@galliera.it (F.F.); gianluca.bottoni@galliera.it (G.B.)
2. Faculty of Biomedical Sciences, University della Svizzera Italiana (USI), 6900 Lugano, Switzerland; giorgio.treglia@usi.ch (G.T.); pierpaolo.trimboli@usi.ch (P.T.)
3. Faculty of Biology and Medicine, University of Lausanne, 1015 Lausanne, Switzerland
4. Academic Education, Research and Innovation Area, General Directorate, Ente Ospedaliero Cantonale, 6500 Bellinzona, Switzerland
5. Clinic of Endocrinology and Diabetology, Lugano and Mendrisio Regional Hospital, Ente Ospedaliero Cantonale, 6500 Bellinzona, Switzerland
* Correspondence: arnoldo.piccardo@galliera.it; Tel.: +39-(0)10-5634541
† These authors contributed equally to this work.

Abstract: ^{18}F-FDG PET/CT is a powerful diagnostic tool in breast cancer (BC). However, it might have a reduced sensitivity in differentiated, oestrogen receptor-positive (ER+) BC. In this setting, specific molecular imaging with fluorine-oestradiol (^{18}F-FES) PET/CT could help in overcoming these limitations; however, the literature on the diagnostic accuracy of this method is limited. We therefore planned this systematic review and meta-analysis to compare ^{18}F-FDG and ^{18}F-FES PET/CT in ER+ BC patients. We performed a literature search to identify all studies performing a head-to-head comparison between the two methods; we excluded review articles, preclinical studies, case reports and small case series. Finally, seven studies were identified (overall: 171 patients; range: 7–49 patients). A patients-based analysis (PBA) showed that ^{18}F-FDG and ^{18}F-FES PET/CT had a similar high pooled sensitivity (97% and 94%, respectively) at the lesion-based analysis (LBA), ^{18}F-FES performed slightly better than ^{18}F-FDG (pooled sensitivity: 95% vs. 85%, respectively). Moreover, when we considered only the studies dealing with the restaging setting (n = 3), this difference in sensitivity was even more marked (98% vs. 81%, respectively). In conclusion, both tracers feature an excellent sensitivity in ER+ BC; however, ^{18}F-FES PET/CT could be preferred in the restaging setting.

Keywords: PET/CT; FDG; FES; breast cancer; oestrogen receptor; diagnosis; nuclear medicine

Citation: Piccardo, A.; Fiz, F.; Treglia, G.; Bottoni, G.; Trimboli, P. Head-to-Head Comparison between ^{18}F-FES PET/CT and ^{18}F-FDG PET/CT in Oestrogen Receptor-Positive Breast Cancer: A Systematic Review and Meta-Analysis. *J. Clin. Med.* 2022, 11, 1919. https://doi.org/10.3390/jcm11071919

Academic Editors: Arutselvan Natarajan and Moritz Wildgruber

Received: 11 February 2022
Accepted: 28 March 2022
Published: 30 March 2022

Publisher's Note: MDPI stays neutral with regard to jurisdictional claims in published maps and institutional affiliations.

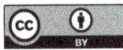

Copyright: © 2022 by the authors. Licensee MDPI, Basel, Switzerland. This article is an open access article distributed under the terms and conditions of the Creative Commons Attribution (CC BY) license (https://creativecommons.org/licenses/by/4.0/).

1. Introduction

^{18}F-FDG PET/CT is a very useful imaging tool in staging breast cancer (BC) patients with locally advanced disease [1–3] or in restaging patients with biochemical relapse without evidence of structural recurrence on conventional imaging procedures [4,5]. However, the ^{18}F-FDG avidity of BC is associated with histopathological features and can thus show relevant variations [6,7]. In particular, patients with less differentiated, triple-negative BC often present with ^{18}F-FDG avid metastases and, in this setting, ^{18}F-FDG PET/CT can provide relevant additional information when compared with morphological imaging modalities or with surgical staging [8]. Conversely, well-differentiated and oestrogen receptor-positive (ER+) BCs often present metastases with relatively low glucose consumption and thus inconstant positivity on ^{18}F-FDG PET/CT. Therefore, in this particular field of patients, more specific PET/CT agents, such as receptor tracers, still represent an unmet diagnostic need.

Fluorine-oestradiol ^{18}F-FES PET/CT has been introduced as an effective imaging procedure in patients with metastatic BC and previous histological confirmation of ER+ status on the primary tumour, to assess whether ERs are also expressed in loco-regional or distant metastases [9]. Indeed, ^{18}F-FES PET/CT provides excellent whole-body information about heterogeneity in ER expression in BC metastases, thus allowing to predict the response to endocrine therapy [10]. However, little can be said about the diagnostic role of this receptor-specific tracer and, although some studies proved its low sensitivity in detecting BC liver metastases [11,12], others showed its relevant diagnostic impact on BC bone metastases [11,13]. Overall, it is not clear yet whether ^{18}F-FES PET/CT could be proposed as a core imaging procedure in ER+ BC patients with suspected distant metastases and whether it could be preferred to ^{18}F-FDG PET/CT, at least in some specific instances.

To clarify this diagnostic issue, we performed a systematic search of the literature to identify original studies reporting a diagnostic head-to-head comparison of ^{18}F-FES PET/CT and ^{18}F-FDG PET/CT in detecting ER+ BC metastases. We also carried out a meta-analysis of the available data using sensitivity as a diagnostic outcome measure.

2. Materials and Methods

The systematic review was conducted according with the PRISMA statement [14].

2.1. Search Strategy

Two authors (A.P. and G.B.) searched the available literature independently. The search and selection process consisted of four separate steps.

In the first step, so-called "sentinel" studies were identified in PubMed by entering various combinations of the following keywords: ^{18}F-FES, ^{18}F-FDG, PET/CT, breast cancer and oestrogen receptor. In the second step, the results were used to identify specific MeSH terms in PubMed. In the third step, PubMed, CENTRAL, Scopus, Web of Science and the web were searched using the selected MeSH terms. In the final step, we evaluated the studies that compared the sensitivity of ^{18}F-FES PET/CT and ^{18}F-FDG PET/CT in identifying disease localization in patients affected by ER+ BC. All initially eligible articles were screened, and those reporting a head-to-head comparison of ^{18}F-FES PET/CT and ^{18}F-FDG PET/CT in BC patients were included. Review articles, studies based on preclinical data, phantom studies, case reports, small case series and studies with overlapping data were excluded.

The references of the included studies were searched to identify further potential matches. The search process was concluded on 21 December 2021.

2.2. Data Extraction

The two authors (A.P. and G.B.) extracted independently:

1. General characteristics of the studies (authors, year of publication, country, study design, population).
2. Technical parameters (mode of acquisition, fasting before ^{18}F-FDG injection and premedication, mean injected activity, uptake time, interval elapsed between the two imaging procedures, PET/CT scan field of view, PET/CT image analysis and use of reference standard).
3. Sensitivity of the two imaging procedures: this parameter was computed as a patient-based analysis (PBA) and a lesion-based analysis (LBA).
4. Standard of reference (SOR).

In the evaluation phase, full-text articles and their supplementary materials were included; in case of missing data, the responsible corresponding authors were contacted via e-mail. The extracted data were cross-checked and any discrepancy was discussed through a consensus meeting.

2.3. Study Quality Assessment

The risk of bias of included studies was assessed by one author (F.F.) using the QUADAS-2 method [15]. Briefly, for each study, an evaluation of the seven QUADAS-2 items was performed and each point was scored as having high, low or unclear risk of bias. High and unclear risk of bias were assigned 1 and 0.5 points, respectively; studies that totalled four or more points were excluded from the meta-analysis.

2.4. Statistical Analysis

A proportion meta-analysis was carried out using a random- effects statistical model. Pooled data are presented with their 95% confidence interval (95% CI) values. Heterogeneity across studies was assessed with the I-square statistic (I^2): a value of 50% or higher was considered as a high heterogeneity. Publication bias was evaluated with Egger's test [16].

The multidisciplinary follow-up was used as SOR to be able to compute the sensitivity of both image modalities (PBA/LBA). The OpenMeta[Analyst] statistical software (CEBM, Providence, RI, USA) was used for the statistical analyses.

3. Results

3.1. Literature Search Outcome

A total of 55 records were initially identified after duplicate removal, and their titles and abstracts were assessed; 12 articles had to be excluded since they reported single cases or small cases series. Out of the remaining 43 records, 36 were excluded because they did not meet the set inclusion criteria. Therefore, seven articles were finally selected [12,17–22], including 171 ER+ BC patients (Figure 1).

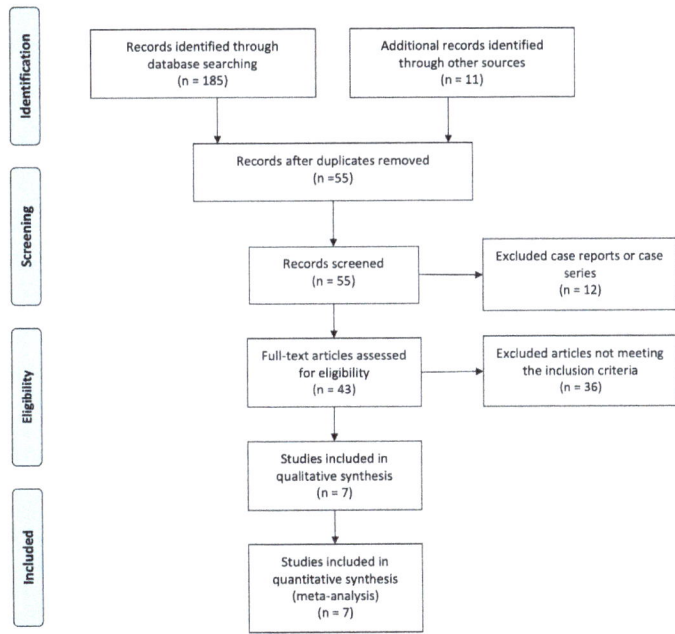

Figure 1. PRISMA flowchart, depicting the studies selection criteria.

3.2. Qualitative Analysis (Systematic Review)

The seven articles included in the systematic review had been published between 2013 and 2021. All of them had a retrospective design. Three studies were carried out in China, while India, Republic of Korea, USA and Italy, contributed one study each. The characteristics of the studies and their patients' populations are summarized in Table 1.

3.2.1. Technical Aspects

The imaging modality consisted of PET/CT with low-dose computed tomography settings in all cases. Information on fasting before ^{18}F-FDG (4–6 h) injection were available in all articles. On the other hand, fasting was not required before ^{18}F-FES injection.

The injected radiotracer activity ranged from 185 to 370 MBq for ^{18}F-FDG PET/CT and from 111 to 222 for ^{18}F-FES PET/CT. The time interval between radiotracer injection and PET/CT image acquisition was similar across the studies, being 60 min for both tracers in the majority of cases but one [19] in which ^{18}F-FES PET/CT acquisition started 80–100 min after the tracer injection.

In all studies, PET image analysis was performed by a combination of qualitative (visual) and semi-quantitative analysis through the calculation of the maximum standardized uptake values (SUV_{max}).

On visual analysis, ^{18}F-FDG focal uptake greater than the surrounding normal tissue that could not be explained by physiological activity was considered as positive in five studies [12,18,20,22,23]. In the remaining two studies, the criteria to classify ^{18}F-FDG PET findings as positive were not clearly specified [17,21]. When ^{18}F-FES PET/CT was considered, in three studies a SUV_{max} cut-off was introduced to interpret as positive each focal tracer uptake [18,20,22]. On the other hand, a visual interpretation (i.e., uptake higher than surrounding background) was used in another study [12], and in a further three analyses, the criteria were not reported [17,19,21]. All technical aspects are summarized in Table 2.

3.2.2. Diagnostic Performance

The seven articles selected for the systematic review were published between 2013 and 2021 and included populations consisting of 7 to 49 patients affected by ER+ BC (Table 1). Table 3 details the rate of positive cases at the PBA and LBA.

Overall, ^{18}F-FDG PET/CT and ^{18}F-FES PET/CT showed very high sensitivity in detecting sites of disease in ER+ BC patients. Indeed, in two studies, ^{18}F-FDG PET/CT identified more patients with BC lesions/metastases than ^{18}F-FES PET/CT [19,22]. Conversely, in one study, ^{18}F-FES PET/CT showed more BC lesions than ^{18}F-FDG PET/CT [21]. In the other four studies [12,17,18,20], both diagnostic procedures identified at least one BC lesion in the 75 patients analysed. Overall, no significant differences between the two methods were reported.

When the ability for detecting each single lesion/metastasis was considered (i.e., LBA), ^{18}F-FES PET/CT identified more BC lesions in three studies [18,21,22] and ^{18}F-FDG PET/CT identified more BC lesions in another three studies [12,19,20]. In one study, including only patients with primary BC, both modalities identified the same number of lesions [17]. As the main finding, we can point out that the studies reporting a higher number of ^{18}F-FDG-positive lesions included patients often affected by ductal carcinoma (i.e., 96%) [19] among which were also included those with ER+ HER2 + BC (11%) [19] and those with liver metastases (>10%) [12]. In addition, these patients were studied at a time of suspicious relapse when heterogeneity, due to the comparison of metastatic ER-clones, is more frequent [12,20]. On the other hand, studies showing a higher number of ^{18}F-FES-positive lesions often analysed patients affected by lobular BC [21] or patients with a high prevalence of bone metastases [22]. Moreover, patients were predominantly affected by ER+ HER- BC [18,22] and were often studied at the time of their first staging [18].

When the impact on clinical decision making was considered, only one study [18] reported that ^{18}F-FES PET/CT was able to change therapeutic strategies in 5 out of the 19 (26.5%) patients analysed at the time of first staging. Indeed, this diagnostic procedure was able to properly downstage two patients and upstage three when compared with ^{18}F-FDG PET/CT.

Table 1. Study and patient characteristics.

Authors	Year	Country	Study Design	Patients	ER+ BC *	Ductal/Lobular	HER2+	Pre/Post-Menopause	Staging/Restaging	Liver Metastases Analysed	SOR
Yang et al. [17]	2013	China	R	18	11	11/0	10	NR	11/0	No	Histopathology *
Gupta et al. [12]	2017	India	R	10	10	NR	N.R.	NR	5/5	Yes	N.R. *
Liu et al. [18]	2019	China	R	19	19	NR	N.R.	NR	19/0	No	Histopathology *
Chae et al. [19]	2020	Korea	R	46	40	38/2	5	13/33	0/40	No	Histopathology *
Liu et al. [20]	2020	China	R	35	35	29/4 **	0	7/28	0/35	No	Multidisciplinary ***
Ulaner et al. [21]	2021	USA	R	7	7	0/7	0	NR	0/7	Yes	Multidisciplinary ***
Bottoni et al. [22]	2021	Italy	R	49	40	N.R.	0	NR	0/49	No	Multidisciplinary ***

* Legend: R = retrospective; NR = not reported; SOR = standard of reference. ** Two patients were affected by mucinous and tubular BC, respectively. *** Clinical and imaging-based follow-up.

Table 2. Technical aspects of PET imaging in the included studies.

Authors	Hybrid Imaging Modality	PET/CT Tomograph	Patient Preparation	Mean Radiotracer Injected Activity	Time Interval between Radiotracer Injection and Image Acquisition	Timeframe between the Two PET/CT	Image Analysis	18F-FES PET/CT Interpreted as Positive When
Yang et al. (2013) [17]	PET/CT with low-dose CT	Siemens Biograph 16 HR	For 18F-FDG fasting (4 h)	18F-FDG: 7.4 MBq/Kg 18F-FES:222 MBq	60 min for both tracers	Up to 7 days	Visual and semi-quantitative (SUV_{max})	NR
Gupta et al. (2017) [12]	PET/CT with low-dose CT	Siemens Biograph TruePoint 40	For 18F-FDG fasting (4 h)	18F-FDG: 4–5 MBq/Kg 18F-FES: 200 MBq	60 min for both tracers	Up to 7 days	Visual and semi-quantitative (SUV_{max})	18F-FES uptake higher than surrounding background
Liu et al. (2019) [18]	PET/CT with low-dose CT	Siemens Biograph 16 HR	For 18F-FDG fasting (6 h)	18F-FDG: 7.4 MBq/Kg 18F-FES: 222 MBq	60 min for both tracers	Up to 7 days	Visual and semi-quantitative (SUV_{max})	18F-FES uptake higher than surrounding background ($SUV_{max} > 1.8$)
Chae et al.(2020) [19]	PET/CT with low-dose CT	Siemens Biograph Sensation 16 or Biograph TruePoint 40, or GE Discovery 690, 690 Elite, or 710	For 18F-FDG fasting	18F-FDG: 5.2–7.4 MBq/Kg 18F-FES:111–222 MBq	80–100 min for 18F-FES 50–70 min for 18F-FDG	Median 10 days	Visual and semi-quantitative (SUV_{max})	NR

Table 2. Cont.

Authors	Hybrid Imaging Modality	PET/CT Tomograph	Patient Preparation	Mean Radiotracer Injected Activity	Time Interval between Radiotracer Injection and Image Acquisition	Timeframe between the Two PET/CT	Image Analysis	^{18}F-FES PET/CT Interpreted as Positive When
Liu et al. (2020) [20]	PET/CT with low-dose CT	Siemens Biograph 16 HR or mCT Flow	For ^{18}F-FDG fasting (6 h)	^{18}F-FDG: 3.7–7.4 MBq/Kg ^{18}F-FES: 222 MBq	60 min for both tracers	Up to 28 days	Visual and semi-quantitative (SUV_{max})	^{18}F-FES uptake higher than surrounding background ($SUV_{max} > 1.8$)
Ulaner et al. (2021) [21]	PET/CT with low-dose CT	NR	For ^{18}F-FDG fasting (6h)	^{18}F-FDG: 444–555 MBq ^{18}F-FES: 185 MBq	60 min for both tracers	Up to 35 days	Visual and semi-quantitative (SUV_{max})	NR
Bottoni et al. (2021) [22]	PET/CT with low-dose CT	GE Discovery ST, Discovery LS or Siemens Biograph mCT Flow	For ^{18}F-FDG fasting (4–6 h)	^{18}F-FDG: according to the patient's body weight (Boellaard R. et al. EJNMMI 2014) ^{18}F-FES: 200 MBq	60 min for both tracers	Up to 10 days	Visual and semi-quantitative (SUV_{max})	^{18}F-FES uptake higher than surrounding background ($SUV_{max} > 2$)

Legend: CT = computed tomography; MBq = megabecquerel; NR = not reported; PET/CT = positron emission tomography; SUV_{max} = maximal standardized uptake value.

Table 3. Data available in the seven studies included in the present systematic review.

First Author [ref]	Patients	^{18}F-FES PET/CT	^{18}F-FDG PET/CT	Lesions	^{18}F-FES PET/CT	^{18}F-FDG PET/CT
	n (tot)	+ve	+ve	n (tot)	+ve	+ve
Yang et al. (2013) [17]	11	11	11	11	11	11
Gupta et al. (2017) [12]	10	10	10	146	116	134
Liu et al. (2019) [18]	19	19	19	238	216	197
Chae et al. (2020) [19]	40	32	36	45	32	36
Liu et al. (2020) [20]	35	35	35	235	218	235
Ulaner et al. (2021) [21]	7	7	6	254	254	111
Bottoni et al. (2021) [22]	49	42	46	1536	1532	912

Legend. +ve: positive.

3.2.3. Quality Assessment of the Studies

The risk of bias was assessed according to seven items, which are listed in Table 4. The overall bias score ranged from none to 2.5; therefore, no study had to be excluded because of high bias risk. The most frequent sources of possible bias were the "study test" and "reference standard categories" since, in some studies, it was unclear whether a blinded evaluation of the two methods had been performed. In particular, in the study by Ulaner et al. [21], the same reader assessed both examinations. In opposition to this, risks regarding the feasibility were almost never detected.

Table 4. Quality assessment of the studies and risk of bias in each study considered.

		Risk of Bias				Feasibility		
First Author	Year	Patient Selection	Study Test	Reference Standard	Timing	Patient Selection	Study Test	Reference Standard
Yang et al. [17]	2013	L	L	L	L	L	L	L
Gupta et al. [12]	2017	H	U	L	L	H	L	L
Liu et al. [18]	2019	L	U	U	L	L	L	L
Chae et al. [19]	2020	L	L	L	U	L	L	L
Liu et al. [20]	2020	L	U	U	L	L	L	L
Ulaner et al. [21]	2021	L	H	H	L	L	L	L
Bottoni et al. [22]	2021	L	U	U	L	L	L	L

Legend: H = high, L = low, U = unclear.

3.3. Quantitative Analysis (Meta-Analysis)

The pooled sensitivity of ^{18}F-FES PET/CT and ^{18}F-FDG PET/CT in terms of PBA and LBA was computed (Table 5 and Figures 2–5) based on the available data (see Table 3). Regarding PBA, the pooled sensitivity of ^{18}F-FDG PET/CT and ^{18}F-FES PET/CT was 97% and 94%, respectively, with overlapping 95% confidence intervals. In the LBA, however, we observed a wider difference between the pooled sensitivity of the two methods (95% for ^{18}F-FES vs. 85% for ^{18}F-FDG). Although the 95% confidence intervals of the two methods were overlapping, the values of ^{18}F-FES PET/CT were consistently at the higher end of the spectrum (93–97%), while those of ^{18}F-FDG PET/CT showed a much larger spread (68–100%). In all the analyses, high heterogeneity was found (Table 5).

On the basis of the above results, the heterogeneity of PBA and LBA was explored by using the following covariates: timing of the studies (i.e., PET/CT assessment on staging and on time of relapse), their sample sizes, the prevalence of ductal or lobular BC, and the prevalence of bone and liver metastases.

Table 5. Pooled sensitivity for PBA and LBA of ^{18}F-FES PET/CT and ^{18}F-FDG PET/CT.

	PBA			LBA		
	Sensitivity (95% CI)	I^2	Egger's Test (p)	Sensitivity (95% CI)	I^2 (%)	Egger's Test (p)
^{18}F-FES PET/CT	94% (89–99)	52.7%	$p = 0.048$	95% (93–97)	93.66%	$p < 0.01$
^{18}F-FDG PET/CT	97% (94–99)	0%	$p = 0.62$	85% (68–100)	99.44%	$p < 0.001$

Legend: PBA, patient-based analysis; LBA, lesion-based analysis.

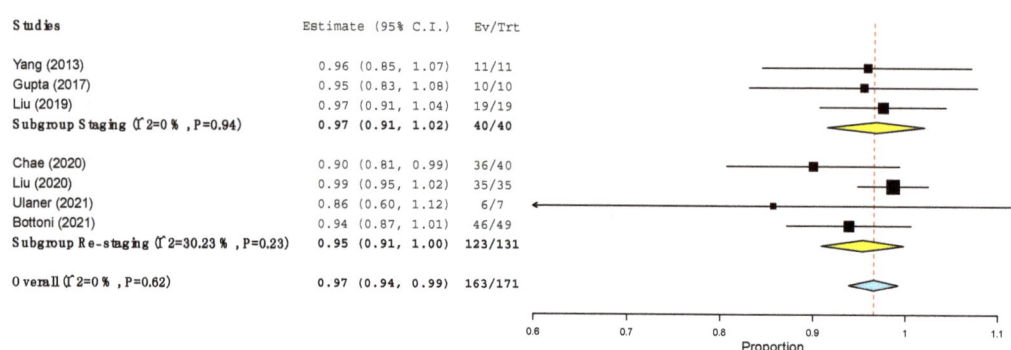

Figure 2. Sensitivity of ^{18}F-FDG PET/CT at the level of patients across studies.

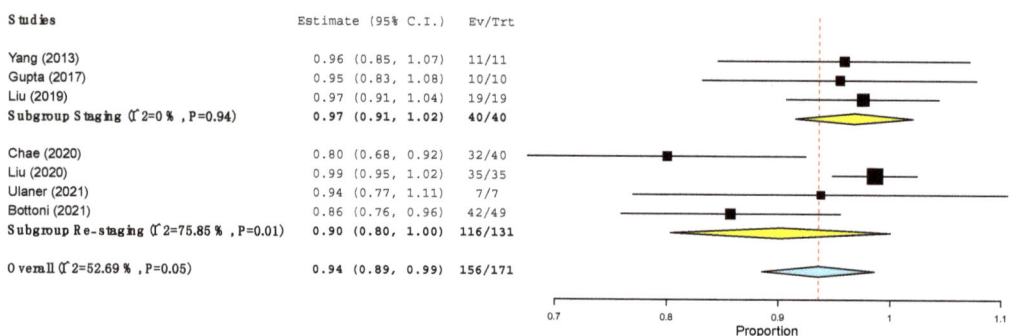

Figure 3. Sensitivity of ^{18}F-FES PET/CT at the level of patients across studies.

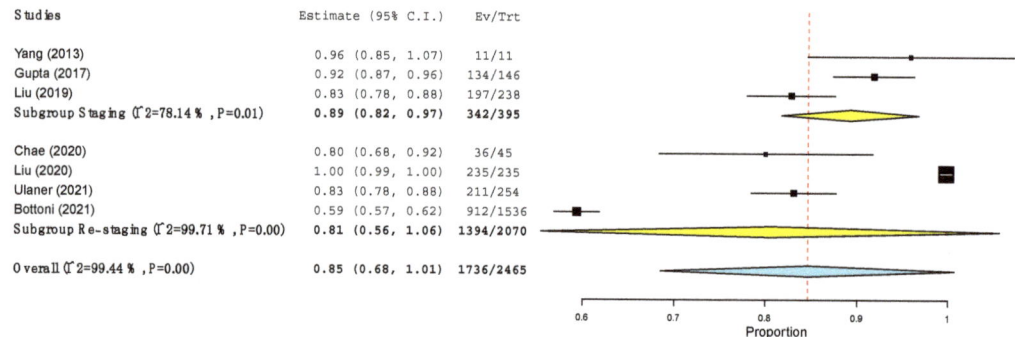

Figure 4. Sensitivity of ^{18}F-FDG PET/CT at the level of the lesions across studies.

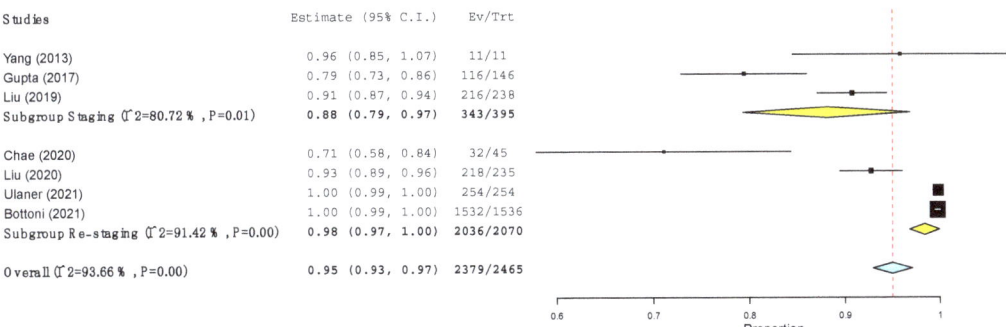

Figure 5. Sensitivity of ^{18}F-FES PET/CT at the level of the lesions across studies.

However, these last variables could not be tested, given incomplete and inconsistent data, and only the variable "timing of the studies" was explored. As illustrated in Figures 2 and 3, the heterogeneity of the ^{18}F-FES PET/CT and ^{18}F-FDG PET/CT results was no longer present in the PBA when we considered these two groups separately. In fact, in the staging scenario, the sensitivity in the PBA of both the ^{18}F-FES PET/CT and ^{18}F-FDG PET/CT was 97% (Figures 2 and 3). Conversely, at the time of restaging, the patient-based sensitivity of ^{18}F-FES PET/CT and ^{18}F-FDG PET/CT was 90% and 95% respectively (Figures 2 and 3).

When LBA was conducted, the sensitivity of ^{18}F-FES PET/CT and ^{18}F-FDG PET/CT at the time of first staging was 88% and 89% respectively, while at the time of restaging it was 81% and 98%, respectively (Figures 4 and 5). Interestingly, the sensitivity of ^{18}F-FES PET/CT at the time of restaging was significantly higher than that of the same procedure at the time of staging (Figure 4).

4. Discussion

In this systematic review and meta-analysis, we aimed to clarify the diagnostic role of ^{18}F-FES PET/CT in BC patients compared to ^{18}F-FDG PET/CT. In fact, ^{18}F-FES PET/CT has gained significant attraction as a non-invasive means to predict the effectiveness of hormone blockade. However, its potential in the mere diagnostic evaluation is still debated [1,8,21]. In this study, we gathered all the available evidence of its sensitivity in ER+ BC patients when compared with the more commonly used ^{18}F-FDG PET/CT.

Our qualitative and quantitative assessment in this particular BC subpopulation showed that there are no significant differences in terms of sensitivity between the two PET tracers at the PBA. Indeed, both molecular imaging modalities proved able to detect patients affected by ER+ BC with similarly high sensitivity. The lack of significant difference between these two modalities can, however, be explained by the selection of patients included in the analysis. These patients were evaluated at the time of first staging for an already known primary tumour or who underwent PET at the time of relapse to evaluate the extension or the ER expression of the metastatic disease. This population is indeed characterized by a very high prevalence of a true positive BC lesion; the probability that at least one these lesions was detected by one of the two molecular imaging procedures was very high. The small diagnostic advantage of the ^{18}F-FDG PET/CT over ^{18}F-FES PET/CT (97% vs. 94%) reported in our analysis seems related to the variability in terms of the clinical characteristics of the patients. Indeed, the high prevalence of metastatic heterogeneity, often present at the time of restaging, can be associated to false negative ^{18}F-FES PET/CT results. When the diagnostic performances of these two imaging procedures at the time of recurrence was explored by means of a PBA, the sensitivity of ^{18}F-FDG PET/CT and that of ^{18}F-FES PET/CT was 95% and 90%, respectively.

Conversely, when we investigated the diagnostic sensitivity of these diagnostic tools by means of an LBA, we found that the sensitivity of ^{18}F-FDG PET/CT and that of ^{18}F-FES

PET/CT was 85% and 95%, respectively. Indeed, when the analysis was focused on the time of disease relapse, ^{18}F-FES PET/CT was more sensitive than ^{18}F-FDG PET/CT (98% vs. 81%) with a trend towards significance (95% CI: 97–100% and 56–100%, respectively).

Overall, the use ^{18}F-FDG PET/CT as a first-line examination appears to be the best strategy to stage and restage the ER+ BC subjects, being able to identify the highest number of true positive patients. However, if this approach is applied to a population of ER+ BC with low metastatic heterogeneity (i.e., lobular breast cancer, or ductal breast cancer with a high percentage of ER positive and HER2 negative cells) it could underestimate the actual disease burden since such a clone could show low glucose avidity. Indeed, although ^{18}F-FES PET/CT has low sensitivity in detecting liver metastases (given the intense background tracer uptake in this organ), it has a very high sensitivity in disclosing peripheral lesions in other organs or tissues, such as bone lesions, which represent the most frequent sites of disease in ER+ BC [22]. In addition, as reported by Gupta et al. [12], one of the diagnostic advantages of this receptor PET tracer is its higher specificity in characterizing cervical, axillary and mediastinal lymph nodes, which may often present unspecific uptake at ^{18}F-FDG PET/CT and thus be misinterpreted on ^{18}F-FDG PET/CT.

Although our systematic review and meta-analysis reported interesting and useful results to understand the weaknesses and strengths of the two imaging procedures, some limitations should also be borne in mind. First, only seven studies, investigating relatively small patient populations, were fit for inclusions in this meta-analysis. In addition, all these seven studies showed a retrospective design, and three out of seven included a low number of ER+ BC patients. However, the selection criteria limited us to studies that tested both ^{18}F-FDG PET/CT and ^{18}F-FES PET/CT within a restricted time frame. Second, a computation of specificity was not possible since none of the studies reported the true negative rate. Third, the absence of histological confirmation of suspected distant metastases detected by both modalities is an important bias that could have affected some of the studies included in this analysis [12,20–22], and we cannot exclude the possibility that some of the metastases detected by PET tracers may have been false-positive findings. However, given the elevated prevalence of patients with disseminated disease, the likelihood of any given finding to be a false negative was relatively low. Moreover, ethical and practical reasons prevented the execution of a biopsy evaluation of each single lesion. In addition, in at least 3 out of 7 studies, a multidisciplinary follow-up (consisting of clinical and imaging evaluation) was available. Fourth, only two out of the seven studies reported information regarding the menopausal status of the patients. Indeed, these data could be of value to correctly estimate the real sensitivity of ^{18}F-FES PET/CT that could theoretically be affected by competitive binding of high oestradiol concentration. However, the exact endogenous oestrogen concentration that can have a measurable effect on tumour ^{18}F-FES uptake remains hitherto unexplored [9]. Statistically significant heterogeneity of the ^{18}F-FES PET/CT pooled heterogeneity was found across studies. Regrettably, the sparse data available in the studies did not allow exploration of the heterogeneity with the exception of the variable "timing of the studies".

Finally, at this time, data about the cost/effectiveness of ^{18}F-FES PET/CT in comparison with that of ^{18}F-FDG PET/CT do not exist. However, it is conceivable that, when the overall expense is considered, the additional information provided by FES might help in optimizing the cost by guiding the choice of the most appropriate therapeutic protocol.

5. Conclusions

The present data show that both ^{18}F-FDG PET/CT and ^{18}F-FES PET/CT represent accurate imaging procedures in patients with ER+ BC, providing comparable results in terms of sensitivity. However, in the field of lesion detection, we observed a non-negligible difference in favour of ^{18}F-FES PET/CT. Thus, the use of ^{18}F-FES PET/CT as a first-line molecular imaging procedure might be considered in lobular breast cancer or ductal breast cancer with a high percentage of ER and HER2 negative. However, larger, multicentre and prospective studies are required to confirm these preliminary indications.

Author Contributions: Conceiving the study and writing the manuscript draft, A.P., G.B., P.T.; performing the literature search and selecting the studies, F.F., G.B.; performing the meta-analysis, P.T.; reviewing the manuscript draft, F.F., G.T. All authors have read and agreed to the published version of the manuscript.

Funding: This research received no external funding.

Institutional Review Board Statement: Not applicable.

Informed Consent Statement: Not applicable.

Data Availability Statement: Not applicable.

Conflicts of Interest: The authors declare no conflict of interest.

References

1. Ulaner, G.A. PET/CT for Patients With Breast Cancer: Where Is the Clinical Impact? *Am. J. Roentgenol.* **2019**, *213*, 254–265. [CrossRef] [PubMed]
2. Alberini, J.-L.; Lerebours, F.; Wartski, M.; Fourme, E.; Le Stanc, E.; Gontier, E.; Madar, O.; Cherel, P.; Pecking, A.P. ^{18}F-fluorodeoxyglucose positron emission tomography/computed tomography (FDG-PET/CT) imaging in the staging and prognosis of inflammatory breast cancer. *Cancer* **2009**, *115*, 5038–5047. [CrossRef] [PubMed]
3. Segaert, I.; Mottaghy, F.; Ceyssens, S.; De Wever, W.; Stroobants, S.; Van Ongeval, C.; Van Limbergen, E.; Wildiers, H.; Paridaens, R.; Vergote, I.; et al. Additional Value of PET-CT in Staging of Clinical Stage IIB and III Breast Cancer. *Breast J.* **2010**, *16*, 617–624. [CrossRef]
4. Champion, L.; Brain, E.; Giraudet, A.-L.; Le Stanc, E.; Wartski, M.; Edeline, V.; Madar, O.; Bellet, D.; Pecking, A.; Alberini, J.-L. Breast cancer recurrence diagnosis suspected on tumor marker rising. *Cancer* **2010**, *117*, 1621–1629. [CrossRef] [PubMed]
5. Hildebrandt, M.G.; Gerke, O.; Baun, C.; Falch, K.; Hansen, J.A.; Farahani, Z.A.; Petersen, H.; Larsen, L.B.; Duvnjak, S.; Buskevica, I.; et al. [^{18}F]Fluorodeoxyglucose (FDG)-Positron Emission Tomography (PET)/Computed Tomography (CT) in Suspected Recurrent Breast Cancer: A Prospective Comparative Study of Dual-Time-Point FDG-PET/CT, Contrast-Enhanced CT, and Bone Scintigraphy. *J. Clin. Oncol.* **2016**, *34*, 1889–1897. [CrossRef] [PubMed]
6. Gil-Rendo, A.; Martínez-Regueira, F.; Zornoza, G.; Garcia-Velloso, M.J.; Beorlegui, C.; Rodriguez-Spiteri, N. Association between [^{18}F]fluorodeoxyglucose uptake and prognostic parameters in breast cancer. *Br. J. Surg.* **2009**, *96*, 166–170. [CrossRef] [PubMed]
7. Kumar, R.; Chauhan, A.; Zhuang, H.; Chandra, P.; Schnall, M.; Alavi, A. Clinicopathologic factors associated with false negative FDG–PET in primary breast cancer. *Breast Cancer Res. Treat.* **2006**, *98*, 267–274. [CrossRef]
8. Ulaner, G.A.; Castillo, R.; Goldman, D.A.; Wills, J.; Riedl, C.; Pinker-Domenig, K.; Jochelson, M.S.; Gönen, M. ^{18}F-FDG-PET/CT for systemic staging of newly diagnosed triple-negative breast cancer. *Eur. J. Pediatr.* **2016**, *43*, 1937–1944. [CrossRef]
9. van Kruchten, M.; de Vries, E.G.E.; Brown, M.; de Vries, E.F.J.; Glaudemans, A.W.J.M.; Dierckx, R.A.J.O.; Schröder, C.P.; Hospers, G.A.P. PET imaging of oestrogen receptors in patients with breast cancer. *Lancet Oncol.* **2013**, *14*, e465–e475. [CrossRef]
10. Kurland, B.F.; Wiggins, J.R.; Coche, A.; Fontan, C.; Bouvet, Y.; Webner, P.; Divgi, C.; Linden, H.M. Whole-Body Characterization of Estrogen Receptor Status in Metastatic Breast Cancer with 16α-^{18}F-Fluoro-17β-Estradiol Positron Emission Tomography: Meta-Analysis and Recommendations for Integration into Clinical Applications. *Oncologist* **2020**, *25*, 835–844. [CrossRef]
11. van Kruchten, M.; Glaudemans, A.; de Vries, E.; Beets-Tan, R.G.; Schröder, C.P.; Dierckx, R.A.; de Vries, E.; Hospers, G. PET Imaging of Estrogen Receptors as a Diagnostic Tool for Breast Cancer Patients Presenting with a Clinical Dilemma. *J. Nucl. Med.* **2012**, *53*, 182–190. [CrossRef]
12. Gupta, M.; Datta, A.; Choudhury, P.S.; Dsouza, M.; Batra, U.; Mishra, A. Can ^{18}F-Fluoroestradiol positron emission tomography become a new imaging standard in the estrogen receptor-positive breast cancer patient: A prospective comparative study with ^{18}F-Fluorodeoxyglucose positron emission tomography? *World J. Nucl. Med.* **2017**, *16*, 133–139. [CrossRef] [PubMed]
13. Nienhuis, H.H.; Van Kruchten, M.; Elias, S.G.; Glaudemans, A.; De Vries, E.F.; Bongaerts, A.H.; Schröder, C.P.; De Vries, E.G.; Hospers, G.A. ^{18}F-Fluoroestradiol Tumor Uptake Is Heterogeneous and Influenced by Site of Metastasis in Breast Cancer Patients. *J. Nucl. Med.* **2018**, *59*, 1212–1218. [CrossRef] [PubMed]
14. McInnes, M.D.F.; Moher, D.; Thombs, B.D.; McGrath, T.A.; Bossuyt, P.M.; Clifford, T.; Cohen, J.F.; Deeks, J.J.; Gatsonis, C.; Hooft, L.; et al. Preferred Reporting Items for a Systematic Review and Meta-analysis of Diagnostic Test Accuracy Studies. The PRISMA-DTA Statement. *JAMA* **2018**, *319*, 388–396. [CrossRef]
15. Whiting, P.F.; Rutjes, A.W.S.; Westwood, M.E.; Mallett, S.; Deeks, J.J.; Reitsma, J.B.; Leeflang, M.M.; Sterne, J.A.; Bossuyt, P.M.; QUADAS-2 Group. QUADAS-2: A Revised Tool for the Quality Assessment of Diagnostic Accuracy Studies. *Ann. Intern. Med.* **2011**, *155*, 529–536. [CrossRef]
16. Sadeghi, R.; Treglia, G. Systematic reviews and meta-analyses of diagnostic studies: A practical guideline. *Clin. Transl. Imaging* **2016**, *5*, 83–87. [CrossRef]
17. Yang, Z.; Sun, Y.; Xue, J.; Yao, Z.; Xu, J.; Cheng, J.; Shi, W.; Zhu, B.; Zhang, Y.; Zhang, Y. Can Positron Emission Tomography/Computed Tomography with the Dual Tracers Fluorine-18 Fluoroestradiol and Fluorodeoxyglucose Predict Neoadjuvant Chemotherapy Response of Breast Cancer?—A Pilot Study. *PLoS ONE* **2013**, *8*, e78192. [CrossRef] [PubMed]

18. Liu, C.; Gong, C.; Liu, S.; Zhang, Y.; Zhang, Y.; Xu, X.; Yuan, H.; Wang, B.; Yang, Z. ^{18}F-FES PET/CT Influences the Staging and Management of Patients with Newly Diagnosed Estrogen Receptor-Positive Breast Cancer: A Retrospective Comparative Study with ^{18}F-FDG PET/CT. *Oncologist* **2019**, *24*, e1277–e1285. [CrossRef]
19. Chae, S.Y.; Son, H.J.; Lee, D.Y.; Shin, E.; Oh, J.S.; Seo, S.Y.; Baek, S.; Kim, J.Y.; Na, S.J.; Moon, D.H. Comparison of diagnostic sensitivity of [^{18}F]fluoroestradiol and [^{18}F]fluorodeoxyglucose positron emission tomography/computed tomography for breast cancer recurrence in patients with a history of estrogen receptor-positive primary breast cancer. *EJNMMI Res.* **2020**, *10*, 1–9. [CrossRef]
20. Liu, C.; Xu, X.; Yuan, H.; Zhang, Y.; Zhang, Y.; Song, S.; Yang, Z. Dual Tracers of 16α-[^{18}F]fluoro-17β-Estradiol and [^{18}F]fluorodeoxyglucose for Prediction of Progression-Free Survival After Fulvestrant Therapy in Patients With HR+/HER2- Metastatic Breast Cancer. *Front. Oncol.* **2020**, *10*, 580467. [CrossRef]
21. Ulaner, G.A.; Jhaveri, K.; Chandarlapaty, S.; Hatzoglou, V.; Riedl, C.C.; Lewis, J.S.; Mauguen, A. Head-to-Head Evaluation of ^{18}F-FES and ^{18}F-FDG PET/CT in Metastatic Invasive Lobular Breast Cancer. *J. Nucl. Med.* **2020**, *62*, 326–331. [CrossRef] [PubMed]
22. Bottoni, G.; Piccardo, A.; Fiz, F.; Siri, G.; Matteucci, F.; Rocca, A.; Nanni, O.; Monti, M.; Brain, E.; Alberini, J.L.; et al. Heterogeneity of bone metastases as an important prognostic factor in patients affected by oestrogen receptor-positive breast cancer. The role of combined [^{18}F]Fluoroestradiol PET/CT and [^{18}F]Fluorodeoxyglucose PET/CT. *Eur. J. Radiol.* **2021**, *141*, 109821. [CrossRef] [PubMed]
23. Chae, S.Y.; Kim, S.-B.; Ahn, S.H.; Kim, H.O.; Yoon, D.H.; Ahn, J.-H.; Jung, K.H.; Han, S.; Oh, S.J.; Lee, S.J.; et al. A Randomized Feasibility Study of ^{18}F-Fluoroestradiol PET to Predict Pathologic Response to Neoadjuvant Therapy in Estrogen Receptor–Rich Postmenopausal Breast Cancer. *J. Nucl. Med.* **2016**, *58*, 563–568. [CrossRef] [PubMed]

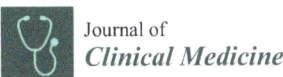

Review

The Current Role of Peptide Receptor Radionuclide Therapy in Meningiomas

Christina-Katharina Fodi [1,2], Jens Schittenhelm [2,3], Jürgen Honegger [1,2], Salvador Guillermo Castaneda-Vega [4,5,†] and Felix Behling [1,2,*,†]

[1] Department of Neurosurgery and Neurotechnology, University Hospital Tübingen, Eberhard-Karls University, 72076 Tübingen, Germany; christina-katharina.fodi@med.uni-tuebingen.de (C.-K.F.); juergen.honegger@med.uni-tuebingen.de (J.H.)
[2] Center for CNS Tumors, Comprehensive Cancer Center Tübingen-Stuttgart, University Hospital Tübingen, Eberhard-Karls-University, 72076 Tübingen, Germany; jens.schittenhelm@med.uni-tuebingen.de
[3] Department of Neuropathology, University Hospital Tübingen, Eberhard-Karls University, 72076 Tübingen, Germany
[4] Department of Nuclear Medicine and Clinical Molecular Imaging, University Hospital Tübingen, Eberhard-Karls University, 72076 Tübingen, Germany; salvador.castaneda@med.uni-tuebingen.de
[5] Werner Siemens Imaging Center, Department of Preclinical Imaging and Radiopharmacy, Eberhard-Karls University, 72076 Tübingen, Germany
* Correspondence: felix.behling@med.uni-tuebingen.de; Tel.: +49-707129-80235; Fax: +49-707129-4549
† These authors contributed equally to this work.

Citation: Fodi, C.-K.; Schittenhelm, J.; Honegger, J.; Castaneda-Vega, S.G.; Behling, F. The Current Role of Peptide Receptor Radionuclide Therapy in Meningiomas. *J. Clin. Med.* **2022**, *11*, 2364. https://doi.org/10.3390/jcm11092364

Academic Editors: Arnoldo Piccardo and Francesco Fiz

Received: 24 March 2022
Accepted: 20 April 2022
Published: 23 April 2022

Publisher's Note: MDPI stays neutral with regard to jurisdictional claims in published maps and institutional affiliations.

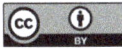

Copyright: © 2022 by the authors. Licensee MDPI, Basel, Switzerland. This article is an open access article distributed under the terms and conditions of the Creative Commons Attribution (CC BY) license (https://creativecommons.org/licenses/by/4.0/).

Abstract: Meningiomas are the most common primary intracranial tumors. The majority of patients can be cured by surgery, or tumor growth can be stabilized by radiation. However, the management of recurrent and more aggressive tumors remains difficult because no established alternative treatment options exist. Therefore, innovative therapeutic approaches are needed. Studies have shown that meningiomas express somatostatin receptors. It is well known from treating neuroendocrine tumors that peptide radioreceptor therapy that targets somatostatin receptors can be effective. As yet, this therapy has been used for treating meningiomas only within individual curative trials. However, small case series and studies have demonstrated stabilization of the disease. Therefore, we see potential for optimizing this therapeutic option through the development of new substances and specific adaptations to the different meningioma subtypes. The current review provides an overview of this topic.

Keywords: meningioma; peptide receptor radionuclide therapy; PRRT; targeted therapy; somatostatin receptor; SSTR

1. Introduction

With an incidence of 8.81/100,000, meningiomas are the most common primary intracranial tumor [1]. These slow-growing tumors develop along the meningeal coverings of the cerebral convexities, skull base, and spine, and in rare cases even within the ventricles. Depending on the size and location, a variety of different symptoms and syndromes can emerge [2]. Treatment is advisable for lesions that show concerning growth, cause symptoms, or have a significant size in a critical location. Most meningiomas can be effectively treated by surgical resection. Radiation therapy can be applied in selected cases but is particularly important in recurrent cases or for meningiomas that are histopathologically graded as more aggressive [3]. Other than surgery and radiation, there are no established treatment modalities outside of previous clinical trials [4]. The management of meningiomas that recur after resection and radiation treatment remains especially challenging, and alternative treatment options are urgently needed. Targeted therapies based on molecular aberrations [5] are currently under investigation in several clinical trials, with a focus on high-grade and recurrent meningiomas (e.g., NCT02648997, NCT03279692, and

NCT03631953). However, an innovative treatment option for recurrent meningiomas has been applied in difficult cases. Peptide receptor radionuclide therapy (PRRT) utilizes the expression of somatostatin receptors (SSTRs) in meningioma tissue. Somatostatin analogs coupled to a radionuclide apply radiation directly to tissue that expresses somatostatin receptor 2A, such as meningioma cells [6,7]. In recent years, this targeted treatment approach has been investigated for use against meningiomas. This review focuses on the current use of PRRT to treat meningiomas and provides an outlook regarding its potential future therapeutic role.

2. Peptide Receptor Radionuclide Therapy

2.1. Somatostatin Receptors

Somatostatin receptors, through which somatostatin exerts its effects, were first described in 1978 by Schonbrunn and Tashjian [8]. Five different subtypes have been discovered in humans and other mammals. The SSTR2 subtype has one intron, which can result in two different receptors, SSTR2A and the SSTR2B, by alternative splicing. The remaining subtypes do not possess introns [9]. However, SSTR2B has only been detected in mouse tissue, and it is unclear whether this subtype is also expressed in humans [10]. These G protein-coupled receptors are composed of glycoproteins [11] and are membrane-bound with seven alpha-helical transmembrane domains [10]. They have an extracellular N-terminal end, which is responsible for binding the specific ligand somatostatin. The C-terminal end is intracellular and transmits signal transduction [10] through a heterotrimeric G protein that consists of an α-, β-, and γ-subunit and triggers different intracellular pathways with the help of GTP. Upon binding of a ligand to the SSTR, the cascade further triggers activation or inhibition of cytoplasmic targets via membrane-bound proteins [12]. Examples of commonly triggered pathways include the adenylate cyclase and the phospholipase C system, which act as signal amplifiers. However, the direct stimulation of potassium or calcium channels can also be triggered to achieve the desired effects [13,14]. Somatostatin is involved in numerous physiological regulatory mechanisms in several different organ systems, including the inhibition of endocrine and exocrine secretions, gastrointestinal motility and nutrient absorption, and neurotransmitter regulation [15].

A central task of SSTR is the inhibition of cell proliferation. The antiproliferative effects of somatostatin and its receptors are mediated through several mechanisms. SSTR2 and SSTR3 can induce apoptosis of single cells via p53 or independently of p53. SSTR1, SSTR4, and SSTR5 can induce cell arrest in the G1 phase of the cell cycle via the modulation of mitogen-activated protein (MAP) kinase [16]. There are numerous other modes of action of SSTRs that are reserved for their respective tissues. SSTRs occur in varying densities and in different expression patterns. They are found in the brain, pituitary gland, and peripheral nervous system. In the gastrointestinal tract, they are found in large numbers in the stomach, duodenum, jejunum, and pancreas. They are also present in the kidneys, adrenal glands, thyroid gland, and immune cells [11,17,18].

An important discovery was the expression of SSTRs in a large variety of tumors, including most neuroendocrine tumors, such as gastroenteropancreatic neuroendocrine tumors (GEP-NETs) and carcinoids. SSTRs also occur in renal cell carcinoma, breast cancer, and lymphoma. Furthermore, SSTRs are expressed in brain tumors, such as glial tumors, pituitary adenomas, and meningiomas [18,19]. Studies conducted on meningiomas have shown the presence of all five different SSTR subtypes in varying degrees of expression. SSTRs could be detected by immunohistochemistry and by mRNA identification with RT-PCR [20–24]. In these studies, SSTR2A showed the strongest expression [20–23,25]. We performed a large retrospective analysis of immunohistochemical expression of all five SSTRs in 726 meningiomas. This large cohort also showed strong expression of SSTR1 and SSTR5 and different expression patterns within various clinical subgroups, such as neurofibromatosis type 2 and WHO grades II and III meningiomas [24].

Whether somatostatin expression is linked to tumor proliferation or progression remains unclear, especially because its main function is essentially antiproliferative.

2.2. History and Development

In 1987, Krenning et al. examined 1000 patients with various tumors by octreotide receptor scintigraphy (Octreoscan) to visualize SSTR expression. It was hypothesized that tumors showing high uptake may respond well to therapy with somatostatin analogs [26] because somatostatin exerts an antiproliferative effect. Furthermore, the idea of combining somatostatin with radiation was developed so that the radiation dose could be directly delivered to the tumor tissue. These so-called "theranostic substances", with diagnostic (peptide receptor scintigraphy) and therapeutic (peptide receptor radionuclide therapy) features, were first used in neuroendocrine tumors [27]. The first instance of PRRT was in the early 1990s for a patient with metastatic glucagonoma, which resulted in tumor growth impairment as well as decreasing levels of circulating glucagon [28].

Initially, 111In-DTPA octreotide, which emits Auger and conversion electrons, was applied for PRRT, with SSTR as the target. However, this compound exhibited affinity exclusively for SSTR2 and was additionally not suitable for commercially available ß-emitters such as ^{90}Y and ^{77}Lu. Therefore, other somatostatin analogs such as DOTATOC and DOTATATE were coupled with the corresponding ß-emitters to form ^{177}Lu-DOTATATE and ^{90}Y-DOTATOC [29] and used in subsequent studies. PRRT was increasingly used in the treatment of neuroendocrine tumors. It is often applied for metastasized tumors for which the usual treatment methods, such as surgery or localized radiation therapy, are no longer suitable options. Often, standard chemotherapy is no longer sufficient or does not achieve adequate symptom control. In these cases, treatment can be carried out with PRRT [29–31]. The phase III NETTER-1 trial demonstrated that PRRT significantly improved the quality of life and progression-free survival of patients with midgut neuroendocrine tumors who received ^{177}Lu-DOTATATE and high-dose octreotide [32]. With the knowledge that several tumor types highly express SSTRs [33], PRRT has also been used therapeutically for other tumor types as an individual curative attempt after the exhaustion of current treatment methods [34–36].

In many cases, meningiomas can be cured by surgical excision or stabilized radiation therapy [3]. However, sometimes these treatments are not sufficient, and it becomes difficult to treat recurrences or multifocal occurrences of meningiomas; for example, a meningiomatosis cerebri. This often affects patients suffering from neurofibromatosis type 2 (NF2) or tumors corresponding to WHO grades II or III. Through various studies, we know that virtually all meningiomas express SSTRs, although to a varying extent [20,22,24,25,37]. This has been recognized as an opportunity to apply PRRT in individual cases of advanced meningioma [29,38].

2.3. Clinical Application and Experience in Meningioma

Certain conditions must be met to perform PRRT. To assess whether there is sufficient receptor expression, the standard procedure prior to therapy is to detect it via peptide receptor positron emission tomography (PET), e.g., with ^{68}Ga. This also includes imaging the kinetics of the therapeutic substance [39]. Once sufficient receptor expression has been determined through PET imaging, the patient becomes a candidate for therapy. Somatostatin analogs, such as DOTATOC or DOTATATE, which bind to SSTRs (particularly SSTR2A), are administered intravenously. The administered peptides are coupled to a ß-emitter, usually ^{90}Yttrium (Y). This coupling allows the systemic delivery of a cytotoxic level of radiation to individual target cells expressing SSTRs [40]. In addition, adjacent tumor cells that do not necessarily express SSTRs are also irradiated. Alternatively, small studies and case reports have shown that intra-arterial administration of the radiopharmaceutical increases the uptake in meningiomas [41–43].

However, there are no specific guidelines regarding this treatment for meningiomas, but general standards for PRRT in NETS are applied. A glomerular filtration rate of at least 40 mL/min or a creatinine value <2.0 mg/dL must be present in order to assure sufficient clearance and to maintain functional organ reserve because the treatment is nephrotoxic. Likewise, there is a risk of hematotoxicity and pretherapeutic cutoffs for platelet and leukocyte count and hemoglobin need to be considered. Therefore, regular monitoring is necessary, which may lead to a pause in treatment [44]. There could also be a risk of acute bone marrow toxicity, particularly in patients who received extended external beam radiation or myelotoxic chemotherapy before PRRT. The number of cycles for non-compromised patients varies from two to five for ^{90}Y-DOTATATE/-DOTATOC and ^{177}Lu-DOTATATE/-DOTATOC. The time interval between cycles ranges between 6 and 12 weeks. The approved activity levels range from 2.78–4.44 GBq for ^{90}Y-DOTATATE/-DOTATOC and from 5.55–7.4 GBq for ^{177}Lu-DOTATATE/-DOTATOC. Therapy needs to be adjusted for patients with restricted renal function or borderline bone marrow capacity [45].

Currently, there are only a few studies on PRRT for meningiomas with small patient cohorts. However, some have shown stabilization of the disease. In one study, 5–15 GBq of ^{90}Y-DOTATOC was administered to a group of 29 patients with recurrent meningiomas, and disease stabilization was observed in 66% of the patients [6]. Another study demonstrated that a combination of external beam radiation therapy (EBRT) and PRRT was well-tolerated in patients with unresectable primary or recurrent meningioma and resulted in disease stabilization in 7 of the 10 patients [46]. These results confirmed the findings of a previous analysis of the outcome of patients treated with EBRT and PRRT in combination. In that study, ten patients with unresectable WHO grades I or II meningiomas experienced disease stabilization [47]. PRRT was also investigated in patients suffering from NF2. They received four cycles of ^{177}Lu-DOTATOC with a median activity of 7.4 GBq. Tumor stabilization occurred in six of eleven patients [48]. A meta-analysis regarding PRRT in meningiomas was performed by Miriam et al. They included 111 patients with treatment-refractory meningiomas, and 63% achieved disease control. The 6-month progression-free survival rates and the 1-year overall survival decreased with higher WHO grades. Explicit guidelines for the treatment of meningioma using SSTR-targeted PRRT have still yet to be internationally established. However, the mentioned comprehensive meta-analysis recently evaluated SSTR-targeted PRRT using ^{90}Y-DOTATOC, ^{177}Lu-DOTATOC, ^{177}Lu-DOTATATE, or combinations in histologically validated meningioma [49]. The evaluated studies in the meta-analysis applied SSTR-targeted PRRT on treatment-refractory meningioma patients with exhausted conventional treatment modalities such as: surgery, fractioned or stereotactic radiotherapy, or chemotherapy prior to SSTR-targeted therapy. Before the start of therapy, intense SSRT-expression was confirmed in the meningiomas using PET/CT. Independent of the tumor grade for up to six cycles of therapy, a median of 12,590 Mbq (range: 1688–29,772) was applied for treatment. Manageable mild transient hematotoxicity (anemia, leukopenia, lymphocytopenia, and thrombocytopenia) was the major side effect co-occurring under PRRT and as such, constant evaluation of hemoglobin, granulocytes, leukocytes, and thrombocytes is warranted before and between PRRT cycles. Overall, PRRT showed a positive treatment effect with manageable side effects. Treatment response was evaluated using different radiological assessment protocols finding favorable overall survival in the combined outcome of all studies [49].

The meta-analysis underlines the small number of cases that have been published so far. At present, no larger controlled trials have been conducted. One randomized trial is currently recruiting patients with recurrent or progressive meningiomas for treatment with the radiolabeled somatostatin antagonist 177Lu-satoreotide (PROMENADE study, NCT04997317). An overview of the studies already conducted can be seen in Table 1.

Table 1. Studies that have investigated the effect of PRRT on meningiomas.

Reference	Type of Study	Cohort	Response	PFS (Months)	OS (Months)	Adverse Events/Toxicity
Bartolomei et al. [6]	prospective	n = 29	stabilization n = 19 progression n = 10	6 (from end of PRRT)	40	white blood cells n = 18 renal n = 1
Hartrampf et al. [46]	prospective	n = 10	stabilization n = 7 progression n = 3	91.1	105	none
Kreissl et al. [47]	prospective	n = 10	stabilization n = 8 Partial remission n = 1 complete remission n = 1	-	-	none
Kertels et al. [48]	retrospective	n = 11	stabilization n = 6 no response n = 5	12	37	temporary leukopenia n = 53 thrombozytopenia n = 15 renal n = 3 liver n = 1
Seystahl et al. [50]	retrospective	n = 20	stabilization n = 10 progression n = 10	5.4	not reached	lymphocytopenia 70%

PFS: progression-free survival. OS: overall survival. PFS and OS are given as mean values.

3. Outlook

3.1. Pretreatment PET Imaging vs. Routine SSTR Expression Assessment

Before PRRT can be considered for meningioma treatment, PET imaging is used to provide important information about the expected treatment efficacy. PET imaging with ^{68}Ga-labeled somatostatin analogs is used to estimate the potential for radionuclide uptake in meningioma tissue during PRRT. Similarly, this method was demonstrated in an imaging study of 11 meningioma patients who underwent several whole-body and single-photon emission computed tomographies (SPECT/CT) during PRRT to assess the radionuclide kinetics [39]. Furthermore, a correlation between the DOTATATE/-TOC PET imaging signal and the response to PRRT was demonstrated in a retrospective analysis of 20 patients suffering from recurrent or high-grade meningioma. The authors also performed immunohistochemical staining of SSTR2A and observed that a high expression signal was associated with improved 6-month progression-free survival [50].

Only a few studies have investigated the expression of the different somatostatin receptors in meningioma tissue, and different methods were applied in these studies. Our recent retrospective analysis described the distribution of the immunohistochemical expression of all five somatostatin receptors in 726 meningiomas, which is the largest analysis of this kind so far [24]. Whether a certain level of SSTR expression is associated with PRRT efficacy is unclear. Currently, SSTR expression as assessed by PET imaging is used to predict treatment efficacy. However, additional immunohistochemical studies on the distribution of SSTRs, and especially their correlation to DOTATATE/DOMITATE PET data, are still warranted. This would allow the definition of an immunohistochemical scoring cutoff that may have predictive value regarding PRRT. Because immunohistochemical staining is easy to perform and analyze, it could be integrated in the routine meningioma workup and possibly replace the more expensive PET imaging for the pre-PRRT assessment. However, the expression of SSTRs may not be homogeneous throughout the entire tumor tissue. Consequently, the immunohistochemical detection of SSTRs and the calculation of total SSTR expression from intraoperative tumor samples may not be representative of the whole tumor. Moreover, SSTR expression may change over time, and the immunohistochemical results from tumor tissue that was resected several years ago may not be representative of the tissue in a recurring tumor later in the disease course. Therefore, a noninvasive assessment of whole-tumor SSTR expression through PET imaging will probably remain a practical, useful, and reliable alternative, despite its costs. Additionally, more experience with grading SSTR expression must be gained, and a standardized scoring system needs to be established.

3.2. Development of New Substances and the Potential of Tailored PRRT

Peptide receptor radionuclide therapy to treat meningiomas is based on its interaction with the somatostatin receptor 2A expressed in meningioma cells. The somatostatin analog applied in PRRT is octreotide, which has a high affinity to SSTR2A [51–53]. Patients who suffer from a meningioma that does not show sufficient SSTR expression through PET imaging should theoretically not be considered for PRRT. Our recent retrospective analysis has demonstrated that SSTR1 and SSTR5 are also highly expressed in many meningiomas. SSTR3 and SSTR4, by contrast, show low immunohistochemical expression [24]. However, there is currently very little knowledge about the link between immunohistochemical somatostatin receptor expression and treatment efficacy. A strong immunohistochemical signal does not necessarily mean that the PRRT will be effective. In our opinion, if the indication of this treatment approach is to be widened, it is crucial to explore the targetability of somatostatin receptors other than SSTR2A. An important factor that supports this idea is the variability of the distribution of SSTR expression among clinical subgroups. For example, SSTR2A expression is significantly lower in neurofibromatosis type 2 meningiomas [24]. Therefore, alternative substances to octeotride should be considered as a vehicle for PRRT. For example, pasireotide has a high affinity to somatostatin receptors 1, 2, 3, and 5 [54], making it a potential candidate for a more efficacious PRRT. In addition, it has not yet been shown whether PRRT would be more efficacious if it were directed towards multiple SSTRs. Extending this idea leads to the prospect of applying a patient-tailored mixture of PRRT vehicles designed after a thorough tissue or imaging analysis of the somatostatin receptor profile of an individual meningioma. Routine immunohistochemistry seems to be an ideal tool for this because it is inexpensive and easy to implement. However, standardized scoring is necessary to ensure comparable results. We utilized the scoring system described by Barresi et al., 2008, which incorporates the staining intensity and area of immunopositivity into a product called the intensity distribution score [25]. Computational quantification can potentially eliminate interobserver variance, which is the main limitation of this score.

Another point which could ensure a better efficacy of PRRT is, as already mentioned in the previous chapter, the intra-arterial application of PRRT. Vonken et al. were able to demonstrate a higher tracer accumulation in the tumor tissue [42]. Apart from another case report and a small study [41,43], which also showed a better uptake in meningioma, further studies are missing. It would therefore be desirable to conduct future studies on the effect of intra-arterial application on the difference in efficacy, overall survival and progression-free survival.

3.3. Refining PRRT through Preclinical Models

Preclinical research in animal models may also help to develop novel personalized therapies by refining the in vivo evaluation of receptor expression in multiple tumor entities. For example, high SSTR2A affinity to radiolabeled octreotide has been previously characterized in rats [53]. Moreover, Soto-Montenegro et al. successfully demonstrated the feasibility of imaging somatostatin analogs using PET/CT in a mouse meningioma xenograft model [55]. Our literature review found that although several meningioma animal models have been established [56,57], preclinical PRRT evaluations are still extremely limited. Specifically, the preclinical evaluation of receptor subtypes focusing on affinity and distribution in multiple tumor grades is lacking. We believe that this information would be highly relevant to validate novel radiopeptide candidates.

Preclinical research has focused on improving the current SSTR2A analogs. For example, the theranostic treatment efficacy of ^{67}Cu-CuSarTATE was shown to be similar to that of ^{177}Lu-DOTATATE in a mouse pancreas tumor model, identifying a novel agent for dosimetry calculation in humans [58]. SSTR2 expression has also been demonstrated in tumor models of pheochromocytoma, small cell lung cancer and thyroid cancer in mice [59–61]. Recent work has also focused on the evaluation of SSTR2 using ^{177}Lu-DOTATATE in combination with small-molecule poly (ADP-ribose) polymerase-1 (PARP) inhibitors, which showed an increased antitumor efficacy in mice [62].

In our opinion, more knowledge is needed about the distribution of SSTRs other than SSTR2A, in order to expand the armamentarium of PRRT. At the same time, more data is required regarding the dynamics of receptor expression in the tumor over time and the influence of adjuvant treatments, such as radiotherapy on SSTR expression. This could be easily accomplished preclinically, where noninvasive in vivo PET imaging can be performed longitudinally and be directly corroborated by immunohistochemistry. This could also provide preliminary evidence on treatment efficacy and the receptor expression profile of specific tumor types. At the same time, these experiments would increase the characterization and evaluation of novel theranostic radiotracers poised for clinical application.

4. Conclusions

Peptide receptor radionuclide therapy is an innovative treatment approach for meningiomas, with a large and untapped potential.

Author Contributions: Conceptualization: C.-K.F. and F.B.; writing and original draft preparation: C.-K.F., S.G.C.-V. and F.B.; writing, review and editing: C.-K.F., J.S., J.H., S.G.C.-V. and F.B. All authors have read and agreed to the published version of the manuscript.

Funding: This research received no external funding. We acknowledge support by the Open Access Publishing Fund of the University of Tübingen.

Data Availability Statement: Not applicable.

Conflicts of Interest: The authors declare no conflict of interest.

References

1. Ostrom, Q.T.; Patil, N.; Cioffi, G.; Waite, K.; Kruchko, C.; Barnholtz-Sloan, J.S. CBTRUS statistical report: Primary brain and other central nervous system tumors diagnosed in the United States in 2013–2017. *Neuro-Oncology* **2020**, *22* (Suppl. 2), iv1–iv96. [CrossRef]
2. Louis, D.N.; Perry, A.; Reifenberger, G.; Von Deimling, A.; Figarella-Branger, D.; Cavenee, W.K.; Ohgaki, H.; Wiestler, O.D.; Kleihues, P.; Ellison, D.W. The 2016 World Health Organization classification of tumors of the central nervous system: A summary. *Acta Neuropathol.* **2016**, *131*, 803–820. [CrossRef] [PubMed]
3. Goldbrunner, R.; Minniti, G.; Preusser, M.; Jenkinson, M.D.; Sallabanda, K.; Houdart, E.; von Deimling, A.; Stavrinou, P.; Lefranc, F.; Lund-Johansen, M.; et al. EANO guidelines for the diagnosis and treatment of meningiomas. *Lancet Oncol.* **2016**, *17*, e383–e391. [CrossRef]
4. Kaley, T.; Barani, I.; Chamberlain, M.; McDermott, M.; Panageas, K.; Raizer, J.; Rogers, L.; Schiff, D.; Vogelbaum, M.; Weber, D.; et al. Historical benchmarks for medical therapy trials in surgery- and radiation-refractory meningioma: A RANO review. *Neuro-Oncology* **2014**, *16*, 829–840. [CrossRef]
5. Brastianos, P.K.; Galanis, E.; Butowski, N.; Chan, J.W.; Dunn, I.F.; Goldbrunner, R.; Herold-Mende, C.; Ippen, F.M.; Mawrin, C.; McDermott, M.W.; et al. Advances in multidisciplinary therapy for meningiomas. *Neuro-Oncology* **2019**, *21* (Suppl. 1), i18–i31. [CrossRef]
6. Bartolomei, M.; Bodei, L.; De Cicco, C.; Grana, C.M.; Cremonesi, M.; Botteri, E.; Baio, S.M.; Aricò, D.; Sansovini, M.; Paganelli, G. Peptide receptor radionuclide therapy with (90)Y-DOTATOC in recurrent meningioma. *Eur. J. Nucl. Med. Mol. Imaging* **2009**, *36*, 1407–1416. [CrossRef] [PubMed]
7. Gerster-Gilliéron, K.; Forrer, F.; Maecke, H.; Mueller-Brand, J.; Merlo, A.; Cordier, D. 90Y-DOTATOC as a therapeutic option for complex recurrent or progressive meningiomas. *J. Nucl. Med.* **2015**, *56*, 1748–1751. [CrossRef]
8. Schonbrunn, A.; Tashjian, H., Jr. Characterization of functional receptors for somatostatin in rat pituitary cells in culture. *J. Biol. Chem.* **1978**, *253*, 6473–6483. [CrossRef]
9. Benali, N.; Ferjoux, G.; Puente, E.; Buscail, L.; Susini, C. Somatostatin receptors. *Digestion* **2000**, *62* (Suppl. 1), 27–32. [CrossRef]
10. Reisine, T.; Bell, G.I. Molecular biology of somatostatin receptors. *Endocr. Rev.* **1995**, *16*, 427–442.
11. Chadwick, D.J.; Cardew, G. *Somatostatin and Its Receptors*; John Wiley & Sons: Hoboken, NJ, USA, 2008; Volume 190.
12. Theodoropoulou, M.; Stalla, G.K. Somatostatin receptors: From signaling to clinical practice. *Front. Neuroendocrinol.* **2013**, *34*, 228–252. [CrossRef] [PubMed]
13. Møller, L.N.; Stidsen, C.E.; Hartmann, B.; Holst, J.J. Somatostatin receptors. *Biochim. Biophys. Acta* **2003**, *1616*, 1–84. [CrossRef]
14. Patel, Y.; Greenwood, M.; Panetta, R.; Demchyshyn, L.; Niznik, H.; Srikant, C. The somatostatin receptor family. *Life Sci.* **1995**, *57*, 1249–1265. [CrossRef]
15. Lahlou, H.; Guillermet-Guibert, J.; Hortala, M.; Vernejoul, F.; Pyronnet, S.; Bousquet, C.; Susini, C. Molecular signaling of somatostatin receptors. *Ann. N. Y. Acad. Sci.* **2004**, *1014*, 121–131. [CrossRef] [PubMed]

16. Ferjoux, G.; Bousquet, C.; Cordelier, P.; Benali, N.; Lopez, F.; Rochaix, P.; Buscail, L.; Susini, C. Signal transduction of somatostatin receptors negatively controlling cell proliferation. *J. Physiol. Paris* **2000**, *94*, 205–210. [CrossRef]
17. Patel, Y.C. Somatostatin and its receptor family. *Front. Neuroendocrinol.* **1999**, *20*, 157–198. [CrossRef]
18. Reubi, J.-C.; Laissue, J.A. Multiple actions of somatostatin in neoplastic disease. *Trends Pharmacol. Sci.* **1995**, *16*, 110–115. [CrossRef]
19. Reubi, J.C.; Schaer, J.C.; Waser, B.; Mengod, G. Expression and localization of somatostatin receptor SSTR1, SSTR2, and SSTR3 messenger RNAs in primary human tumors using in situ hybridization. *Cancer Res.* **1994**, *54*, 3455–3459.
20. Pauli, S.U.; Schulz, S.; Händel, M.; Dietzmann, K.; Firsching, R.; Höllt, V. Immunohistochemical determination of five somatostatin receptors in meningioma reveals frequent overexpression of somatostatin receptor subtype sst2A. *Clin. Cancer Res.* **2000**, *6*, 1865–1874.
21. Dutour, A.; Kumar, U.; Panetta, R.; Ouafik, L.; Fina, F.; Sasi, R.; Patel, Y.C. Expression of somatostatin receptor subtypes in human brain tumors. *Int. J. Cancer* **1998**, *76*, 620–627. [CrossRef]
22. Silva, C.B.; Ongaratti, B.R.; Trott, G.; Haag, T.; Ferreira, N.P.; Leães, C.G.; Pereira-Lima, J.F.; Oliveira Mda, C. Expression of somatostatin receptors (SSTR1-SSTR5) in meningiomas and its clinicopathological significance. *Int. J. Clin. Exp. Pathol.* **2015**, *8*, 13185–13192. [PubMed]
23. Arena, S.; Barbieri, F.; Thellung, S.; Pirani, P.; Corsaro, A.; Villa, V.; Dadati, P.; Dorcaratto, A.; Lapertosa, G.; Ravetti, J.-L.; et al. Expression of somatostatin receptor mRNA in human meningiomas and their implication in in vitro antiproliferative activity. *J. Neuro-Oncol.* **2004**, *66*, 155–166. [CrossRef] [PubMed]
24. Behling, F.; Fodi, C.; Skardelly, M.; Renovanz, M.; Castaneda, S.; Tabatabai, G.; Honegger, J.; Tatagiba, M.; Schittenhelm, J. Differences in the expression of SSTR1–5 in meningiomas and its therapeutic potential. *Neurosurg. Rev.* **2022**, *45*, 467–478. [CrossRef] [PubMed]
25. Barresi, V.; Alafaci, C.; Salpietro, F.; Tuccari, G. Sstr2A immunohistochemical expression in human meningiomas: Is there a correlation with the histological grade, proliferation or microvessel density? *Oncol. Rep.* **2008**, *20*, 485–492. [CrossRef]
26. Krenning, E.P.; Kwekkeboom, D.J.; Bakker, W.H.; Breeman, W.A.; Kooij, P.P.; Oei, H.Y.; van Hagen, M.; Postema, P.T.; de Jong, M.; Reubi, J.C.; et al. Somatostatin receptor scintigraphy with [111In-DTPA-d-Phe1]- and [123I-Tyr3]-octreotide: The Rotterdam experience with more than 1000 patients. *Eur. J. Nucl. Med. Mol. Imaging* **1993**, *20*, 716–731. [CrossRef] [PubMed]
27. Levine, R.; Krenning, E.P. Clinical history of the theranostic radionuclide approach to neuroendocrine tumors and other types of cancer: Historical review based on an interview of Eric P. Krenning by Rachel Levine. *J. Nucl. Med.* **2017**, *58* (Suppl. 2), 3S–9S. [CrossRef]
28. Krenning, E.P.; Kooij, P.P.M.; Bakker, W.H.; Breeman, W.A.P.; Postema, P.T.E.; Kwekkeboom, D.J.; Oei, H.Y.; Jong, M.; Visser, T.J.; Reijs, A.E.M.; et al. Radiotherapy with a Radiolabeled Somatostatin Analogue, [^{111}In-DTPA-d-Phe^{1}]-Octreotide. *Ann. N. Y. Acad. Sci.* **1994**, *733*, 496–506. [CrossRef]
29. Reubi, J.C.; Mäcke, H.R.; Krenning, E.P. Candidates for peptide receptor radiotherapy today and in the future. *J. Nucl. Med.* **2005**, *1* (Suppl. 1), 67S–75S.
30. Ito, T.; Lee, L.; Jensen, R.T. Treatment of symptomatic neuroendocrine tumor syndromes: Recent advances and controversies. *Expert Opin. Pharmacother.* **2016**, *17*, 2191–2205. [CrossRef]
31. Werner, R.A.; Weich, A.; Kircher, M.; Solnes, L.B.; Javadi, M.S.; Higuchi, T.; Buck, A.K.; Pomper, M.G.; Rowe, S.P.; Lapa, C. The theranostic promise for Neuroendocrine Tumors in the late 2010s—Where do we stand, where do we go? *Theranostics* **2018**, *8*, 6088–6100. [CrossRef]
32. Strosberg, J.; Wolin, E.; Chasen, B.; Kulke, M.; Bushnell, D.; Caplin, M.; Baum, R.P.; Kunz, P.; Hobday, T.; Hendifar, A.; et al. Health-related quality of life in patients with progressive midgut neuroendocrine tumors treated with 177Lu-Dotatate in the Phase III NETTER-1 Trial. *J. Clin. Oncol.* **2018**, *36*, 2578–2584. [CrossRef] [PubMed]
33. Reubi, J.C. Peptide receptors as molecular targets for cancer diagnosis and therapy. *Endocr. Rev.* **2003**, *24*, 389–427. [CrossRef] [PubMed]
34. Salavati, A.; Puranik, A.; Kulkarni, H.R.; Budiawan, H.; Baum, R.P. Peptide receptor radionuclide therapy (PRRT) of medullary and nonmedullary thyroid cancer using radiolabeled somatostatin analogues. *Semin. Nucl. Med.* **2016**, *46*, 215–224. [CrossRef] [PubMed]
35. Hasan, O.K.; Kumar, A.R.; Kong, G.; Oleinikov, K.; Ben-Haim, S.; Grozinsky-Glasberg, S.; Hicks, R. Efficacy of peptide receptor radionuclide therapy for esthesioneuroblastoma. *J. Nucl. Med.* **2020**, *61*, 1326–1330. [CrossRef] [PubMed]
36. Sollini, M.; Farioli, D.; Froio, A.; Chella, A.; Asti, M.; Boni, R.; Grassi, E.; Roncali, M.; Versari, A.; Erba, P.A. Brief report on the use of radiolabeled somatostatin analogs for the diagnosis and treatment of metastatic small-cell lung cancer patients. *J. Thorac. Oncol.* **2013**, *8*, 1095–1101. [CrossRef] [PubMed]
37. Reubi, J.C.; Kappeler, A.; Waser, B.; Laissue, J.; Hipkin, R.W.; Schonbrunn, A. Immunohistochemical localization of somatostatin receptors sst2A in human tumors. *Am. J. Pathol.* **1998**, *153*, 233–245. [CrossRef]
38. Sherman, W.J.; Raizer, J.J. Medical management of meningiomas. *CNS Oncol.* **2013**, *2*, 161–170. [CrossRef]
39. Hänscheid, H.; Sweeney, R.A.; Flentje, M.; Buck, A.; Löhr, M.; Samnick, S.; Kreissl, M.; Verburg, F.A. PET SUV correlates with radionuclide uptake in peptide receptor therapy in meningioma. *Eur. J. Nucl. Med. Mol. Imaging* **2012**, *39*, 1284–1288. [CrossRef]
40. Baum, R.; Söldner, J.; Schmücking, M.; Niesen, A. Peptidrezeptorvermittelte Radiotherapie (PRRT) neuroendokriner Tumoren. *Der Onkologe* **2004**, *10*, 1098–1110. [CrossRef]

41. Braat, A.J.A.T.; Snijders, T.J.; Seute, T.; Vonken, E.P.A. Will 177Lu-DOTATATE treatment become more effective in salvage meningioma patients, when boosting somatostatin receptor saturation? A promising case on intra-arterial administration. *Cardiovasc. Interv. Radiol.* **2019**, *42*, 1649–1652. [CrossRef]
42. Vonken, E.P.A.; Bruijnen, R.C.G.; Snijders, T.J.; Seute, T.; Lam, M.G.E.H.; Keizer, B.; Braat, A.J.A.T. Intra-arterial administration boosts (177)Lu-HA-DOTATATE accumulation in salvage meningioma patients. *J. Nucl. Med.* **2021**, *63*, 406–409. [CrossRef] [PubMed]
43. Verburg, F.A.; Wiessmann, M.; Neuloh, G.; Mottaghy, F.M.; Brockmann, M.-A. Intraindividual comparison of selective intraarterial versus systemic intravenous 68Ga-DOTATATE PET/CT in patients with inoperable meningioma. *Nukl. -Nucl.* **2019**, *58*, 23–27. [CrossRef] [PubMed]
44. Haug, A.; Bartenstein, P. Peptidradiorezeptortherapie neuroendokriner Tumoren. *Der Onkologe* **2011**, *17*, 602–608. [CrossRef]
45. Bodei, L.; Mueller-Brand, J.; Baum, R.P.; Pavel, M.E.; Hörsch, D.; O'Dorisio, M.S.; O'Dorisio, T.M.; Howe, J.R.; Cremonesi, M.; Kwekkeboom, D.J.; et al. The joint IAEA, EANM, and SNMMI practical guidance on peptide receptor radionuclide therapy (PRRNT) in neuroendocrine tumours. *Eur. J. Nucl. Med. Mol. Imaging* **2013**, *40*, 800–816. [CrossRef]
46. Hartrampf, P.E.; Hänscheid, H.; Kertels, O.; Schirbel, A.; Kreissl, M.C.; Flentje, M.; Sweeney, R.A.; Buck, A.K.; Polat, B.; Lapa, C. Long-term results of multimodal peptide receptor radionuclide therapy and fractionated external beam radiotherapy for treatment of advanced symptomatic meningioma. *Clin. Transl. Radiat. Oncol.* **2020**, *22*, 29–32. [CrossRef]
47. Kreissl, M.C.; Hänscheid, H.; Löhr, M.; Verburg, F.A.; Schiller, M.; Lassmann, M.; Reiners, C.; Samnick, S.S.; Buck, A.K.; Flentje, M.; et al. Combination of peptide receptor radionuclide therapy with fractionated external beam radiotherapy for treatment of advanced symptomatic meningioma. *Radiat. Oncol.* **2012**, *7*, 99. [CrossRef]
48. Kertels, O.; Breun, M.; Hänscheid, H.; Kircher, M.; Hartrampf, P.; Schirbel, A.; Monoranu, C.; Ernestus, R.; Buck, A.; Löhr, M.; et al. Peptide receptor radionuclide therapy in patients with neurofibromatosis type 2: Initial experience. *Clin. Nucl. Med.* **2021**, *46*, e312–e316. [CrossRef]
49. Mirian, C.; Duun-Henriksen, A.K.; Maier, A.D.; Pedersen, M.M.; Jensen, L.R.; Bashir, A.; Graillon, T.; Hrachova, M.; Bota, D.; van Essen, M.; et al. Somatostatin receptor–targeted radiopeptide therapy in treatment-refractory meningioma: Individual patient data meta-analysis. *J. Nucl. Med.* **2021**, *62*, 507–513. [CrossRef]
50. Seystahl, K.; Stoecklein, V.; Schüller, U.; Rushing, E.; Nicolas, G.; Schäfer, N.; Ilhan, H.; Pangalu, A.; Weller, M.; Tonn, J.-C.; et al. Somatostatin-receptor-targeted radionuclide therapy for progressive meningioma: Benefit linked to68Ga-DOTATATE/-TOC uptake. *Neuro-Oncology* **2016**, *18*, 1538–1547. [CrossRef]
51. Casar-Borota, O.; Heck, A.; Schulz, S.; Nesland, J.M.; Ramm-Pettersen, J.; Lekva, T.; Alafuzoff, I.; Bollerslev, J. Expression of SSTR2a, but not of SSTRs 1, 3, or 5 in somatotroph adenomas assessed by monoclonal antibodies was reduced by octreotide and correlated with the acute and long-term effects of octreotide. *J. Clin. Endocrinol. Metab.* **2013**, *98*, E1730–E1739. [CrossRef]
52. Hofland, L.J.; Lamberts, S.W. Somatostatin receptors and disease: Role of receptor subtypes. *Baillière's Clin. Endocrinol. Metab.* **1996**, *10*, 163–176. [CrossRef]
53. Laznicek, M.; Laznickova, A.; Maecke, H.R. Receptor affinity and preclinical biodistribution of radiolabeled somatostatin analogs. *Anticancer Res.* **2012**, *32*, 761–766. [PubMed]
54. Öberg, K.; Lamberts, S.W.J. Somatostatin analogues in acromegaly and gastroenteropancreatic neuroendocrine tumours: Past, present and future. *Endocr. -Relat. Cancer* **2016**, *23*, R551–R566. [CrossRef] [PubMed]
55. Soto-Montenegro, M.L.; Peña-Zalbidea, S.; Mateos-Pérez, J.M.; Oteo, M.; Romero, E.; Morcillo, M.Á.; Desco, M. Meningiomas: A Comparative Study of 68Ga-DOTATOC, 68Ga-DOTANOC and 68Ga-DOTATATE for molecular imaging in mice. *PLoS ONE* **2014**, *9*, e111624. [CrossRef]
56. Boetto, J.; Peyre, M.; Kalamarides, M. Mouse models in meningioma research: A systematic review. *Cancers* **2021**, *13*, 3712. [CrossRef]
57. Kalamarides, M.; Peyre, M.; Giovannini, M. Meningioma mouse models. *J. Neuro-Oncol.* **2010**, *99*, 325–331. [CrossRef]
58. Cullinane, C.; Jeffery, C.M.; Roselt, P.D.; van Dam, E.M.; Jackson, S.; Kuan, K.; Jackson, P.; Binns, D.; van Zuylekom, J.; Harris, M.J.; et al. Peptide receptor radionuclide therapy with (67)Cu-CuSarTATE is highly efficacious against a somatostatin-positive neuroendocrine tumor model. *J. Nucl. Med.* **2020**, *61*, 1800–1805. [CrossRef]
59. Lewin, J.; Cullinane, C.; Akhurst, T.; Waldeck, K.; Watkins, D.N.; Rao, A.; Eu, P.; Mileshkin, L.; Hicks, R.J. Peptide receptor chemoradionuclide therapy in small cell carcinoma: From bench to bedside. *Eur. J. Nucl. Med. Mol. Imaging* **2015**, *42*, 25–32. [CrossRef]
60. Ullrich, M.; Bergmann, R.; Peitzsch, M.; Zenker, E.F.; Cartellieri, M.; Bachmann, M.; Ehrhart-Bornstein, M.; Block, N.L.; Schally, A.V.; Eisenhofer, G.; et al. Multimodal somatostatin receptor theranostics using [(64)Cu]Cu-/[(177)Lu]Lu-DOTA-(Tyr(3))octreotate and AN-238 in a mouse pheochromocytoma model. *Theranostics* **2016**, *6*, 650–665. [CrossRef]
61. Thakur, S.; Daley, B.; Millo, C.; Cochran, C.; Jacobson, O.; Lu, H.; Wang, Z.; Kiesewetter, D.O.; Chen, X.; Vasko, V.V.; et al. 177Lu-DOTA-EB-TATE, a radiolabeled analogue of somatostatin receptor type 2, for the imaging and treatment of thyroid cancer. *Clin. Cancer Res.* **2021**, *27*, 1399–1409. [CrossRef]
62. Cullinane, C.; Waldeck, K.; Kirby, L.; Rogers, B.E.; Eu, P.; Tothill, R.W.; Hicks, R.J. Enhancing the anti-tumour activity of 177Lu-DOTA-octreotate radionuclide therapy in somatostatin receptor-2 expressing tumour models by targeting PARP. *Sci. Rep.* **2020**, *10*, 10196. [CrossRef] [PubMed]

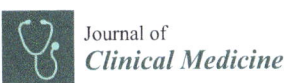

Review

Intracranial Solitary Fibrous Tumor: A "New" Challenge for PET Radiopharmaceuticals

Angela Sardaro [1], Paolo Mammucci [2], Antonio Rosario Pisani [2,*], Dino Rubini [2], Anna Giulia Nappi [2], Lilia Bardoscia [3] and Giuseppe Rubini [2]

[1] Section of Radiology and Radiation Oncology, Interdisciplinary Department of Medicine, University of Bari "Aldo Moro", 70124 Bari, Italy
[2] Section of Nuclear Medicine, Interdisciplinary Department of Medicine, University of Bari Aldo Moro, Piazza Giulio Cesare 11, 70124 Bari, Italy
[3] Radiation Oncology Unit, S. Luca Hospital, Healthcare Company Tuscany Nord Ovest, 55100 Lucca, Italy
* Correspondence: apisani71@libero.it; Tel.: +39-080-5594388

Abstract: Solitary fibrous tumor (SFT) of the central nervous system, previously named and classified with the term hemangiopericytoma (HPC), is rare and accounts for less than 1% of all intracranial tumors. Despite its benign nature, it has a malignant behavior due to the high rate of recurrence and distant metastasis, occurring in up to 50% of cases. Surgical resection of the tumor is the treatment of choice. Radiotherapy represents the gold standard in the case of post-surgery residual disease, relapse, and distant metastases. In this context, imaging plays a crucial role in identifying the personalized therapeutic decision for each patient. Although the referring imaging approach in SFT is morphologic, an emerging role of positron emission tomography (PET) has been reported in the literature. However, there is still a debate on which radiotracers have the best accuracy for studying these uncommon tumors because of the histological or biological heterogeneity of SFT.

Keywords: solitary fibrous tumor; hemangiopericytoma; PET/CT; fluorodeoxyglucose; fluorocholine; non-FDG radiopharmaceuticals

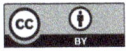

1. Introduction

In 2021, the latest and most recent version of the 5th edition of WHO Classification of Tumors of the Central Nervous System (CNS5) was published. One of the most important innovations is the introduction of a new classification of tumor types and subtypes, thanks to novel diagnostic technologies such as DNA methylome profiling. Focusing on mesenchymal, non-meningothelial tumors, the hybrid term solitary fibrous tumor/hemangiopericytoma (SFT/HPC), previously used in the 2016 WHO classification, has been abandoned in favor of the use of the term solitary fibrous tumor (SFT) alone to fully comply with the nomenclature of soft-tissue pathology [1].

SFTs are rare mesenchymal malignancies of soft-tissue cells with a high percentage of recurrence. In particular, intracranial SFTs constitute 2.5% of meningeal neoplasms and less than 1% of all intracranial tumors [2]. At present, magnetic resonance imaging has a well-established role in the identification and diagnosis of this rare tumor. However, because of SFTs' high tendency to have locoregional recurrences and distant metastases, in recent years, multimodality imaging, particularly positron emission tomography/computed tomography (PET/CT), has shown an increasingly significant role, thanks to the possibility of obtaining both metabolic and morphological information in a single scan. Furthermore, it is a non-invasive and total-body examination, with high sensitivity and specificity [3,4].

We aimed to present a brief critical overview of the role of PET/CT in diagnosing, local disease relapse, or distant metastases evaluation in the treatment response to surgery and/or radiotherapy and in the follow-up of patients affected by intracranial SFT.

2. Solitary Fibrous Tumor

SFT is a very rare and uncommon neoplasm, accounting for only 1.6% of all central nervous system (CNS) tumors. In the 2016 World Health Organization (WHO) classification of CNS tumors, SFTs and HPCs constituted a single disease entity, known as SFT/HPC. However, in the last recent update of WHO CNS5, the term "hemangiopericytoma" was deleted to emphasize the biological similarities within tumor types and to align with the soft-tissue pathology nomenclature [1].

This tumor was firstly known by the term hemangiopericytoma, coined by Stout and Murray in 1942, to highlight the origin from the capillary and postcapillary venules of pericytes. It can occur in any anatomical body region with the presence of capillaries and a typical localization involves the meninges of the dura mater, with an incidence of 16–33% of SFTs in the head or neck [5]. From a histological point of view, these tumors are characterized by spindle mesenchymal cells with a rich vascular component. Usually, the presence of hypercellularity, hemorrhage and/or necrosis, pleomorphic nuclei, and foci of dedifferentiation suggests a malignant behavior [6]. The tumor immunophenotype can be characterized by CD34 and smooth-muscle-actin positivity and by S100 protein, CK pool, and desmin negativity [7]. In accordance with previous immunohistochemical features, the new WHO CNS5 reported that STFs show NAB2 and STAT6 gene fusion as well as STAT6 overexpression [2].

Even many years after the end of the first (line) treatment, locoregional relapses, as well as distant metastases, are very common, and a prompt diagnosis could be crucial for better patient management. However, probably due to SFTs' rarity, there are no clear recommendations on the best imaging method to evaluate them [8]. The literature is characterized by small-sample-size studies and case series, showing that complete surgical resection with clear margins is the treatment of choice. However, one year after the stand-alone surgery option, a very high percentage of disease relapse, rating from 88 to 100%, may occur as a result of tumor infiltration in adjacent vascular structures with a worsening of survival [9]. Stereotaxic radiosurgery has emerged as a promising adjuvant treatment to reduce the relapse rate of the disease [2]. In an updated overview on radiation therapy options for intracranial HPC, Ciliberti and colleagues showed that postoperative radiotherapy (RT) can lead to a consistent decrease in local recurrences, moving from 88% to 12.5%, and longer relapse-free survival [9]. In addition, when the lesion is close to critical anatomical structures, stereotactic radiotherapy can be considered. However, even after a wide surgical resection or a combined surgery–radiotherapy treatment, recurrences and metastases can subsequently occur in up to 50% of cases [10,11].

In this scenario, imaging can play a crucial role in potentially guiding the best therapeutic decision and in establishing tailored treatment.

Although the referring imaging approach in SFTs is morphologic, it may fail in differentiating between scar tissue and viable tumor in post-treatment evaluation. For this purpose, PET has demonstrated a promising role [12,13].

3. Search Strategy

A literature search was conducted on the Medline (PubMed) database including all articles published up to 30 June 2022. The following keywords were entered to rule the search: "intracranial solitary fibrous tumor" AND "positron emission tomography", AND "PET" AND "nuclear medicine", "hemangiopericytoma" AND "positron emission tomography" AND "PET" AND "nuclear medicine", "intracranial hemangiopericytoma" AND "positron emission tomography" AND "PET" AND "nuclear medicine". Only articles edited in English in the last 10 years were included in this review. After reading the abstracts, some articles were excluded because they did not meet the goal of our review in evaluating the use of PET/CT in patients affected by intracranial SFT/HPC. For the same reason, some articles were not considered in the final draft after reading the full text. To identify supplementary eligible articles, additional references were searched from the retrieved review articles. Due to the rarity of SFT, most of the articles in the literature are represented by case reports and interesting images. The main characteristics of the included studies are detailed in Table 1.

Table 1. Main characteristics of the included studies of intracranial SFTs/HPCs with probable distant metastases studied using PET/CT or scintigraphy with ^{111}In-Pentreotide (n = 16).

Case	Authors	Year	Age, Sex	Intracranial Primitive Site	Metastatic Sites	Radiopharmaceuticals	Qualitative and Semiquantitative Uptake Level
1	Z. Wu et al. [14]	2015	25, M	Right occipital lobe	Lungs, bones	^{18}F-FDG	Mild–moderate SUVmean 4.9—SUVmax 8.1
2	H. Cheung et al. [15]	2018	67, F	Right posterior occipital calvary	Paravertebral, bones, lymph nodes	^{18}F-FDG	Mild *
3	K.P. Cheng et al. [8]	2017	41, F	Intracranial meninges	Bones	^{18}F-FDG	Intense *
4	T. Hiraide et al. [16]	2012	41, M	Cerebellum	Kidneys, lungs, pancreas	^{18}F-FDG	Intense *
5	X. Liu et al. [17]	2021	40, M	Fronto-parietal	Kidney	^{18}F-FDG	Mild, SUVmax 3.17
6	H. N. Hayenga et al. [18]	2019	34, F	Right cerebellopontine angle	Thoracic spine	^{18}F-FDG	Low *
7	A. Yasen et al. [19]	2020	62, F	Frontal cerebral convex, parafalx	Liver	^{18}F-FDG	Absent
8	H. Grunig et al. [20]	2021	46, F	Intracranial dura	Liver, muscles	^{18}F-FDG	High-moderate SUVmax 9.0
9	Sardaro et al. [7]	2021	69, M	Left orbit	/	^{18}F-FDG	Absent
						^{18}F-FCH	Intense, SUVmax 6.8
10	Jehanno et al. [21]	2019	50, M	Right spheno-orbital region	/	^{18}F-FDG	Low, SUVmax 3.5
						^{18}F-FCH	Intense, SUVmax 5.9
11	Lavacchi et al. [22]	2020	64, F	Posterior fossa	Liver, kidneys, lungs	^{111}In-Pentreotide	Intense *
			35, M	Falx cerebri	Liver	^{18}F-FDG	Intense *
12	G. Kota et al. [23]	2013	54, F	Right optic nerve sheath	Bones	^{18}F-FDG	Low *
						^{111}In-Pentreotide	Intense *
13	T. Hung et al. [24]	2016	68, F	Not specified	Lungs	^{18}F-FDG	Minimal *
						^{68}GA-DOTATATE	Intense *
14	K.C. Patro et al. [25]	2018	53, F	Right posterior cranial fossa	Bones, liver	^{18}F-FDG	Low *
						^{68}Ga-PSMA	Intense *
15	Zhang et al. [26]	2021	23, F	Right frontal lobe	/	^{18}F-FDG	Low, SUVmax 1.6
						^{68}GA-FAPI	Intense, SUVmax 30.9
16	I. Jong et al. [27]	2013	47, M	Not specified	Bones	^{18}F-FDG	Mild *
						^{11}C-Acetate	Intense *

Abbreviations: FDG = fluorodeoxyglucose; SUVmean = average standardized uptake value; SUVmax = maximum standardized uptake value; FCH = fluorocholine; PSMA = prostate-specific membrane antigen; DOTATATE = dodecane tetra-acetic acid tyrosine-3-octreotate; FAPI = fibroblast-activation-protein inhibitor. Annotation: * = semiquantitative parameters not known.

4. Evidence-Based Medicine of PET/CT in Intracranial Solitary Fibrous Tumor/Hemangiopericytoma

In the last decade, PET/CT emerged as a non-invasive, whole-body diagnostic tool with an important role in diagnosis, staging, detecting possible disease relapses and distant metastases, differentiating between scar and viable tissues, and in the follow-up of patients affected by SFT. To the best of our knowledge, this is the first literature review that focuses on the role of PET/CT in intracranial SFTs. This topic could reveal to be great interest in identifying the best accurate PET radiopharmaceutical to diagnose and follow up this rare tumor. Indeed, despite its benign nature, SFT has a malignant behavior, with a characteristic high rate of locoregional relapse and of distant metastases due to its hypervascularity.

To date, most of the authors referred to ^{18}F-FDG as the main PET radiotracer used in this oncological field to assess glucose metabolism activity, usually increased in neoplastic cells. ^{18}F-FDG is intracellularly trapped after GLUT-transporter uptake and hexokinase phosphorylation in glucose-6-phosphate. The hypercellularity of SFT lesions may support its application in these cases. However, the intense physiological uptake of the brain makes adequate ^{18}F-FDG PET imaging of intracranial tumors a challenge [21]. In some cases of SFT/HPC, ^{18}F-FDG PET may be helpful to differentiate necrotic from viable tumors, with both hypoenhancing on CT but with different metabolic activities on PET, significantly influencing the treatment decision [28]. Generally, FDG uptake in SFT/HPC cells is decreased compared with the surrounding tissue, while intense ^{18}F-FDG hypermetabolism may suggest the presence of a more malignant variety of SFT, with a significant impact on prognosis [22]. The relatively low SUVmax values in ^{18}F-FDG PET studies could help to differentiate SFT from other malignancies. In addition, a differential diagnosis with respect to other tumors may be facilitated by a dual-tracer technique to compare different image patterns developed by two PET radiotracers. For example, low glucose metabolism in contrast to high ^{11}C-Methionine uptake may help to differentiate HPC from meningioma [29].

The high probability of developing metastases linked to the malignant behavior of this mesenchymal tumor makes ^{18}F-FDG PET/CT a potential ideal tool to ensure adequate whole-body examination and to correctly guide therapeutic decision making with a tailored approach [8].

In Wu et al.'s case report, ^{18}F-FDG PET/CT was performed to restage a 25-year-old man affected by a malignant SFT of the right occipital lobe primarily treated with multiple craniotomies and postoperative conformal RT. PET/CT showed both intracranial disease recurrence and, above all, massive bilateral pulmonary lesions and multiple bone metastases [14].

Cheung et al. confirmed the fundamental role of ^{18}F-FDG PET/CT in identifying distant metastases from SFT/HPC describing a case of a 67-year-old woman treated with the resection of a paravertebral soft-tissue mass with histological diagnosis of HPC. After eight years, MRI detected three histologically proven SFT/HPC lesions of the right posterior occipital calvarium, while ^{18}F-FDG PET/CT showed multiple hypermetabolic lesions involving lymph nodes and bone from the calvarium to the sacrum [15].

Furthermore, the literature reports a case of 41-year-old man surgically treated for a cerebellar HPC. After twenty-two years, the patient experienced multiple renal and pulmonary metastases, pathologically proven to be HPC, and a local intracranial recurrence, all of them surgically treated. Two years later, abdominal CT revealed a pancreatic tumor, confirmed with whole-body ^{18}F-FDG PET/CT with intense radiopharmaceutical uptake. This lesion was surgically removed and histopathological examination confirmed the diagnosis of HPC, with similar pathological findings to those of the original cerebellum HPC [16].

However, in some cases, ^{18}F-FDG PET/CT may not prove to be adequately reliable in accurately detecting all SFT/HPC lesions, since low–moderate glucose metabolism in both primary and metastatic lesions can be observed. Recently, Liu Xiao et al. reported a case of a 40-year-old patient affected by intracranial STF/HPC with a left renal metastatic lesion showing only mild ^{18}F-FDG uptake and homogeneous contrast enhancement after contrast-medium administration [17].

Similarly, Hayenga and his colleagues reported a case of a 34-year-old woman affected by HPC of the right cerebellopontine angle (CPA) who underwent surgical treatment combined with postoperative RT. After 3 years of disease-free interval, ^{18}F-FDG PET/CT was performed showing low FDG avidity both in intracranial and extracranial recurrences of the spinal canal [18]. Consistent with these reports, Yasen and colleagues reported negative FDG uptake in the presence of HPC recurrence and metastasis. Namely, a woman with bilateral-frontal-cerebral-convex and parafalx HPC was surgically treated and underwent ^{18}F-FDG PET/CT six years later, demonstrating high-density lesions on CT images without FDG uptake and low-density solid lesions without FDG uptake in the frontal lobe parafalx and in the right posterior and left outer lobes of the liver, respectively. The histological examination of calvarium and hepatic lesions showed homogeneous features of HPC tumor [19]. These are examples of SFT/HPC lesions with low glucose metabolism, almost similar to background FDG activity, suggesting that ^{18}F-FDG PET/CT should not be the only diagnostic tool to be used in this set of patients, especially for the detection of craniospinal-axis SFT/HPC [18].

Another issue that deserves consideration and that may limit ^{18}F-FDG PET/CT performance is the FDG heterogenous uptake between primitive SFT/HPC and metastatic lesions. In this regard, Grunig and colleagues reported a case of a 46-year-old patient with high FDG uptake in primary-dura HPC and liver metastases, but moderate radiopharmaceutical uptake in a leg-muscle tissue lesion [20].

In relation to these ^{18}F-FDG PET/CT limitations, current literature debates which is the most accurate PET radiopharmaceutical to adequately study this rare benign, but with malignant behavior, tumor with possible histological or biological heterogeneity.

Some authors highlighted that SFT/HPC shows different spectral patterns on MR spectroscopy, with dominant Choline expression [30,31]. This feature suggested the potential usefulness of radiolabeled Choline as an ideal PET radiopharmaceutical in SFT/HPC detection [21,32,33]. Choline is a precursor of the biosynthesis of cell-membrane phospholipids, which is increased in the most malignant tumors, including SFTs. In fact, once intracellular uptake is performed by specific transporters, Choline is phosphorylated by choline-kinase in phosphorylcholine and incorporated into the cell membrane [34–36]. Considering the anatomical proximity with brain parenchyma, a further advantage of ^{18}F-FCH PET/CT is the very low brain uptake with a favorable tumor-to-background ratio with a better image contrast. The low physiological distribution of Choline in normal white and grey matter may help to distinguish different brain tumors with increased uptake from benign lesions and radiation necrosis with the lowest uptake [36]. In the case report by Sardaro et al., ^{18}F-Fluorocholine (^{18}F-FCH) PET/CT showed superior performance compared with ^{18}F-FDG PET/CT in a 69-year-old patient with two local recurrences of malignant orbital SFT, playing a crucial role in differentiating between small recurrences/pathological lesions and scar tissue in brain parenchyma (Figure 1) [7]. The favorable Choline tumor-to-background ratio [37] allows better and well-defined visualization of the lesion with intracranial localization to be obtained [38].

Similarly, Jehanno et al. reported a case of a 50-year-old male with a previous history of surgically treated intracranial HPC who experienced a local recurrence eighteen months later. After partial resection, the authors performed both preoperative ^{18}F-FDG PET/CT and ^{18}F-FCH PET/CT for the treatment planning of residual disease located along the optic nerve. ^{18}F-FDG PET/CT did not show any significant uptake. Conversely, ^{18}F-FCH PET/CT precisely detected an intense radiopharmaceutical uptake of residual disease in the retro-orbital region, more properly guiding the following RT [21].

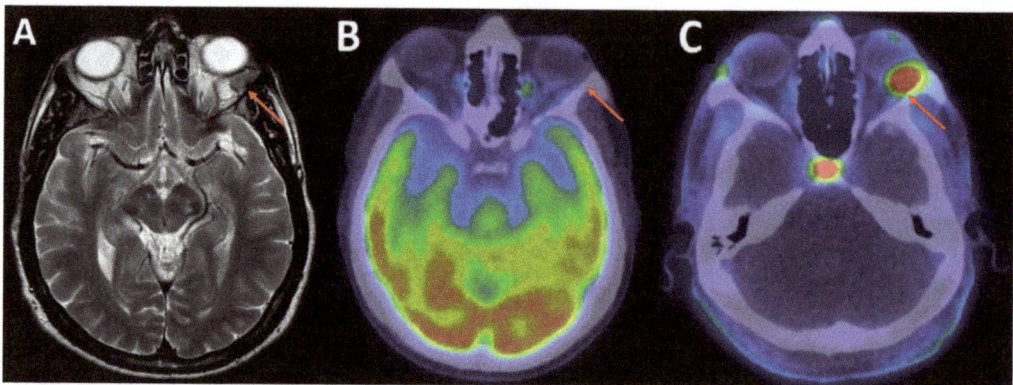

Figure 1. A 69-year-old male patient with a second loco-regional recurrence of left supraorbital solitary fibrous tumor. (**A**) A brain MRI scan revealed on axial MRI T2c+ a rounded lesion on the lateral side of the left orbit, strongly suspected of disease relapse (red arrow). (**B**) Two weeks later, ^{18}F-FDG PET/CT showed no radiopharmaceutical uptake in the left supraorbital region (red arrow). (**C**) Conversely, after seven days, ^{18}F-FCH PET/CT showed intense uptake in the aforementioned lesion (red arrow; SUVmax 6.8).

Some authors reported SFT lesions immunohistochemically and histologically characterized by a high expression of somatostatin receptor (SSRs), especially subtype 2, well studied with somatostatin-receptor molecular imaging methods. Lavacchi and colleagues reported a case of an intracranial SFT/HPC with distant metastasis studied with ^{111}In Pentetreotide, a gamma-emitter radiolabeled somatostatin analogue, able to target the highly expressed SSRs in anecdotal SFT lesions, with potential theragnostic implication. In Lavacchi et al.'s case, high radiopharmaceutical uptake was observed both in primitive and distant metastases. Namely, a 64-year-old female affected by cranial-posterior-fossa SFT was restaged 18 years after surgical treatment due to an ^{111}In Pentetreotide scan having detected multiple intracranial recurrences and hepatic, renal, and pulmonary metastases with avid tracer uptake [22]. Similarly, high SSR expression in intracranial and extracranial lesions was detected with a ^{111}In-Pentreotide scan in a 54-year-old woman with intracranial HPC of the right optic nerve sheath and bone distant metastases. In the same patient, low FDG uptake in the aforementioned sites confirmed the unreliability of ^{18}F-FDG PET/CT in some cases [23]. Furthermore, ^{68}Ga -Dodecane tetra-acetic acid tyrosine-3-octreotate (^{68}Ga-DOTATATE) is a PET radiopharmaceutical usually used for neuroendocrine-tumor imaging and now increasingly considered as an adjunctive imaging tracer for multiple solid neoplasms, including mesenchymal tumors [39]. Similarly to ^{111}In-Pentetreotide, ^{68}Ga-DOTATATE is a positron-emitter radiolabeled somatostatin analogue able to reveal a high concentration of surface SSRs, with the advantages of superior spatial resolution and accuracy, faster acquisition and lower radiation exposure [24]. In particular, Hung et al. found negligible FDG uptake but intense ^{68}Ga-DOTATATE avidity of pulmonary metastases in a 68-year-old woman affected by primitive intracranial HPC [24].

In addition to FDG and choline, the literature reports the use of other PET radiotracers for the identification of this uncommon neoplasm. In some cases, HPC/SFTs may show high ^{68}Ga-Prostate-Specific Membrane Antigen (^{68}Ga-PSMA) avidity [40]. PSMA is a type II integral transmembrane glycoprotein, known as folate-hydrolase 1 or glutamate-carboxypeptidase II, with neuropeptidase activity. It was found to be surprisingly overexpressed in the neovasculature endothelium of some brain tumors, such as gliomas with significant angiogenic activity, whereas low PSMA expression can be found in tumor cells or healthy brain. Low PSMA uptake in the normal brain parenchyma and its high tumor-to-background ratio allows an accurate localization of intracranial lesions with PSMA overexpression to be performed, which seems not to be related to the type of brain malignancy. The literature reports higher PSMA-uptake in high-grade gliomas and metastatic brain tumors than in central-nervous-system lymphoma and radiation necrosis, while there are no data about the differential diagnosis with SFT/HPC because of the rarity of this tumor [25,36,41]. Patro and colleagues described intense ^{68}Ga-PSMA avidity in all hepatic and bones metastases in a 53-year-old woman with primitive right-posterior-cranial-fossa HPC, in contrast with the low glucose metabolism of these lesions, probably due to PSMA overexpression in tumor neovasculature [25].

Interestingly, Zhang et al. showed an intense ^{68}Ga-Fibroblast-activation-protein inhibitor (^{68}Ga-FAPI) (compared with low ^{18}F-FDG uptake) in a 23-year-old female patient with SFT/HPC of the right frontal lobe. Fibroblast activation protein (FAP) is strongly overexpressed in the stroma of human cancers, including SFTs, and its quinoline-based FAP inhibitor can be internalized after binding to the FAP enzymatic domain. This suggests the potential role of this new PET radiotracer with a specific target for FAP, which can be overexpressed in this mesenchymal tumor [26,42]. The Acetate property of being a fatty acid precursor and thus an indirect biomarker of fatty acid synthesis can be exploited. In fact, ACT is converted to Acetyl Co-A, which is incorporated into cholesterol and fatty acids. Jong et al. reported a single case of dual-tracer ^{11}C-acetate (^{11}C-ACT) and ^{18}F-FDG PET/CT in a 47-year-old male patient with intracranial HPC, showing significantly higher ^{11}C-ACT uptake of bone metastases than FDG uptake, probably due to the over-expression of fatty acid synthase in this kind of tumors [27,43].

5. Conclusions

PET/CT could play a fundamental role in diagnosis, staging, post-treatment evaluation (surgery, radiotherapy, chemotherapy), disease relapses and distant metastases detection, and follow-up of patients affected by intracranial SFT, a benign but inherently aggressive tumor.

However, the literature still debates which type of PET radiopharmaceutical could guarantee the best accuracy for correctly and promptly guiding the management of this set of patients.

^{18}F-FDG PET/CT shows an extremely heterogeneous behavior, with modest or low radiopharmaceutical uptake in most cases of single- or dual-tracer studies, variable sensitivity and low reliability.

Compared with ^{18}F-FDG PET/CT, ^{18}F-FCH PET/CT appears to be superior in detecting intracranial SFTs thanks to the histological and biological features of SFT and a favorable tumor-to-background ratio.

Other radiopharmaceuticals labeled with Gallium 68 also demonstrate a promising role in SFT-relapse or distant-metastases detection.

The current literature shows that ^{18}F-FDG is the most widely used radiopharmaceutical in this set of patients. However, although fully aware that numerous studies are needed to identify which radiotracer to use based on the biological and histological characteristics of this rare tumor, our limited experience unquestionably reveals the superiority of ^{18}F-FCH PET/CT, compared with ^{18}F-FDG PET/CT, for the study of patients with intracranial SFT. ^{18}F-FCH PET/CT can play a significant role in providing information for both local recurrence and distant metastases.

Therefore, for all the aforementioned reasons, it would be desirable to include PET/CT as a diagnostic, sensitive, non-invasive method in the guidelines for the management of SFT.

Author Contributions: Conceptualization, P.M.; methodology, P.M. and A.G.N.; validation, A.S.; formal analysis, A.R.P. and L.B.; investigation, P.M. and D.R.; data curation, A.R.P. and L.B.; writing—original draft preparation, D.R. and A.G.N.; writing—review and editing, A.S. and P.M.; supervision, G.R. All authors have read and agreed to the published version of the manuscript.

Funding: This research study received no external funding.

Institutional Review Board Statement: Not applicable.

Informed Consent Statement: Informed consent was obtained from the subject included in the analysis.

Data Availability Statement: Not applicable.

Conflicts of Interest: The authors declare no conflict of interest.

References

1. Louis, D.N.; Perry, A.; Wesseling, P.; Brat, D.J.; Cree, I.A.; Figarella-Branger, D.; Hawkins, C.; Ng, H.K.; Pfister, S.M.; Reifenberger, G.; et al. The 2021 WHO Classification of Tumors of the Central Nervous System: A summary. *Neuro Oncol.* **2021**, *23*, 1231–1251. [CrossRef] [PubMed]
2. Allen, A.J.; Labella, D.A.; Richardson, K.M.; Sheehan, J.P.; Kersh, C.R. Recurrent Solitary Fibrous Tumor (Intracranial Hemangiopericytoma) Treated with a Novel Combined-Modality Radiosurgery Technique: A Case Report and Review of the Literature. *Front. Oncol.* **2022**, *12*, 907324. [CrossRef] [PubMed]
3. Altini, C.; Lavelli, V.; Ruta, R.; Ferrari, C.; Nappi, A.G.; Pisani, A.; Sardaro, A.; Rubini, G. Typical and atypical PET/CT findings in non-cancerous conditions. *Hell. J. Nucl. Med.* **2020**, *23*, 48–59. [CrossRef]
4. Altini, C.; Asabella, A.N.; Lavelli, V.; Bianco, G.; Ungaro, A.; Pisani, A.; Merenda, N.; Ferrari, C.; Rubini, G. Role of 18F-FDG PET/CT in comparison with CECT for whole-body assessment of patients with esophageal cancer. *Recenti Prog. Med.* **2019**, *110*, 144–150. [CrossRef] [PubMed]
5. Stout, A.P.; Murray, M.R. Hemangiopericytoma: A vascular tumor featuring Zimmermann's pericytes. *Ann. Surg.* **1942**, *116*, 26–33. [CrossRef] [PubMed]
6. Demicco, E.G.; Park, M.S.; Araujo, D.M.; Fox, P.S.; Bassett, R.L.; Pollock, R.E.; Lazar, A.J.; Wang, W.L. Solitary fibrous tumor: A clinicopathological study of 110 cases and proposed risk assessment model. *Mod. Pathol.* **2012**, *25*, 1298–1306. [CrossRef]
7. Sardaro, A.; Ferrari, C.; Mammucci, P.; Piscitelli, D.; Rubini, D.; Maggialetti, N. The significant role of multimodality imaging with 18 Fluorocholine PET/CT in relapsed intracranial hemangiopericytoma. *Rev. Esp. Med. Nucl. Imagen Mol.* **2021**, in press. [CrossRef]
8. Cheng, K.P.; Wong, W.J.; Hashim, S.; Mun, K.S. Hemangiopericytoma 11 years later: Delayed recurrence of a rare soft tissue sarcoma. *J. Thorac. Dis.* **2017**, *9*, E752–E756. [CrossRef]
9. Ciliberti, M.P.; D'Agostino, R.; Gabrieli, L.; Nikolaou, A.; Sardaro, A. The radiation therapy options of intracranial hemangiopericytoma: An overview and update on a rare vascular mesenchymal tumor. *Oncol. Rev.* **2018**, *12*, 63–68. [CrossRef]
10. Ramsey, H.J. Fine structure of hemangiopericytoma and hemangio-endothelioma. *Cancer* **1966**, *19*, 2005–2018. [CrossRef]
11. d'Amore, E.S.G.; Manivel, J.C.; Sung, J.H. Soft-tissue and meningeal hemangiopericytomas: An immunohistochemical and ultrastructural study. *Hum. Pathol.* **1990**, *21*, 414–423. [CrossRef]
12. Purandare, N.C.; Dua, S.G.; Rekhi, B.; Shah, S.; Sharma, A.R.; Rangarajan, V. Metastatic recurrence of an intracranial hemangiopericytoma 8 years after treatment: Report of a case with emphasis on the role of PET/CT in follow-up. *Cancer Imaging* **2010**, *10*, 117–120. [CrossRef] [PubMed]
13. Jacobs, A.H.; Kracht, L.W.; Gossmann, A.; Rüger, M.A.; Thomas, A.V.; Thiel, A.; Herholz, K. Imaging in neurooncology. *NeuroRx* **2005**, *2*, 333–347. [CrossRef] [PubMed]
14. Wu, Z.; Yang, H.; Weng, D.; Ding, Y. Rapid recurrence and bilateral lungs, multiple bone metastasis of malignant solitary fibrous tumor of the right occipital lobe: Report of a case and review. *Diagn. Pathol.* **2015**, *10*, 91. [CrossRef] [PubMed]
15. Cheung, H.; Lawhn-Heath, C.; Lopez, G.; Vella, M.; Aparici, C.M. Metastatic cervical paravertebral solitary fibrous tumor detected by fluorodeoxyglucose positron emission tomography-computed tomography. *Radiol. Case Rep.* **2018**, *13*, 464–467. [CrossRef] [PubMed]
16. Hiraide, T.; Sakaguchi, T.; Shibasaki, Y.; Morita, Y.; Suzuki, A.; Inaba, K.; Tokuyama, T.; Baba, S.; Suzuki, S.; Konno, H. Pancreatic metastases of cerebellar hemangiopericytoma occurring 24 years after initial presentation: Report of a case. *Surg. Today* **2014**, *44*, 558–563. [CrossRef]
17. Xiao, L.; Li, L. Bilateral renal metastasis from intracranial solitary fibrous tumor/hemangiopericytoma revealed on 18 F-FDG PET/CT and contrast-enhanced CT. *Hell. J. Nucl. Med.* **2021**, *24*, 272–273. [CrossRef] [PubMed]
18. Hayenga, H.N.; Bishop, A.J.; Wardak, Z.; Sen, C.; Mickey, B. Intraspinal Dissemination and Local Recurrence of an Intracranial Hemangiopericytoma. *World Neurosurg.* **2019**, *123*, 68–75. [CrossRef]
19. Yasen, A.; Ran, B.; Jiang, T.; Maimaitinijiati, Y.; Zhang, R.; Guo, Q.; Shao, Y.; Aji, T.; Wen, H. Liver metastasis and local recurrence of meningeal hemangiopericytoma: A case report. *Transl. Cancer Res.* **2020**, *9*, 1278–1283. [CrossRef]
20. Grünig, H.; Skawran, S.; Stolzmann, P.; Messerli, M.; Huellner, M.W. A Rare Case of Metastatic Solitary Fibrous Tumor (Hemangiopericytoma) of the Dura on 18F-FDG PET/CT. *Clin. Nucl. Med.* **2021**, *46*, 768–769. [CrossRef]
21. Jehanno, N.; Cassou-Mounat, T.; Mammar, H.; Luporsi, M.; Huchet, V. 18F-Choline PET/CT Imaging for Intracranial Hemangiopericytoma Recurrence. *Clin. Nucl. Med.* **2019**, *44*, e305–e307. [CrossRef]
22. Lavacchi, D.; Antonuzzo, L.; Briganti, V.; Berti, V.; Abenavoli, E.M.; Linguanti, F.; Messerini, L.; Giaccone, G. Metastatic intracranial solitary fibrous tumors/hemangiopericytomas: Description of two cases with radically different behaviors and review of the literature. *Anti-Cancer Drugs* **2020**, *31*, 646–651. [CrossRef] [PubMed]
23. Kota, G.; Gupta, P.; Lesser, G.J.; Wilson, J.A.; Mintz, A. Somatostatin receptor molecular imaging for metastatic intracranial hemangiopericytoma. *Clin. Nucl. Med.* **2013**, *38*, 984–987. [CrossRef]

24. Hung, T.J.; MacDonald, W.; Muir, T.; Celliers, L.; Al-Ogaili, Z. 68Ga DOTATATE PET/CT of Non-FDG-Avid pulmonary metastatic hemangiopericytoma. *Clin. Nucl. Med.* **2016**, *41*, 779–780. [CrossRef] [PubMed]
25. Patro, K.C.; Palla, M.; Kashyap, R. Unusual Case of Metastatic Intracranial Hemangiopericytoma and Emphasis on Role of 68Ga-PSMA PET in Imaging. *Clin. Nucl. Med.* **2018**, *43*, e331–e333. [CrossRef] [PubMed]
26. Zhang, Y.; Cai, J.; Wu, Z.; Yao, S.; Miao, W. Intense [68 Ga] Ga-FAPI-04 uptake in solitary fibrous tumor/hemangiopericytoma of the central nervous system. *Eur. J. Nucl. Med. Mol. Imaging* **2021**, *48*, 4103–4104. [CrossRef] [PubMed]
27. Jong, I.; Chen, S.; Leung, Y.L.; Cheung, S.K.; Ho, C.-L. ^{11}C-acetate PET/CT in a case of recurrent hemangiopericytoma. *Clin. Nucl. Med.* **2014**, *39*, 478–479. [CrossRef]
28. Chan, W.S.W.; Zhang, J.; Khong, P.L. 18F-FDG-PET-CT imaging findings of recurrent intracranial haemangiopericytoma with distant metastases. *Br. J. Radiol.* **2010**, *83*, e172–e174. [CrossRef] [PubMed]
29. Kracht, L.W.; Bauer, A.; Herholz, K.; Terstegge, K.; Friese, M.; Schröder, R.; Heiss, W.D. Positron emission tomography in a case of intracranial hemangiopericytoma. *J. Comput. Assist. Tomogr.* **1999**, *23*, 365–368. [CrossRef]
30. Cho, Y.D.; Choi, G.H.; Lee, S.P.; Kim, J.K. ^{1}H-MRS metabolic patterns for distinguishing between meningiomas and other brain tumors. *Magn. Reson. Imaging* **2003**, *21*, 663–672. [CrossRef]
31. Mama, N.; Ben Abdallah, A.; Hasni, I.; Kadri, K.; Arifa, N.; Ladib, M.; Tlili-Graiess, K. MR imaging of intracranial hemangiopericytomas. *J. Neuroradiol.* **2014**, *41*, 296–306. [CrossRef] [PubMed]
32. Ito, S.; Yokoyama, J.; Yoshimoto, H.; Yazawa, M.; Kazuo, K.; Hanaguri, M.; Ohba, S.; Fujimaki, M.; Ikeda, K. Usefulness of Choline-PET for the detection of residual hemangiopericytoma in the skull base: Comparison with FDG-PET. *Head Face Med.* **2012**, *8*, 3. [CrossRef] [PubMed]
33. Cuccurullo, V.; Di Stasio, G.D.; Evangelista, L.; Castoria, G.; Mansi, L. Biochemical and Pathophysiological Premises to Positron Emission Tomography with Choline Radiotracers. *J. Cell. Physiol.* **2017**, *232*, 270–275. [CrossRef] [PubMed]
34. Glunde, K.; Penet, M.F.; Jiang, L.; Jacobs, M.A.; Bhujwalla, Z.M. Choline metabolism-based molecular diagnosis of cancer: An update. *Expert Rev. Mol. Diagn.* **2015**, *15*, 735–747. [CrossRef] [PubMed]
35. Lockman, P.R.; Allen, D.D. The transport of choline. *Drug Dev. Ind. Pharm.* **2002**, *28*, 749–771. [CrossRef] [PubMed]
36. Alongi, P.; Quartuccio, N.; Arnone, A.; Kokomani, A.; Allocca, M.; Nappi, A.G.; Santo, G.; Mantarro, C.; Laudicella, R. Brain PET/CT using prostate cancer radiopharmaceutical agents in the evaluation of gliomas. *Clin. Transl. Imaging* **2020**, *8*, 433–448. [CrossRef]
37. Khan, N.; Oriuchi, N.; Ninomiya, H.; Higuchi, T.; Kamada, H.; Endo, K. Positron emission tomographic imaging with 11C-choline in differential diagnosis of head and neck tumors: Comparison with 18F-FDG PET. *Ann. Nucl. Med.* **2004**, *18*, 409–417. [CrossRef] [PubMed]
38. Dunet, V.; Pomoni, A.; Hottinger, A.; Nicod-Lalonde, M.; Prior, J.O. Performance of 18F-FET versus 18F-FDG-PET for the diagnosis and grading of brain tumors: Systematic review and meta-analysis. *Neuro Oncol.* **2016**, *18*, 426–434. [CrossRef] [PubMed]
39. Veldhuijzen van Zanten, S.E.M.; Bos, E.M.; Verburg, F.A.; van Doormaal, P.J. Intracranial hemangiopericytoma showing excellent uptake on arterial injection of [68 Ga] DOTATATE. *Eur. J. Nucl. Med. Mol. Imaging* **2021**, *48*, 1673–1674. [CrossRef] [PubMed]
40. Hammes, J.; Kobe, C.; Hilgenberg, U.; Lieb, W.E.; Drzezga, A. Orbital Hemangiopericytoma in 68Ga-Prostate-Specific Membrane Antigen-HBED-CC PET/CT. *Clin. Nucl. Med.* **2017**, *42*, 812–814. [CrossRef]
41. Matsuda, M.; Ishikawa, E.; Yamamoto, T.; Hatano, K.; Joraku, A.; Iizumi, Y.; Masuda, Y.; Nishiyama, H.; Matsumura, A. Potential use of prostate specific membrane antigen (PSMA) for detecting the tumor neovasculature of brain tumors by PET imaging with 89 Zr-Df-IAB2M anti-PSMA minibody. *J. Neurooncol.* **2018**, *138*, 581–589. [CrossRef] [PubMed]
42. Giesel, F.L.; Adeberg, S.; Syed, M.; Lindner, T.; Jiménez-Franco, L.D.; Mavriopoulou, E.; Staudinger, F.; Tonndorf-Martini, E.; Regnery, S.; Rieken, S.; et al. FAPI-74 PET/CT Using Either 18 F-AlF or Cold-Kit 68 Ga Labeling: Biodistribution, Radiation Dosimetry, and Tumor Delineation in Lung Cancer Patients. *J. Nucl. Med.* **2021**, *62*, 201–207. [CrossRef] [PubMed]
43. Schuster, D.M.; Nanni, C.; Fanti, S. PET Tracers Beyond FDG in Prostate Cancer. *Semin. Nucl. Med.* **2016**, *46*, 507–521. [CrossRef] [PubMed]

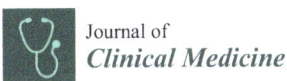

Article

Multiparametric Dual-Time-Point [18F]FDG PET/MRI for Lymph Node Staging in Patients with Untreated FIGO I/II Cervical Carcinoma

Matthias Weissinger [1,2,3], Stefan Kommoss [4], Johann Jacoby [5], Stephan Ursprung [3], Ferdinand Seith [3], Sascha Hoffmann [4], Konstantin Nikolaou [3,6,7], Sara Yvonne Brucker [4], Christian La Fougère [1,6,7,*] and Helmut Dittmann [1]

1. Department of Nuclear Medicine and Clinical Molecular Imaging, University Hospital Tuebingen, 72076 Tuebingen, Germany
2. Department of Diagnostic and Interventional Radiology, Eberhard-Karls-University Tuebingen, Hoppe Seyler-Straße 3, 72076 Tuebingen, Germany
3. Department of Diagnostic and Interventional Radiology, University Hospital Tuebingen, 72076 Tuebingen, Germany
4. Department of Women's Health, University Hospital Tuebingen, 72076 Tuebingen, Germany
5. Institute for Clinical Epidemiology and Applied Biometry, University Hospital Tuebingen, 72076 Tuebingen, Germany
6. iFIT-Cluster of Excellence, Eberhard Karls University Tuebingen, 72074 Tuebingen, Germany
7. German Cancer Consortium (DKTK), Partner Site Tuebingen, 69120 Heidelberg, Germany
* Correspondence: christian.lafougere@med.uni-tuebingen.de; Tel.: +49-7071-2986553; Fax: +49-7071-29-4601

Abstract: [18F]FDG PET/MRI was shown to have limited sensitivity for N-staging in FIGO I/II cervical carcinoma. Therefore, this prospective study aimed to investigate the additional value of multiparametric dual-time-point PET/MRI and to assess potential influencing factors for lymph node metastasis (LNM) detection. A total of 63 patients underwent whole-body dual-time-point [18F]FDG PET/MRI 60 + 90 min p.i., and 251 LN were evaluated visually, quantified multiparametrically, and correlated with histology. Grading of the primary tumor (G2/G3) had a significant impact on visual detection (sens: 8.3%/31%). The best single parameter for LNM detection was SUVavg, however, with a significant loss of discriminatory power in G2 vs. G3 tumors (AUC: 0.673/0.901). The independent predictors SUVavg, ΔSUVpeak, LN sphericity, ADC, and histologic grade were included in the logistic-regression-based malignancy score (MS) for multiparametric analysis. Application of MS enhanced AUCs, especially in G2 tumors (AUC: G2:0.769; G3:0.877) and improved the accuracy for single LNM from 34.5% to 55.5% compared with the best univariate parameter SUVavg. Compared with visual analysis, the use of the malignancy score increased the overall sensitivity from 31.0% to 79.3% (Youden optimum) with a moderate decrease in specificity from 98.3% to 75.6%. These findings indicate that multiparametric evaluation of dual-time-point PET/MRI has the potential to improve accuracy compared with visual interpretation and enables sufficient N-staging also in G2 cervical carcinoma.

Keywords: [18F]FDG PET/MRI; multiparametric imaging; dual-time-point kinetic; cervical carcinoma; lymph node metastases

Citation: Weissinger, M.; Kommoss, S.; Jacoby, J.; Ursprung, S.; Seith, F.; Hoffmann, S.; Nikolaou, K.; Brucker, S.Y.; La Fougère, C.; Dittmann, H. Multiparametric Dual-Time-Point [18F]FDG PET/MRI for Lymph Node Staging in Patients with Untreated FIGO I/II Cervical Carcinoma. *J. Clin. Med.* **2022**, *11*, 4943. https://doi.org/10.3390/jcm11174943

Academic Editors: Arnoldo Piccardo and Francesco Fiz

Received: 15 July 2022
Accepted: 17 August 2022
Published: 23 August 2022

Publisher's Note: MDPI stays neutral with regard to jurisdictional claims in published maps and institutional affiliations.

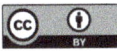

Copyright: © 2022 by the authors. Licensee MDPI, Basel, Switzerland. This article is an open access article distributed under the terms and conditions of the Creative Commons Attribution (CC BY) license (https://creativecommons.org/licenses/by/4.0/).

1. Introduction

Cervical cancer is the fourth most common cancer in women worldwide [1]. It affects young women starting in their 20s with the highest incidence at the age of 40 in the US and EU (of 15.1/100,000) [1,2]. Lymphatic spread occurs frequently already in early-stage cervical cancer, which mostly presents with (micro-) metastases [3,4]. These small metastases are hard to detect by CT or MRI, but the presence of lymph node metastases (LNM) is the most important prognostic factor in early tumor stages [2–7], and decisions on primary treatment (surgery vs. radiochemotherapy) depend on nodal involvement.

As cervical carcinoma is staged using the clinical FIGO classification, systematic lymphadenectomy, despite being associated with high morbidity, is still the gold standard for N-staging [2,7–9]. To reduce morbidity, sentinel lymph node (SLN) biopsy was introduced in 1999 for cervical carcinomas, proving to be safe for early-stage cancer in the case of successful SLN labeling [2,7,10–13]. However, even with correct tracer injection, SLN mapping can fail owing to strong venous tracer outflow or a transformation of the tumoral lymphatic drainage in pre-existing lymphatic tumor spread [14–16]. In addition, parametrial infiltration, while increasing the risk of LNM from 1% to 5–20% and fundamentally changing clinical management, often remains undetected until surgery [17,18]. Furthermore, the SLN technique was reported to be insufficient for the evaluation of the para-aortic LN status [16,19].

As a consequence, efforts have been made in recent years towards enabling more accurate and noninvasive N-staging by means of new imaging techniques, contrast agents, and tracers [20]. In this context, MRI reaches a very high specificity of about 95%, but only unsatisfying sensitivity of about 50% in early tumor stages [21]. However, the combination of MRI and [^{18}F]FDG PET ([^{18}F]FDG PET/MRI) improves the diagnostic accuracy in detecting pelvic and para-aortic LNM as well as distant metastases significantly [22]. Nevertheless, the sensitivity of the visual assessment of [^{18}F]FDG PET/MRI in cervical carcinoma, even by experts, is limited owing to the low tumor-to-background ratio, especially of small LNM [16]. As histological ultrastaging revealed a much higher prevalence of isolated tumor cells in the LN or micro-LNM in early tumor stages than hitherto expected [23], the performance of [^{18}F]FDG PET/MRI has to be improved.

Therefore, this study aimed to analyze the additional value of multiparametric PET/MR imaging comprising a dual-time-point [^{18}F]FDG PET/MRI for N-staging in early tumor stages compared with expert reading using a swift, clinically applicable imaging protocol.

2. Materials and Methods

This prospective trial was registered in the German Clinical Trial Register (DRKS-ID: DRKS00014346) and approved by the institutional review board (registry no. 173/2015BO01) [24]. All participants provided written informed consent. A total of 69 consecutive patients with histopathologically confirmed cervical carcinoma and clinically determined stage ≤ FIGO IIB underwent whole-body dual-time-point [^{18}F]FDG PET/MRI. A total of 63 of 69 participants underwent preoperative SLN mapping with SPECT/CT, followed by intraoperative SLN detection with a gamma probe and surgical staging between March 2016 and October 2020, and were included in the analysis (Figure 1).

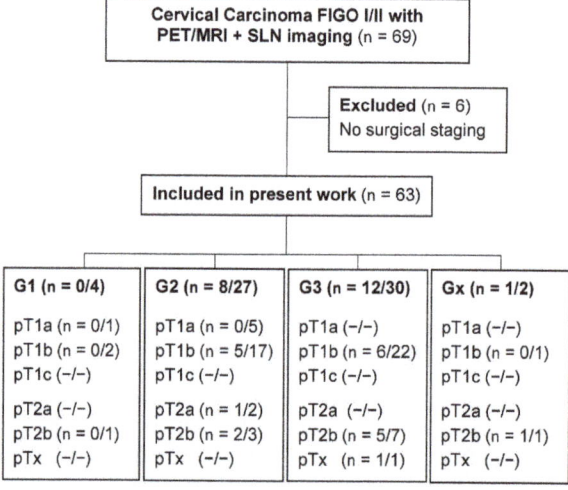

Figure 1. Consort flow diagram. Data are given as numbers of patients with LNM/all patients in subgroups.

2.1. PET/MRI Protocol

All patients underwent whole-body dual-time-point PET/MR after injection of about 3 MBq [^{18}F]FDG per kg body weight (150–250 MBq, Biograph mMR®, (Siemens Healthineers, Erlangen, Germany), axial field of view: 258 mm, 4 × 4 × 20 mm LSO crystals, sensitivity: 14.1 cps/kBq, full width at half maximum @1 cm: 4.6 mm, no time-of-flight). Patients were asked to fast for at least 8 h, and blood sugar levels had to be below 150 mg/dl at injection. The early PET/MRI scan started with the first pass from midthigh to skull base 64.7 ± 11.7 min p.i., immediately followed by the delayed scan covering the inguinal and pelvic LN levels 90.6 ± 12.6 min p.i. An MRI contrast agent (8 mL Gadovist®) was applied except when contraindicated. Detailed MRI parameters are presented in Supplementary Table S1.

PET and MRI acquisitions were performed simultaneously, and the images were fused for further analysis. Acquisition time was defined by the MRI sequences and was BMI-adapted at 4–6 min/bed position for the first scan and 12–16 min/bed position for the delayed pelvic scan. Imaging data were reconstructed applying an iterative ordered subset expectation maximization algorithm (256 × 256 matrix) with a 4 mm Gaussian filter. Attenuation correction was performed using an MRI-based µ-map (SyngoMR E11®, Siemens Numaris/4, Siemens Healthineers, Erlangen, Germany).

2.2. SLN SPECT/CT

LN mapping was performed 3–5 h after intracervical injection of ≈ 200 MBq [^{99m}Tc]Tc-Nanocolloide at the 3, 6, 9, and 12 o'clock positions. Imaging was performed with a hybrid SPECT/CT scanner (Discovery 670 Pro®, GE Healthcare, Chicago, IL, USA), as described previously [16]. An SLN was defined as focal activity enrichment in SPECT in a plausible anatomical region.

2.3. Histological Validation

Histological validation of LN was performed by removing the SLN, followed by a systematic pelvic lymphadenectomy. Para-aortic LN were removed if intraoperatively conspicuous or malignant SLN. [^{99m}Tc]Tc-Nanocolloide-labeled SLN were localized and identified intraoperatively through a laparoscopic gamma probe (Neoprobe®, Models 1017 and 1100, Devicor Medical Products, Inc., Cincinnati, OH, USA), resected separately, and sent for frozen sectioning. SLN were further ultrastaged with the preparation of the entire LN in 200 µm slices.

2.4. Image Evaluation and Data Quantification

The evaluation of PET/MRI images with malignancy assessment of LN was performed prospectively in consensus by one radiology and one nuclear medicine specialist each with at least 8 years of experience in PET and MRI imaging. Anatomical positions of resected LN were identified on PET/MRI images based on their position in SLN SPECT/CT and the surgeon's description of the localization intraoperatively.

Multiparametric data were collected using a dedicated software (syngo.via® 8.2; Siemens Healthineers) and matched retrospectively with histology. Volumes of interest (VOI) were placed manually around every histologically confirmed LN on early and (standardized uptake value = SUV_e) and delayed PET (SUV_d). Quantification was performed as SUVmax and SUVpeak as well as SUVmean (50% isocontour). Blood pool correction (bpc) for SUV measurements (bpcSUV) was performed by dividing the lesions SUV by the SUVmean (without isocontour) of an ROI placed in a large venous vessel in the same PET bed position.

$$bpcSUV = \frac{SUV\ VOI}{SUV\ blood\ pool} \qquad (1)$$

Dual-time-point [^{18}F]FDG kinetics were calculated using a retention index (RI), as described by Nogami et al. [25], and extended with a blood pool correction.

$$\text{RI} = \frac{\text{bpcSUVd} - \text{bpcSUVe}}{\text{bpcSUVe}} \times 100\% \qquad (2)$$

In addition, the absolute difference of the bpcSUV between the early and delayed scan was defined as SUVΔ.

$$\Delta\text{SUV} = \text{bpcSUVd} - \text{bpcSUVe} \qquad (3)$$

LN diameters were measured in the perpendicular short and long axis in the transaxial plane. Sphericity was defined as the ratio of short- to long-axes diameter. Diffusion was quantified manually using an ROI in the apparent diffusion coefficient (ADC) maps in LN $\geq$ 4 mm.

2.5. Statistical Analysis

Statistical analysis was performed using the SPSS Statistics 25.0 software (IBM Inc., Armonk, NY, USA), MedCalc v20.009 (MedCalc Software Ltd., Ostend, Belgium), and R 4.0.3 (R Foundation for Statistical Computing, Vienna, Austria). All parameters acquired were benchmarked against the gold standard histology. Differences in prevalence were tested for significance using the Chi^2 test. Differences between the means of groups were analyzed using the two-tailed *t*-test.

Listwise deletion was performed in case of missing values. Optimal cut-off values in ROC analyses were set at the Youden optimum.

The newly defined malignancy score (MS) predicts the probability of a lymph node exhibiting malignant histology based on a mixed logistic regression model, including the multiparametric imaging measures. This model uses the optimally weighted combination given the included predictors and covariances in the sample predicting the histological findings and incorporates random intercepts for patients within which the individual nodes account for dependencies. The probabilities are predicted for the current sample without using these random effects as these will not be known in future cases or samples for which one may wish to use the procedure. The criterion for statistical significance was set at $\alpha = 0.05$.

3. Results

3.1. Patient Cohort

In total, 251 LN from 63 patients were assessed histologically and quantified multi-parametrically with [^{18}F]FDG PET/MRI. A total of 211 of 251 LN were located within the FOV of the delayed scan, enabling dual-time-point [^{18}F]FDG kinetic calculation. A total of 219 of 251 LN had a sufficient size for ADC calculation. A total of 79 of 251 LN from 54 of 63 patients met the criteria for SLN in [^{99m}Tc]Tc-Nanocolloide SPECT/CT. Detailed patient characteristics are presented in Table 1.

Table 1. Patient characteristics (*n* = 63).

	Average ± SD	Range
Age at PET/MR (years)	46.8 ± 11.5	28–72
Patient height (cm)	166 ± 6.6	152–187
Patient weight (kg)	71.0 ± 16.2	44–117
BMI (kg/m^2)	25.7 ± 5.4	15–40
Time between PET/MR and LN histology (days)	22.4 ± 16.7	1–89 *

* One outlier with 89 d but no LNM at histology.

3.2. Prevalence of LNM Dependent on Stage and Grade of Primary Tumors

In 2 patients and 6 LN, respectively, no grading of the primary tumor was reported owing to conizations performed at other centers and no tumor was left when performing the (radical) hysterectomy in our center. The prevalence of LNM increased with the T-stage of the primary tumor (Figure 1). The patient-based prevalence of LNM was not significantly higher in patients with G3 (40%) than G2 (29.6%) tumors ($p = 0.35$). No LNM occurred in patients with G1 tumors.

3.3. Interrelationships of Histology and PET/MRI Parameters

LNM demonstrated a higher SUV, larger diameters, higher RI, and ΔSUV than benign LN, as detailed in Supplementary Table S2.

Moreover, these differences were amplified by the grade of the primary tumor, as presented in Figure 2 and Supplementary Table S2. In particular, LNM from G3 tumors presented with significantly higher SUV and FDG dynamics between early and delayed scan measured with RI-SUVavg ($p = 0.03$) and ΔSUVavg ($p = 0.02$) compared with LNM from G2 tumors ($p < 0.01$; Supplementary Table S3). Furthermore, G3 LNM presented with a greater short-axis diameter vs. G2 LNM ($p < 0.01$) and a slight increase in sphericity ($p = 0.08$), while ADC revealed no significant difference.

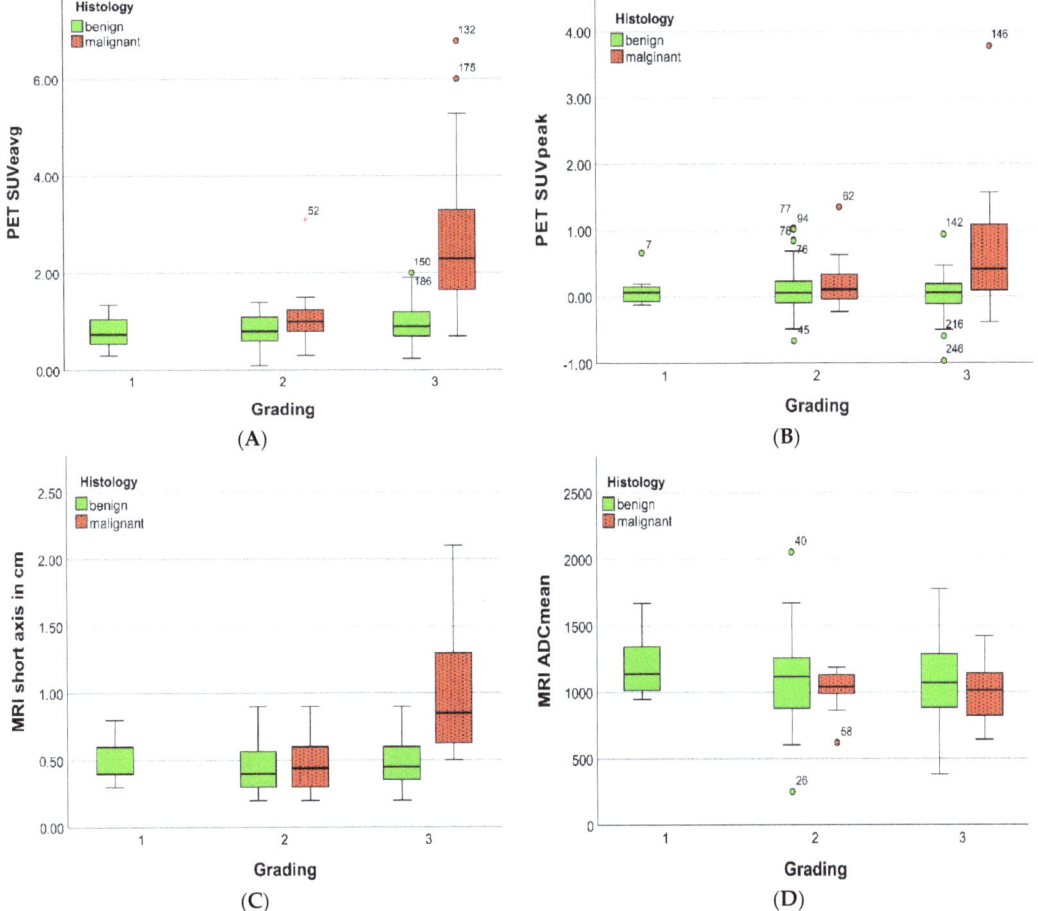

Figure 2. Boxplots presenting [^{18}F]FDG PET (**A**,**B**) and MRI (**C**,**D**) parameters of lymph nodes dependent on the tumor grade of the primary tumor derived from biopsy before PET/MRI. No LNM were present in G1 carcinomas.

LN short-axis diameter correlated significantly with SUV_e, SUV_d, $_{BPC}SUV_e$, $_{BPC}SUV_d$, and ΔSUVpeak ($p < 0.01$, r: 0.477–0.716) but not with RI-SUVpeak (r = 0.085) or ADC (r = 0.241).

G3 LNM revealed an increase in [^{18}F]FDG uptake between early and delayed scans compared with benign LN (RI-SUVpeak and ΔSUVpeak: $p < 0.01$ and 0.02), as presented for representative cases in Figure 3a,b. A similar trend was observed for RI-SUVpeak in G2 LNM, though not reaching significance ($p = 0.19$).

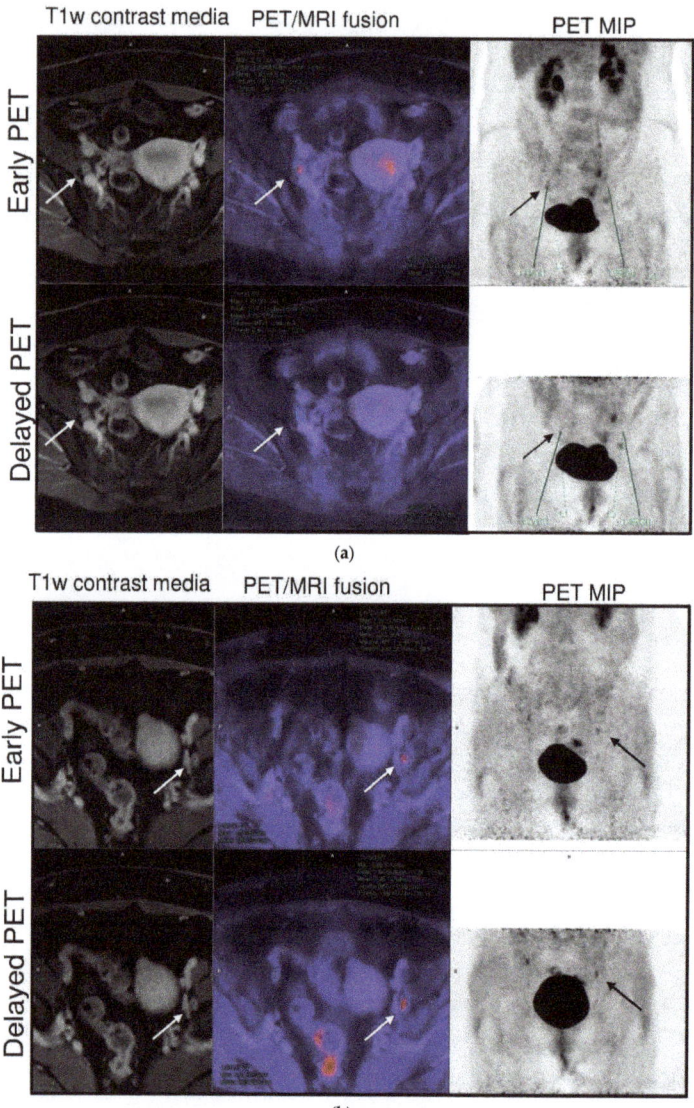

Figure 3. (**a**). Case of a 49-year-old patient with pT1b2 G3 cervical cancer. Focal [^{18}F]FDG uptake (arrow) of the right interiliac LN decreased by 33% between early (60 min, SUVavg 1.8) and delayed PET scan (88 min, SUVavg 1.2) and was histologically confirmed as lymphofollicular hyperplasia. (**b**). Case of a 41-year-old patient with pT2b G3 cervical cancer. The left iliac extern LNM (arrow) presents an ongoing [^{18}F]FDG trapping between the early (60 min, SUVavg 2.1) and delayed scan (82 min, SUVavg 2.5) and a slight decrease in blood pool activity.

3.4. PET/MRI Parameter Evaluation

PET demonstrated high accuracy in differentiating between LNM and benign LN using an SUV-based quantification with an AUC of up to 0.809 (Figure 4 and Supplementary Table S2) without significant differences between the SUV quantification parameters $SUV_e max$, $SUV_e peak$, and $SUV_e mean$ ($p \geq 0.54$).

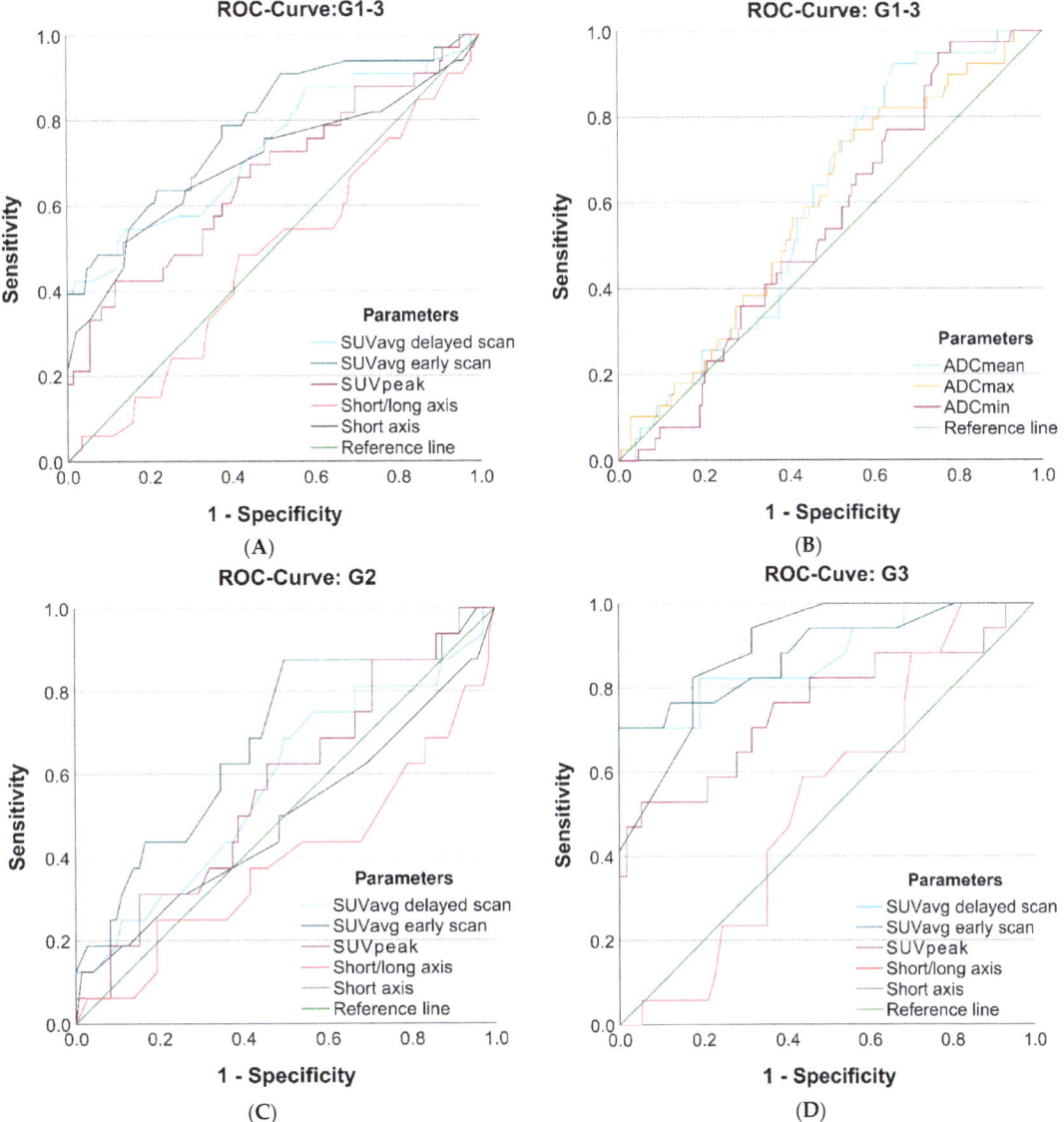

Figure 4. ROC analysis for the detection of lymph node metastases of selected [^{18}F]FDG PET/MRI parameters for G 1-3 tumors (**A**) and (**B**) as well es G2 tumors (**C**) and G3 tumors (**D**) separately.

The delayed PET scan did not result in a significantly higher AUC than the early PET scan ($p \geq 0.55$). Blood pool correction improved the AUC in the delayed PET slightly but nonsignificantly ($SUV_e avg$: 0.784 vs. 0.766; $SUV_d avg$: 0.741 vs. 0.767, $p = 0.73$).

The primary tumor grade crucially impacted the accuracy of LNM detection in PET with a significant decrease in discriminatory power in G2 versus G3 tumors (SUV$_e$avg G2: 0.673; G3: 0.901, $p < 0.01$). The error rate (ER = false-positive + false-negative rate = 1-accuracy) was more than twice as high for G2 LNM (65.5%) as for G3 LNM (30.4%) at their individual optimal SUV$_e$avg cut-off (Supplementary Figure S1), while the prevalence was comparable (G2: 17.5% vs. G3: 23.0%).

Dual-time-point kinetics calculated with RI and ΔSUV significantly correlated with malignancy, especially in G3 tumors with an AUC up to 0.791 ($p < 0.01$). The SUVpeak quantification method achieved the highest AUCs but required blood pool correction. Overall, the ΔSUV calculation method was comparable to the RI-SUV but performed slightly and nonsignificantly better in G3 tumors (G3 SUVavg: 0.791 vs. 0.718, $p = 0.48$).

LN diameters revealed a significant discriminatory power for short-axis (0.741) and long-axis (0.777) measurements and performed best in LNM from G3 tumors (AUC: 0.904 and 0.881). LN sphericity was not a significant stand-alone predictor of LNM, neither in G2 nor G3 tumors ($p \geq 0.269$).

ADC presented a borderline significant discriminatory power (AUC 0.600, $p = 0.05$), with a significantly lower AUC compared with the SUVavg and short-axis diameter ($p < 0.01$ and $p = 0.03$, $n = 162$).

3.5. Multiparametric Approach

The parameters ADC, sphericity, bpcSUV$_e$avg, and tumor grade of the primary tumor were identified as independent predictors of LNM and were included in the calculation of the MS, as described above. The response variable of the model were the probabilities of being malignant predicted by the model, calculated as a sum of the predictor values weighted according to their (fixed effect) regression coefficients. After listwise exclusion of cases with missing parameters, the sample size was 171 LN with 21.1% prevalence of metastases.

Using MS resulted in a high discriminatory power between malignant and benign LN (AUC: 0.820, 95% CI: 0.736–0.879). At the optimal cut-off value (Youden optimum: 0.042), the MS improved sensitivity from 63.5% to 72.2% compared with SUV$_e$avg at a specificity of 80.7%.

Furthermore, error rates could be lowered (47.0%) and kept constant over a wider cut-off range compared with the best single parameter SUV$_e$avg (52.7%), as presented in Supplementary Figure S1.

Further subgroup analysis focusing on the grade of the primary tumor revealed a significantly ($p < 0.01$) better prediction of LNM in G3 tumors (AUC 0.850, 95% CI: 0.755–0.945) compared with G2 tumors (AUC 0.695, 95% CI: 0.526–0.863). In particular, the parameter SUV$_e$ showed a markedly different predictivity for LNM in G2 compared with G3 tumors (log-odds: SUV: 1.5/17.7, $p = 0.01$).

3.6. Additional Value of Dual-Time-Point [^{18}F]FDG Kinetic

The implementation of dual-time-point parameters significantly improved the model fit. The most predictive parameters were ΔSUVpeak (log-likelihood: −42.66; χ^2 difference = 7.11; $p < 0.01$) and RI-SUVpeak (log-likelihood: −43.44; χ^2 difference = 5.20; $p = 0.02$; log-likelihood of the comparison model without these dual-time-point parameters: −46.21, $n = 144$).

Implementing the dual-time-point [^{18}F]FDG kinetic parameter ΔSUVpeak in the MS lowered error rates in G2 tumors by one-third from 65.5% to 44.5% compared with the best single parameter SUVavg (Supplementary Figure S1).

Inclusion of ΔSUVpeak and RI-SUVpeak resulted in a slightly but not significantly increased discriminatory power (MS + ΔSUVpeak: AUC: 0.837; sensitivity: 79.3%; specificity: 75.7%) compared with the standard MS model (AUC: 0.820; sensitivity: 72.2%; specificity: 80.7%).

3.7. Visual vs. Multiparametric Evaluation

Specificity was set by the visual evaluation, and corresponding sensitivity was compared between visual and multiparametric LN evaluation using MS. Applying MS increased the overall sensitivity from 31.0% to 37.9% compared with the expert consensus at a set specificity of 98.3% (*n* = 144, prevalence: 20.1%), although the defined specificity was far from the Youden optimum of the MS (sensitivity: 79.3%; specificity: 75.6% at cut-off of 0.0042).

For G3 tumors, MS revealed a higher sensitivity (47.1% vs. 58.8%) compared with the human reader at a set specificity of 96.3% (*n* = 71, prevalence 23.9%), which was close to the Youden optimum (sensitivity of 76.4% at a specificity of 85.1%; cut-off: 0.0908).

For G2 LNM, using MS, resulted in an identical sensitivity of 8.3% at a set specificity of 100% (*n* = 73, prevalence: 16.4%). However, sensitivity increased from 8.3% to 83.3% if adjusted to the Youden optimum at a specificity of 72.1% (cut-off: 0.0435).

4. Discussion

To our knowledge, this is the first prospective study analyzing the additional diagnostic value of a multiparametric [^{18}F]FDG PET/MRI analysis compared with expert consensus reading for N-staging with histology as the gold standard in FIGO I/II cervical carcinomas. A multiparametric malignancy score was introduced, which integrates dual-time-point [^{18}F]FDG kinetics and biopsy-based grading of the primary tumor in addition to established PET and MRI parameters. Using [^{99m}Tc]Tc-Nanocolloide for SLN labeling provided accurate transfer of LN positions via SLN SPECT/CT to PET/MRI, resulting in high data quality, which is a strength of this study.

Our results indicate that multiparametric analysis using the MS may double the sensitivity in LNM detection in FIGO I/II cervical cancer in G2 tumors compared with visual evaluation. As PET/MRI has already been shown to improve T- and M-staging, enhancing the accuracy in N-staging is the next big step in optimizing noninvasive staging for cervical carcinoma. This is of high clinical relevance, as surgical LN staging is currently the first step of surgery in advanced cervical cancer (in contrast to early cancer, where radical hysterectomy is usually the first step, followed by (sentinel-) LN dissection) [2]. Furthermore, preoperative assessment and evaluation of nodal involvement have a direct therapeutic impact as the presence of LNM leads to a change from radical hysterectomy to radiochemotherapy according to current guidelines [2].

4.1. Impact of Tumor Grade

Another key finding of this study was the strong influence of tumor grade on [^{18}F]FDG uptake and [^{18}F]FDG kinetics of LNM, which fundamentally affects their visibility in PET. As grading is usually assessed by biopsy as part of the initial gynecological examination, this is available when PET/MRI scan is performed.

The integration of histological characteristics into a multiparametric imaging-based analysis adds complementary information. In particular, primary tumor histology changed both the weighting of the individual parameters and their cut-off values in our study.

The present data indicate that the low sensitivity of [^{18}F]FDG PET/MRI for G2 LNM might rather be due to smaller size, low SUV, and discreet [^{18}F]FDG kinetics compared with their hitherto often assumed lower prevalence. In fact, LNM prevalence in G2 was not significantly different from that in G3 tumors using ultrastaging as the gold standard [26]. This finding is of high clinical relevance, as a solely visual assessment of [^{18}F]FDG PET comes with insufficient sensitivity for N-staging in G2 tumors. Under consideration of early data, it can be hypothesized that the SLN technique may achieve more accurate N-staging than visual evaluation of [^{18}F]FDG PET/MRI in early-stage G2 carcinoma [16,27]. This is even more important as, currently, in stage T1B1 and lower (i.e., early cervical cancer below 2 cm), LN dissection of only the SLN is currently considered state of the art [2]. Thus, preoperative knowledge of positive LN has a direct impact on the surgical procedure.

4.2. Dual-Time-Point [^{18}F]FDG PET

In contrast to previous studies, we introduced a short-period dual-time-point imaging protocol using an interval of 30 min instead of 1–2.5 h [25,27,28], which enables continuous scanning without the need for repositioning patients. Even for this short time interval, a significant increase in tumoral [^{18}F]FDG uptake was found—calculated as RI as proposed by Nogami et al. [25]—which was a significant independent predictor of malignancy. Furthermore, it was shown for the first time that the increase in [^{18}F]FDG uptake over time was only significant for G3 LNM but not for G2 LNM. G2 LNM presented with a slight decrease in SUV analogous to the decline of blood pool activity, which might be explained by lower metabolic activity and tumor cell density [29].

Blood pool correction was crucial for dual-time-point dynamic measurements owing to a decreasing blood pool and increasing scatter correction artefacts caused by rising activity concentrations in the bladder. Although the dual-time-point kinetics were a significant factor, delayed PET images did not outperform the early scans. This might be due to LNM with increasing SUV dynamics already showing increased uptake on early PET scans.

4.3. Experts vs. Malignancy Score

Visual evaluation of LNM by expert readers was highly specific but accompanied by poor sensitivity, which runs counter to the principle of presurgical screening.

By using the MS with a cut-off value at the Youden optimum, the sensitivity could be improved substantially, especially in G2. The moderate loss of specificity would be acceptable, as false-positive pelvic LN are re-evaluated during surgery.

The sensitivity of visual evaluation was even lower than described in previous studies (31% vs. 45–88%) [30,31]. This might be due to our cohort of solely early-stage carcinomas and the higher number of micrometastases detectable by ultrastaging, as discussed above.

4.4. Limitations

The results presented here only pertain to G2 and G3 tumors as no LNM occurred in the small number of G1 tumors in our cohort.

The smaller FOV of the delayed [^{18}F]FDG PET/MRI scan limited the dual-time-point analysis to pelvic LN.

In order to avoid further strain on the information extracted from the data, a listwise exclusion of cases was applied throughout the analyses; however, this resulted in a varying number of LNM in the results.

Furthermore, the multiparametric evaluation was based on histology and, therefore, was performed retrospectively in contrast to prospective reading of the experts. Consequently, the multiparametric analysis was subjected to accommodation of random effects to keep the diagnostic performance of MS comparable to the expert reading and other cohorts.

Prior to a broader clinical application, the presented MS should be validated prospectively in a comparable setting, which is planned for the second half of this ongoing clinical trial.

5. Conclusions

G2 vs. G3 tumor grade was identified as a crucial factor for limited visual detectability of LNM on [^{18}F]FDG PET/MRI in early cervical carcinoma.

Multiparametric evaluation of dual-time-point [^{18}F]FDG PET/MRI has the potential to considerably improve the accuracy of LNM detection and to extend sufficient N-staging also to G2 tumors.

Supplementary Materials: The following supporting information can be downloaded at: https://www.mdpi.com/article/10.3390/jcm11174943/s1, Figure S1. Error rates for the detection of lymph node metastases by single parameter and multiparametric malignancy score in dependence of tumor grading. The multiparametric malignancy score (MS) (D) lowers the error rate (ER = false positive rate FNR + false negative rate FPR) about 5 percentage points and stabilizes the ER over a wider range compared to the best single parameter SUV$_e$avg (A). Implementing dual timepoint kinetics (E) further enhances this effect and lowers the summed error rate ER by another 2 percentage points compared to the standard MS (D). In G2 tumors, this effect is most evident with a significant reduction in summed error rate ER of 21 percentage points from 65.5% (C) to 44.5% (F). Grade of primary tumor has an huge impact on detectability of lymph note metastases with an doubling of error rates in G2 LNM (C) compared to G3 LNM (B) with a sharp increase in FNR starting at an SUV of 1. Table S1. MRI imaging parameters. Table S2. Survey table of AUC analysis of the dual-time-point PET/MRI parameters for G2 and G3 cervical carcinoma. No lymph node present in G1 tumors. Table S3. Effect of the tumor grade on PET/MR parameters of lymph node metastases.

Author Contributions: Conceptualization, M.W.; data curation, M.W. and S.H.; formal analysis, M.W. and J.J.; funding acquisition, S.K., K.N. and C.L.F.; investigation, M.W. and H.D.; methodology, M.W., J.J., C.L.F. and H.D.; project administration, M.W., S.K. and C.L.F.; resources, S.K., K.N., S.Y.B. and C.L.F.; software, J.J.; supervision, K.N., S.Y.B. and H.D.; visualization, M.W.; writing – original draft, M.W.; writing—review & editing, S.K., J.J., S.U., F.S., S.H., K.N., S.Y.B., C.L.F. and H.D. All authors have read and agreed to the published version of the manuscript.

Funding: Funded by the Deutsche Forschungsgemeinschaft (DFG, German Research Foundation) under Germany's Excellence Strategy (EXC 2180–390900677).

Institutional Review Board Statement: The study was conducted in accordance with the Declaration of Helsinki, and approved by the Institutional Review Board of University Hospital Tübingen (protocol code 173/2015BO01) on 28 October 2015.

Informed Consent Statement: Informed consent was obtained from all subjects involved in the study.

Data Availability Statement: The data presented in this study are available on request from the corresponding author. The data are not publicly available due to data protection regulations.

Acknowledgments: Special thanks to technicians Carsten Groeper, Hans Volz, and Gerd Zeger for the enthusiastic and accurate performance of PET/MRI examinations. We acknowledge the financial support for publication fees by Open Access Publishing Fund of the University of Tübingen.

Conflicts of Interest: The authors declare no conflict of interest.

References

1. Arbyn, M.; Weiderpass, E.; Bruni, L.; de Sanjose, S.; Saraiya, M.; Ferlay, J.; Bray, F. Estimates of incidence and mortality of cervical cancer in 2018: A worldwide analysis. *Lancet Glob. Health* **2020**, *8*, e191–e203. [CrossRef]
2. Leitlinienprogramm Onkologie (Deutsche Krebsgesellschaft, Deutsche Krebshilfe, AWMF): S3-Leitlinie Diagnostik, Therapie und Nachsorge der Patientin mit Zervixkarzinom, Langversion, 2.2, 2022, AWMF-Registernummer: 032/033OL. Available online: https://www.leitlinienprogramm-onkologie.de/leitlinien/zervixkarzinom/ (accessed on 15 August 2022).
3. Marchiole, P.; Buenerd, A.; Benchaib, M.; Nezhat, K.; Dargent, D.; Mathevet, P. Clinical significance of lympho vascular space involvement and lymph node micrometastases in early-stage cervical cancer: A retrospective case-control surgico-pathological study. *Gynecol. Oncol.* **2005**, *97*, 727–732. [CrossRef] [PubMed]
4. Bats, A.S.; Mathevet, P.; Buenerd, A.; Orliaguet, I.; Mery, E.; Zerdoud, S.; Le Frere-Belda, M.A.; Froissart, M.; Querleu, D.; Martinez, A.; et al. The sentinel node technique detects unexpected drainage pathways and allows nodal ultrastaging in early cervical cancer: Insights from the multicenter prospective SENTICOL study. *Ann. Surg. Oncol.* **2013**, *20*, 413–422. [CrossRef]
5. Kim, S.M.; Choi, H.S.; Byun, J.S. Overall 5-year survival rate and prognostic factors in patients with stage IB and IIA cervical cancer treated by radical hysterectomy and pelvic lymph node dissection. *Int. J. Gynecol. Cancer* **2000**, *10*, 305–312. [CrossRef] [PubMed]
6. Tanaka, Y.; Sawada, S.; Murata, T. Relationship between lymph node metastases and prognosis in patients irradiated postoperatively for carcinoma of the uterine cervix. *Acta. Radiol. Oncol.* **1984**, *23*, 455–459. [CrossRef]
7. Koh, W.J.; Abu-Rustum, N.R.; Bean, S.; Bradley, K.; Campos, S.M.; Cho, K.R.; Chon, H.S.; Chu, C.; Clark, R.; Cohn, D.; et al. Cervical Cancer, Version 3.2019, NCCN Clinical Practice Guidelines in Oncology. *J. Natl. Compr. Cancer Netw.* **2019**, *17*, 64–84. [CrossRef]
8. Bhatla, N.; Berek, J.S.; Cuello Fredes, M.; Denny, L.A.; Grenman, S.; Karunaratne, K.; Kehoe, S.T.; Konishi, I.; Olawaiye, A.B.; Prat, J.; et al. Revised FIGO staging for carcinoma of the cervix uteri. *Int. J. Gynaecol. Obstet.* **2019**, *145*, 129–135. [CrossRef]
9. Marth, C.; Landoni, F.; Mahner, S.; McCormack, M.; Gonzalez-Martin, A.; Colombo, N.; Committee, E.G. Cervical cancer: ESMO Clinical Practice Guidelines for diagnosis, treatment and follow-up. *Ann. Oncol.* **2018**, *29*, iv262. [CrossRef]
10. van de Lande, J.; Torrenga, B.; Raijmakers, P.G.; Hoekstra, O.S.; van Baal, M.W.; Brolmann, H.A.; Verheijen, R.H. Sentinel lymph node detection in early stage uterine cervix carcinoma: A systematic review. *Gynecol. Oncol.* **2007**, *106*, 604–613. [CrossRef]
11. Niikura, H.; Tsuji, K.; Tokunaga, H.; Shimada, M.; Ishikawa, M.; Yaegashi, N. Sentinel node navigation surgery in cervical and endometrial cancer: A review. *Jpn. J. Clin. Oncol.* **2019**, *49*, 495–500. [CrossRef]
12. Tax, C.; Rovers, M.M.; de Graaf, C.; Zusterzeel, P.L.; Bekkers, R.L. The sentinel node procedure in early stage cervical cancer, taking the next step; a diagnostic review. *Gynecol. Oncol.* **2015**, *139*, 559–567. [CrossRef] [PubMed]
13. Echt, M.L.; Finan, M.A.; Hoffman, M.S.; Kline, R.C.; Roberts, W.S.; Fiorica, J.V. Detection of sentinel lymph nodes with lymphazurin in cervical, uterine, and vulvar malignancies. *South Med. J.* **1999**, *92*, 204–208. [CrossRef] [PubMed]

14. Balaya, V.; Bresset, A.; Guani, B.; Magaud, L.; Montero Macias, R.; Delomenie, M.; Bonsang-Kitzis, H.; Ngo, C.; Bats, A.S.; Mathevet, P.; et al. Risk factors for failure of bilateral sentinel lymph node mapping in early-stage cervical cancer. *Gynecol. Oncol.* **2020**, *156*, 93–99. [CrossRef] [PubMed]
15. Sahbai, S.; Taran, F.A.; Staebler, A.; Wallwiener, D.; la Fougere, C.; Brucker, S.; Dittmann, H. Sentinel lymph node mapping using SPECT/CT and gamma probe in endometrial cancer: An analysis of parameters affecting detection rate. *Eur. J. Nucl. Med. Mol. Imaging* **2017**, *44*, 1511–1519. [CrossRef]
16. Weissinger, M.; Taran, F.A.; Gatidis, S.; Kommoss, S.; Nikolaou, K.; Sahbai, S.; Fougere, C.; Brucker, S.Y.; Dittmann, H. Lymph Node Staging with a Combined Protocol of (18)F-FDG PET/MRI and Sentinel Node SPECT/CT: A Prospective Study in Patients with FIGO I/II Cervical Carcinoma. *J. Nucl. Med.* **2021**, *62*, 1062–1067. [CrossRef]
17. Sakuragi, N.; Satoh, C.; Tanaka, T.; Horikawa, I.; Nishiya, M.; Ohkubo, H.; Hirahatake, K.; Ohkochi, T.; Iwakawa, Y.; Fujimoto, S. The incidence and clinical significance of paraaortic lymph node metastases in patients with uterine cervical cancer. *Nihon Sanka Fujinka Gakkai Zasshi* **1990**, *42*, 60–66.
18. Tsunoda, A.T.; Marnitz, S.; Soares Nunes, J.; de Cunha Andrade, C.E.M.; Scapulatempo Neto, C.; Blohmer, J.U.; Herrmann, J.; Kerr, L.M.; Martus, P.; Schneider, A.; et al. Incidence of Histologically Proven Pelvic and Para-Aortic Lymph Node Metastases and Rate of Upstaging in Patients with Locally Advanced Cervical Cancer: Results of a Prospective Randomized Trial. *Oncology* **2017**, *92*, 213–220. [CrossRef]
19. Diaz-Feijoo, B.; Perez-Benavente, M.A.; Cabrera-Diaz, S.; Gil-Moreno, A.; Roca, I.; Franco-Camps, S.; Fernandez, M.S.; Garcia-Jimenez, A.; Xercavins, J.; Martinez-Palones, J.M. Change in clinical management of sentinel lymph node location in early stage cervical cancer: The role of SPECT/CT. *Gynecol. Oncol.* **2011**, *120*, 353–357. [CrossRef]
20. Wang, X.; Zhong, X.; Lei, H.; Yang, N.; Gao, X.; Cheng, L. Tumor microenvironment-responsive contrast agents for specific cancer imaging: A narrative review. *J. Bio-X Res.* **2020**, *3*, 144–156. [CrossRef]
21. Liu, B.; Gao, S.; Li, S. A Comprehensive Comparison of CT, MRI, Positron Emission Tomography or Positron Emission Tomography/CT, and Diffusion Weighted Imaging-MRI for Detecting the Lymph Nodes Metastases in Patients with Cervical Cancer: A Meta-Analysis Based on 67 Studies. *Gynecol. Obstet. Investig.* **2017**, *82*, 209–222. [CrossRef]
22. Sarabhai, T.; Schaarschmidt, B.M.; Wetter, A.; Kirchner, J.; Aktas, B.; Forsting, M.; Ruhlmann, V.; Herrmann, K.; Umutlu, L.; Grueneisen, J. Comparison of (18)F-FDG PET/MRI and MRI for pre-therapeutic tumor staging of patients with primary cancer of the uterine cervix. *Eur. J. Nucl. Med. Mol. Imaging* **2018**, *45*, 67–76. [CrossRef] [PubMed]
23. Cysouw, M.C.F.; Kramer, G.M.; Hoekstra, O.S.; Frings, V.; de Langen, A.J.; Smit, E.F.; van den Eertwegh, A.J.; Oprea-Lager, D.E.; Boellaard, R. Accuracy and Precision of Partial-Volume Correction in Oncological PET/CT Studies. *J. Nucl. Med.* **2016**, *57*, 1642–1649. [CrossRef] [PubMed]
24. German Clinical Trials Register (DRKS). Available online: https://www.drks.de/drks_web/setLocale_EN.do (accessed on 27 August 2020).
25. Nogami, Y.; Banno, K.; Irie, H.; Iida, M.; Masugi, Y.; Murakami, K.; Aoki, D. Efficacy of 18-FDG PET-CT dual-phase scanning for detection of lymph node metastasis in gynecological cancer. *Anticancer Res.* **2015**, *35*, 2247–2253. [PubMed]
26. Minig, L.; Fagotti, A.; Scambia, G.; Salvo, G.; Patrono, M.G.; Haidopoulos, D.; Zapardiel, I.; Domingo, S.; Sotiropoulou, M.; Chisholm, G.; et al. Incidence of Lymph Node Metastases in Women with Low-Risk Early Cervical Cancer (<2 cm) without Lymph-Vascular Invasion. *Int. J. Gynecol. Cancer* **2018**, *28*, 788–793. [CrossRef]
27. Collarino, A.; Garganese, G.; Valdes Olmos, R.A.; Stefanelli, A.; Perotti, G.; Mirk, P.; Fragomeni, S.M.; Ieria, F.P.; Scambia, G.; Giordano, A.; et al. Evaluation of Dual-Timepoint (18) F-FDG PET/CT Imaging for Lymph Node Staging in Vulvar Cancer. *J. Nucl. Med.* **2017**, *58*, 1913–1918. [CrossRef]
28. Ma, S.Y.; See, L.C.; Lai, C.H.; Chou, H.H.; Tsai, C.S.; Ng, K.K.; Hsueh, S.; Lin, W.J.; Chen, J.T.; Yen, T.C. Delayed (18) F-FDG PET for detection of paraaortic lymph node metastases in cervical cancer patients. *J. Nucl. Med.* **2003**, *44*, 1775–1783.
29. Peppicelli, S.; Andreucci, E.; Ruzzolini, J.; Bianchini, F.; Calorini, L. FDG uptake in cancer: A continuing debate. *Theranostics* **2020**, *10*, 2944–2948. [CrossRef]
30. Stecco, A.; Buemi, F.; Cassara, A.; Matheoud, R.; Sacchetti, G.M.; Arnulfo, A.; Brambilla, M.; Carriero, A. Comparison of retrospective PET and MRI-DWI (PET/MRI-DWI) image fusion with PET/CT and MRI-DWI in detection of cervical and endometrial cancer lymph node metastases. *Radiol. Med.* **2016**, *121*, 537–545. [CrossRef]
31. Kim, S.K.; Choi, H.J.; Park, S.Y.; Lee, H.Y.; Seo, S.S.; Yoo, C.W.; Jung, D.C.; Kang, S.; Cho, K.S. Additional value of MR/PET fusion compared with PET/CT in the detection of lymph node metastases in cervical cancer patients. *Eur. J. Cancer* **2009**, *45*, 2103–2109. [CrossRef]

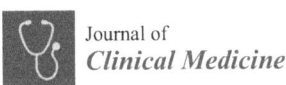

Article

Primary Staging of Prostate Cancer Patients with [^{18}F]PSMA-1007 PET/CT Compared with [^{68}Ga]Ga-PSMA-11 PET/CT

Manuela A. Hoffmann [1,2,*], Jonas Müller-Hübenthal [3], Florian Rosar [4], Nicolas Fischer [5], Finn Edler von Eyben [6], Hans-Georg Buchholz [2], Helmut J. Wieler [7] and Mathias Schreckenberger [2]

1 Department of Occupational Health & Safety, Federal Ministry of Defense, 53123 Bonn, Germany
2 Clinic of Nuclear Medicine, Johannes Gutenberg-University, 55101 Mainz, Germany
3 Practice of Radiology and Nuclear Medicine, Praxis im KölnTriangle, 50679 Cologne, Germany
4 Department of Nuclear Medicine, Saarland University Medical Center, 66421 Homburg, Germany
5 Clinic of Urology, Medical Center of Leverkusen, 51375 Leverkusen, Germany
6 Center for Tobacco Control Research, DK-5230 Odense, Denmark
7 Medical Center, University of Dusseldorf, 40225 Dusseldorf, Germany
* Correspondence: manhoffm@uni-mainz.de

Citation: Hoffmann, M.A.; Müller-Hübenthal, J.; Rosar, F.; Fischer, N.; von Eyben, F.E.; Buchholz, H.-G.; Wieler, H.J.; Schreckenberger, M. Primary Staging of Prostate Cancer Patients with [^{18}F]PSMA-1007 PET/CT Compared with [^{68}Ga]Ga-PSMA-11 PET/CT. *J. Clin. Med.* 2022, 11, 5064. https://doi.org/10.3390/jcm11175064

Academic Editors: Arnoldo Piccardo and Francesco Fiz

Received: 29 July 2022
Accepted: 23 August 2022
Published: 29 August 2022

Publisher's Note: MDPI stays neutral with regard to jurisdictional claims in published maps and institutional affiliations.

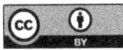

Copyright: © 2022 by the authors. Licensee MDPI, Basel, Switzerland. This article is an open access article distributed under the terms and conditions of the Creative Commons Attribution (CC BY) license (https://creativecommons.org/licenses/by/4.0/).

Abstract: Background: Hybrid imaging with prostate-specific membrane antigen (PSMA) is gaining importance as an increasingly meaningful tool for prostate cancer (PC) diagnostics and as a guide for therapy decisions. This study aims to investigate and compare the performance of [^{18}F]PSMA-1007 (^{18}F-PSMA) and [^{68}Ga]Ga-PSMA-11 positron emission tomography/computed tomography (^{68}Ga-PSMA) in the initial staging of PC patients. Methods: The data of 88 biopsy-proven patients were retrospectively evaluated. PSMA-avid lesions were compared with the histopathologic Gleason Score (GS) for prostate biopsies, and the results were plotted by receiver operating characteristic (ROC)-curve. Optimal maximum standardized uptake value (SUV_{max}) cut-off values were rated using the Youden index. Results: ^{18}F-PSMA was able to distinguish GS ≤ 7a from ≥7b with a sensitivity of 62%, specificity of 85%, positive predictive value (PPV) of 92%, and accuracy of 67% for a SUV_{max} of 8.95, whereas sensitivity was 54%, specificity 91%, PPV 93%, and accuracy 66% for ^{68}Ga-PSMA (SUV_{max} 8.7). Conclusions: Both methods demonstrated a high concordance of detected PSMA-avid lesions with histopathologically proven PC. ^{18}F-PSMA and ^{68}Ga-PSMA are both suitable for the characterization of primary PC with a comparable correlation of PSMA-avid lesions with GS. Neither method showed a superior advantage. Our calculated SUV_{max} thresholds may represent valuable parameters in clinical use to distinguish clinically significant PC (csPC) from non-csPC.

Keywords: PSMA hybrid imaging; staging of primary prostate cancer; [^{18}F]PSMA-1007; [^{68}Ga]Ga-PSMA-11; SUV_{max} cut-off level; prostate carcinoma

1. Introduction

Prostate carcinoma (PC) is the second most common tumor in men worldwide. Its predicted mortality rate in the European Union for 2020 is 10/100,000, which has decreased by 7.1% since 2015 due to advances in screening and treatment of the disease [1]. In particular, the early detection of PC and the early initiation of therapy have contributed significantly to the reduced mortality rate.

Current conventional imaging for PC, such as multiparametric magnetic resonance imaging (MRI) and computed tomography (CT), show limitations, especially in the primary diagnosis of lymph node metastases (LNM) [2]. Other diagnostic methods, such as positron emission tomography (PET), usually in combination with CT, are therefore used in PC diagnostics. The prospective, randomized multicenter study called "proPSMA" showed that in patients with biopsy-proven high-risk PC, PET/CT with prostate-specific membrane antigen (PSMA PET/CT) imaging is superior to conventional combined CT and bone scintigraphy for primary staging of PC metastases [2,3]. The transmembrane protein PSMA is particularly overexpressed in higher-grade prostate cancer cells and offers an optimal target for radiolabeled ligands [4]. One of the world's most commonly used PSMA inhibitors is the ^{68}Gallium(^{68}Ga)-labeled [^{68}Ga]Ga-HBED-CC-PSMA, also named [^{68}Ga]Ga-PSMA-11, which was also used in the Hofmann study [2,3,5]. Several other PSMA ligands for labeling with ^{68}Ga and ^{18}Fluorine (^{18}F) have been developed in recent years. In particular, the ^{18}F-labeled tracers will be further explored [2,4]. ^{18}F has a half-life of 110 min, whereas ^{68}Ga has one of 68 min, which is an advantage for the delivery of radiopharmaceuticals. An additional advantage of ^{18}F-labeled PSMA ligands is optimal positron energy, which enables higher resolution of PET images with refined image quality [2,4,6]. Currently, according to the European Association of Urology (EAU), European Association of Nuclear Medicine (EANM), European Society for Radiotherapy & Oncology (ESTRO), European Society of Urogenital Radiology (ESUR), the International Society of Urological Pathology (ISUP), and the International Society of Geriatric Oncology (SIOG) there are few comparative data on ^{18}F- with ^{68}Ga-labeled PSMA tracers in a clinical setting [2].

The goal of this study is to investigate and compare [^{18}F]PSMA-1007 PET/CT (^{18}F-PSMA) and [^{68}Ga]Ga-PSMA-11 PET/CT (^{68}Ga-PSMA) for the primary staging of PC patients and to distinguish between low- and intermediate-risk versus (vs.) high-risk PC as well as between low- and intermediate-favorable risk vs. intermediate-unfavorable and high-risk PC, using the best maximum standardized uptake value (SUV$_{max}$) cut-off value to identify clinically significant PC foci.

2. Materials and Methods

2.1. Study Design

Our investigation included 88 consecutive patients with elevated serum PSA levels and with biopsy-confirmed PC who underwent PSMA PET/CT for primary staging and specifically for the detection of possible metastases. For the retrospective analysis of the data, the datasets of patients who had received prior prostate therapy were excluded. The data for the period 2017 to 2021 were collected at a practice for Radiology and Nuclear Medicine in Cologne, Germany. Fifty-two patients underwent ^{18}F-PSMA, and thirty-six patients underwent ^{68}Ga-PSMA. The PSMA uptake of the ^{18}F-PSMA and of the ^{68}Ga-PSMA PET findings were quantified as SUV$_{max}$. The PSMA-positive lesions in the included patients were compared with histopathologic results of the prostate biopsies. A prostate biopsy was performed in all patients. PC was verified histologically with TRUS-guided or multiparametric MRI (mpMRI)-fusion guided prostate biopsy. In all patients, an adenocarcinoma of the prostate was histopathologically proven by biopsy. The biopsy results expressed as Gleason Score (GS) formed the reference basis for the PSMA PET/CT findings. Clinically significant PC (csPC) was defined as GS 7b-tumors or greater (any ISUP grade group $\geq$ 3) (subgroup: csPCa) and as GS 8-tumors or greater (any ISUP grade group $\geq$ 4) (subgroup: csPCb) [2].

2.2. Positron Emission Tomography/Computed Tomography Imaging Protocol and Interpretation

The study was performed using a PET/CT scanner (Gemini TF16; Philips Medical Systems, Best, The Netherlands). PET/CT images were acquired in 3D acquisition mode (matrix 168 × 168) 90 ± 10 min after intravenous injection of 326 ± 51.8 MBq [^{18}F]PSMA-1007 or 60 ± 10 min post injectionem (p.i.) of 257 ± 85.7 MBq [^{68}Ga]Ga-PSMA-11. PET images from the skull base to the proximal thigh were acquired for 3 min per bed position (axial field of view: 21.8 cm). A maximum inspiratory contrast-enhanced CT in the venous phase was performed in all included patients for attenuation correction and anatomical correlation. Decay, random, scatter, and attenuation correction were implemented. PET image reconstruction was carried out by using an ordered-subset expectation maximization (OSEM)-algorithm with 2 iterations and 14 subsets and Gaussian filtering with 4.2 mm transaxial resolution at full width at half maximum. Volumes of interest (VOIs) were drawn on the foci suspected of being malignant due to the PSMA distribution pattern on PET in consensus with CT imaging. Values for tracer uptake expressed as the SUV_{max} measured on the VOIs were plotted on a receiver operating characteristic (ROC) curve. The area under the ROC (AUC) as well as the best cut-off level for SUV_{max} to classify the VOIs were calculated. Two experienced board-certified nuclear medicine physicians and two experienced board-certified radiology physicians, each of them with more than 5 years of experience in PSMA PET/CT hybrid imaging, assessed the images by consensus.

2.3. Statistical Analysis

Numeric data are presented as median or mean ± standard deviation (SD). We evaluated the relationship between PSMA PET/CT positivity (e.g., expressed as SUV_{max}) and clinical parameters such as GS. To compare the two patient cohorts ^{18}F-PSMA and ^{68}Ga-PSMA and identify differences between them, we performed Student's *t*-tests for data that showed a normal distribution or nonparametric Mann–Whitney U tests for sample data that was not normally distributed. Using a ROC curve analyses, the performances of the procedures (^{18}F-PSMA and ^{68}Ga-PSMA) for distinguishing between PC with low- and intermediate-favorable risk vs. intermediate-unfavorable and high-risk as well as between low- and intermediate-risk vs. high-risk were calculated by plotting sensitivity against 1-specificity. Optimal SUV_{max} cut-off values were rated using the Youden index for the separate methods (^{18}F-PSMA and ^{68}Ga-PSMA). A *p* value < 0.05 was considered as statistically significant. We carried out the statistical analyses using SPSS version 27.0 (IBM SPSS Statistics Corporation, Ehningen, Germany).

3. Results

We identified 88 patients who underwent ^{18}F-PSMA (52) or ^{68}Ga-PSMA (36). The median age was 67.5 years (range 51–80 years) in the patient group of ^{18}F-PSMA and 65.5 years (range 48–79 years) in patients whose imaging was conducted with ^{68}Ga-PSMA. Clinical and pathological characteristics of the study population are summarized in Table 1.

Table 1. Patients' characteristics.

Clinical Variable	Value	Clinical Variable	Value
Number of [^{18}F]PSMA-1007 PET/CT patients	52	Number of [^{68}Ga]Ga-PSMA-11 PET/CT patients	36
Age		Age	
Median	67.5	Median	65.5
Range	51–80	Range	48–79
Mean ± SD	67.4 ± 7.7	Mean ± SD	65.8 ± 7.7
Gleason Score (GS)		Gleason Score (GS)	
GS 6 (low-risk + grade group 1)	3 / 5.8%	GS 6 (low-risk + grade group 1)	5 / 13.9%
GS 7a (low–intermediate or intermediate-favorable risk + grade group 2)	10 / 19.2%	GS 7a (low–intermediate or intermediate-favorable risk + grade group 2)	7 / 19.4%
GS 7b (high–intermediate or intermediate-unfavorable risk + grade group 3)	11 / 21.2%	GS 7b (high–intermediate or intermediate-unfavorable risk + grade group 3)	14 / 38.9%
GS 8 (high-risk + grade group 4)	8 / 15.4%	GS 8 (high-risk + grade group 4)	7 / 19.4%
GS > 8 (high-risk + grade group 5)	20 / 38.5%	GS > 8 (high-risk + grade group 5)	3 / 8.3%
PSA (ng/mL)		PSA (ng/mL)	
Median	8.8	Median	13.0
Range	2.68–167	Range	3.1–93
Positivity rate		Positivity rate	
PET/CT positive patients/total	52/52 / 100%	PET/CT positive patients/total	35/36 / 97.2%

Abbreviations: PSMA, prostate-specific membrane antigen; PET/CT, positron emission tomography/computed tomography; SD, standard deviation; y, year; PSA, prostate-specific antigen.

PSMA-avid lesions were found in all 52 study patients in the ^{18}F-PSMA cohort and in 97.2% (35/36) of the ^{68}Ga-PSMA cohort. The ^{18}F-PSMA scans detected prostatic lesions with elevated PSMA avidity in 100% (52/52), LNM in 32.7% (17/52), and bone metastases in 17.3% (9/52) of cases. A total of 35 out of 36 (97.2%) untreated patients, who underwent a ^{68}Ga-PSMA, showed lesions with an elevated tracer uptake in the prostate. ^{68}Ga-PSMA scans also detected LNM in 16.7% (6/36) and bone metastases in 8.4% (3/36) of cases. A total of 33 patients, who underwent ^{18}F-PSMA, demonstrated solitary PSMA tracer-positive prostatic lesions, whereas 26 patients showed them in the ^{68}Ga-PSMA group.

In our study, 5.8% (3/52) of PSMA-positive PET lesions, based on all patients with PSMA-positive findings, in the ^{18}F-PSMA cohort and 11.4% (4/35) in the ^{68}Ga-PSMA cohort were categorized as low-risk PC (GS < 7) with ISUP grade group 1. In one patient with a biopsy finding of GS 6, no increased PSMA avidity was detected in the PET/CT with [^{68}Ga]Ga-PSMA-11. Intermediate-risk PC (GS 7) with ISUP grade groups 2 and 3 occurred in 40.4% (21/52) of ^{18}F-PSMA-positive and in 60% (21/35) of ^{68}Ga-PSMA-positive patients, whereas 53.8% (28/52, ^{18}F-PSMA) and 28.6% (10/35, ^{68}Ga-PSMA) showed high-risk PC lesions with an ISUP grade group 4 to 5 (Table 2, Figures 1 and 2).

Table 2. PSMA-positive scan lesions for staging patients in relation to the Gleason Score (GS).

	GS < 7	GS 7a	GS 7b	GS 8	GS > 8	Chi^2, r
[^{18}F]PSMA-1007 PET/CT patients (52):						
PSMA positive (52/52)	3	10	11	8	20	
Prostatic lesions (52/52)	3/5.8%	10/19.2%	11/21.2%	8/15.4%	20/38.5%	
Metastases (19/52)	0	3/5.8%	3/5.8%	3/5.8%	10/19.2%	p =0.494 * r = 0.252
LNM (17/52)	0	2/3.8%	3/5.8%	3/5.8%	9/17.3%	p = 0.531 * r = 0.266
[^{68}Ga]Ga-PSMA-11 PET/CT patients (36):						
PSMA positive (35/36)	4	7	14	7	3	
Prostatic lesions (35/36)	4/11.4%	7/20%	14/40%	7/20%	3/8.6%	
Metastases (9/36)	0	0	3/8.6%	4/11.4%	2/5.7%	p =0.030 * r = 0.513
LNM (6/36)	0	0	2/5.7%	2/5.7%	2/5.7%	p = 0.086 * r = 0.442

* Fisher exact test. Abbreviations: PSMA, prostate-specific membrane antigen; PET/CT, positron emission tomography/computed tomography; LNM, Lymph node metastases; GS, Gleason Score; $p < 0.05$ is considered significant; r, Pearson correlation coefficient.

The 88 study patients were separately (^{18}F-PSMA and ^{68}Ga-PSMA) grouped into categories by GS and compared as follows: patients with GS 6 and GS 7 vs. patients with GS $\geq$ 8 and with GS 6 and GS 7a vs. patients with GS $\geq$ 7b (Figures 1 and 2).

In the ^{18}F-PSMA cohort, PC prostatic lesions with histopathology of low- and intermediate-favorable risk PC (GS $\leq$ 7a) were shown in 25% (13/52) compared to 75% (39/52) with histopathology of intermediate-unfavorable and high-risk PC (GS $\geq$ 7b) (Figure 1). PSMA-avid metastases and PSMA-positive LNM were shown in 5.8% with GS $\leq$ 7a (3/52) vs. 30.8% with GS $\geq$ 7b (16/52) and in 3.8% with GS $\leq$ 7a (2/52) vs. 28.8% (15/52) with GS $\geq$ 7b (Figure 1).

For the ^{68}Ga-PSMA cohort, the distribution of the PSMA-avid PC lesions in the prostate was as follows: 31.4% (11/35) with GS $\leq$ 7a vs. 68.6% (24/35) with GS $\geq$ 7b, respectively (Figure 2). Neither PSMA-positive metastases nor LNM were shown in the subgroup with GS $\leq$ 7a, whereas the subgroup with GS $\geq$ 7b revealed PSMA-avid metastases in 25.7% (9/35) of cases and positive LNM in 17.1% (6/35) (Figure 2).

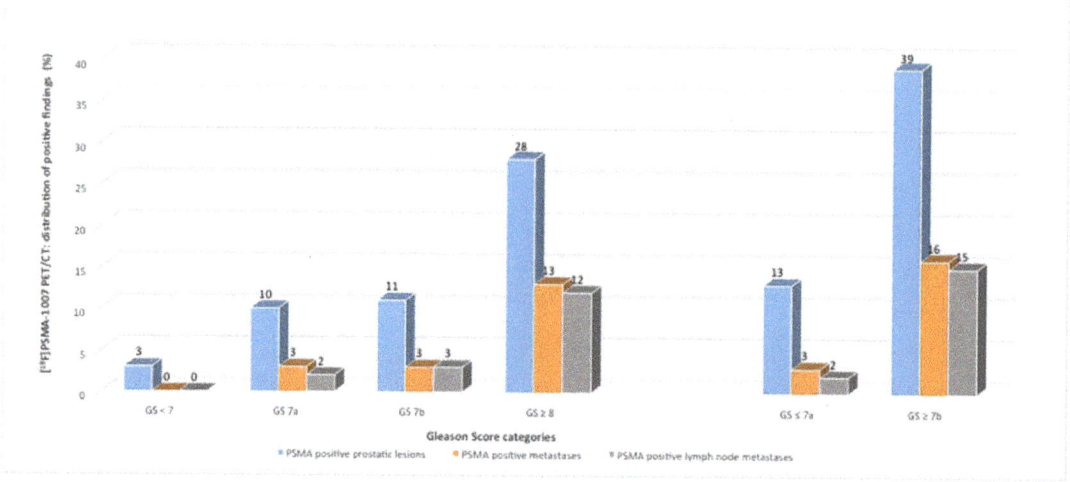

Figure 1. Distribution of positive findings (shown by [^{18}F]PSMA-1007 PET/CT) classified by Gleason Score (GS) categories (patients with GS < 7 to GS ≥ 8 and the comparison of GS ≤ 7a versus patients with GS ≥ 7b).

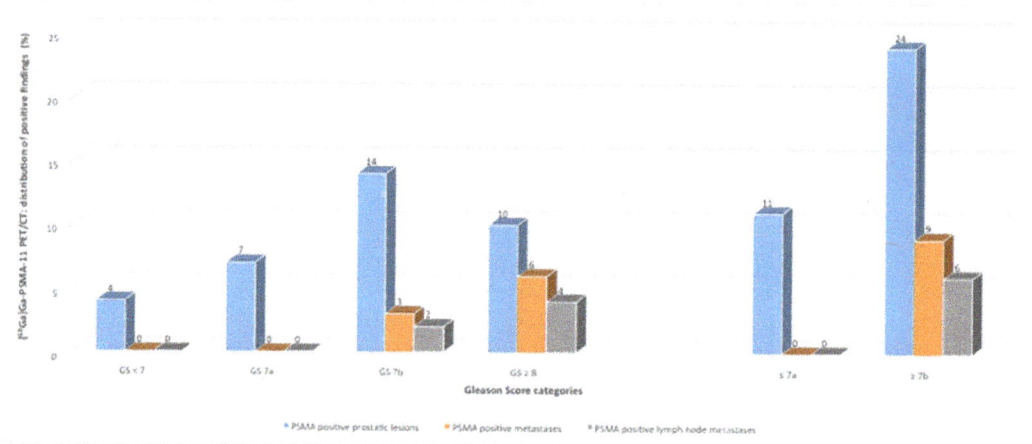

Figure 2. Distribution of positive findings (shown by [^{68}Ga]Ga-PSMA-11 PET/CT) classified by Gleason Score (GS) categories (patients with GS < 7 to GS ≥ 8 and the comparison of GS ≤ 7a versus patients with GS ≥ 7b).

The PSMA uptake of the [^{18}F]PSMA-1007 and of the [^{68}Ga]Ga-PSMA-11 PET findings was quantified as SUV_{max}. Comparing ^{18}F-PSMA and ^{68}Ga-PSMA scanned patients, there was no statistical significance for the differentiation of mean and median SUV_{max} for the most intense prostatic lesions (p = 0.224) (mean SUV_{max} ± SD: 12.2 ± 10.4 vs. 10.0 ± 8.0, median SUV_{max} 9.0 vs. 6.7).

When using a SUV_{max} of 2.5 as the cut-off value between PC lesions in the prostate with low- and intermediate-favorable risk (GS ≤ 7a) vs. with intermediate-unfavorable and high-risk (GS ≥ 7b), ^{18}F-PSMA indicated a sensitivity of 100%, a positive predictive value (PPV) of 76%, and an accuracy of 76% (Table 3). For ^{68}Ga-PSMA, the sensitivity was 97%, the PPV was 75%, and the accuracy was 77%, respectively (Table 3).

Table 3. Test parameters for the staging of prostate cancer with [^{18}F]PSMA-1007 PET/CT and with [^{68}Ga]Ga-PSMA-11 PET/CT; distribution of positive prostatic findings classified by Gleason Score (GS) categories (GS ≤ 7a versus GS ≥ 7b; GS ≤ 7 versus GS ≥ 8).

	GS ≤ 7a vs. ≥7b Cut-Off SUV_{max} 2.5		GS ≤ 7a vs. ≥7b Cut-Off SUV_{max} 8.95/SUV_{max} 8.7 *		GS ≤ 7 vs. ≥8 Cut-Off SUV_{max} 4.75/SUV_{max} 6.2 **	
	[^{18}F]PSMA-1007 PET/CT	[^{68}Ga]Ga-PSMA-11 PET/CT	[^{18}F]PSMA-1007 PET/CT	[^{68}Ga]Ga-PSMA-11 PET/CT	[^{18}F]PSMA-1007 PET/CT	[^{68}Ga]Ga-PSMA-11 PET/CT
Sensitivity	100%	97%	62%	54%	90%	89%
Specificity	10%	27%	85%	91%	52%	33%
NPV	100%	100%	42%	48%	73%	93%
PPV	76%	75%	92%	93%	61%	43%
Accuracy	76%	77%	67%	66%	63%	63%

Abbreviations: SUV_{max}, maximum standardized uptake value; vs., versus; PSMA, prostate-specific membrane antigen; PET/CT, positron emission tomography/computed tomography; NPV, negative predictive value; PPV, positive predictive value. * for [^{18}F]PSMA-1007 PET/CT SUV_{max} 8.95, [^{68}Ga]Ga-PSMA-11 PET/CT SUV_{max} 8.7. ** for [^{18}F]PSMA-1007 PET/CT SUV_{max} 4.75, [^{68}Ga]Ga-PSMA-11 PET/CT SUV_{max} 6.2.

Using the Youden index, the best analyzed cut-off value for ^{18}F-PSMA was a SUV_{max} of 8.95 (subgroup: ^{18}F-7a/b) for distinguishing GS ≤ 7a from GS ≥ 7b prostatic lesions. ROC analysis showed an AUC of 0.750 (95% Cl 0.590; 0.911; SD (AUC) = 0.082; p = 0.007) for the comparison with a SUV_{max} of 8.95 (^{18}F-7a/b). The sensitivity, the specificity, the PPV, and the accuracy for ^{18}F-7a/b was 62%, 85%, 92%, and 67%, respectively. For the differentiation of GS ≤ 7 from GS ≥ 8 (subgroup: ^{18}F-7/8) an AUC of 0.592 (95% Cl 0.539; 0.881; SD (AUC) = 0.055; p = 0.26) with a SUV_{max} of 4.75 (^{18}F-7/8) was evaluated with a sensitivity of 90%, a specificity of 52%, a PPV of 61%, and an accuracy of 63%, respectively (Table 3).

By means of ROC analysis, the best cut-off value for ^{68}Ga-PSMA was a SUV_{max} of 8.7 (subgroup: ^{68}Ga-7a/b) to differentiate GS ≤ 7a and GS ≥ 7b PC lesions (AUC = 0.814; 95% Cl 0.668; 0.961; SD (AUC) = 0.075; p = 0.003) with a sensitivity of 54%, a specificity of 91%, a PPV of 93%, and an accuracy of 66%. The best AUC for distinguishing GS ≤ 7 from GS ≥ 8 PC lesions was 0.710 (95% Cl 0.539; 0.881; SD (AUC) = 0.087; p = 0.055) with a SUV_{max} of 6.2 (subgroup: ^{68}Ga-7/8) and with a sensitivity of 89%, a specificity of 33%, a PPV of 43%, and an accuracy of 63% (Table 3).

Figure 3 shows a ^{18}F-PSMA with a histopathologically confirmed aggressive PC with a GS of 8 (4 + 4), without locoregional LNM and without skeletal metastases, but with three mediastinal LNM of normal size, located infracarinally and bilaterally hilar with a high PSMA avidity, and Figure 4 shows a ^{68}Ga-PSMA with a histopathologically confirmed aggressive PC with a GS of 8 (4 + 4) with locoregional LNM and without distant LNM and without skeletal metastases.

(a)

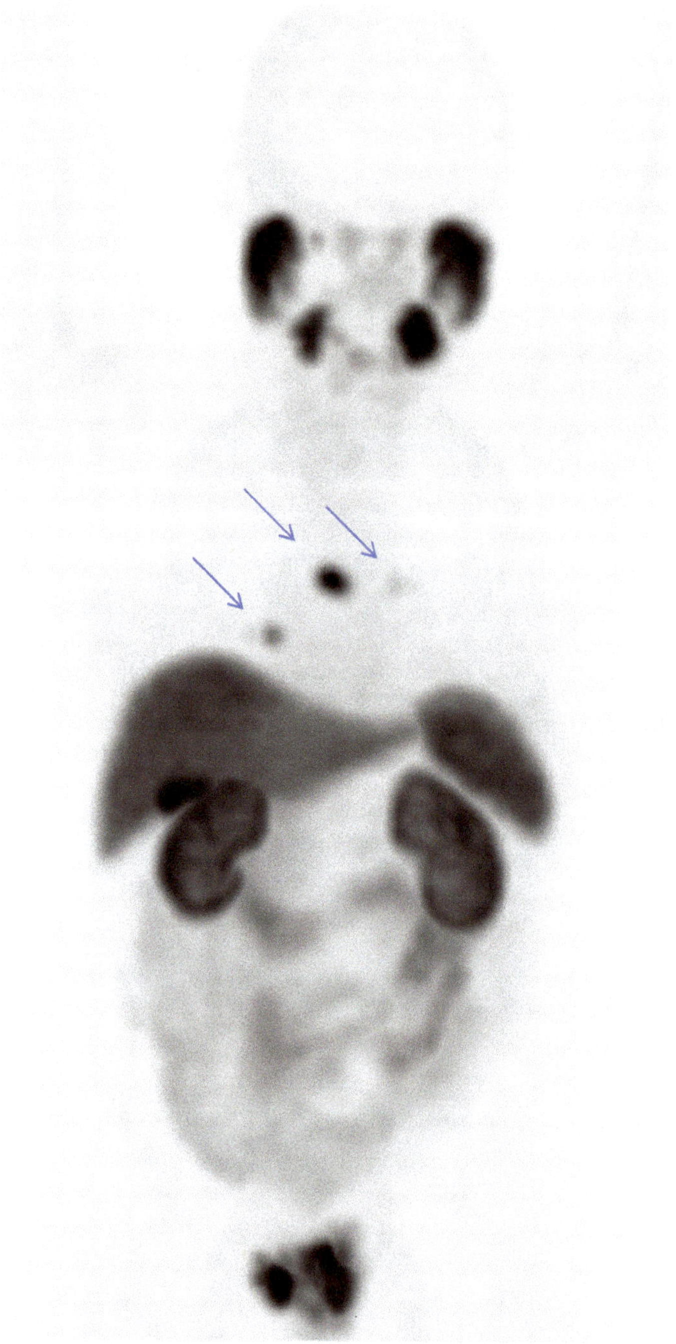

Figure 3. *Cont.*

(b)

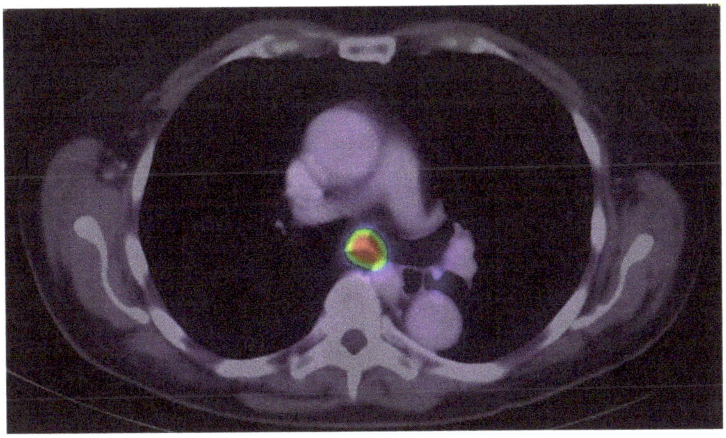

(c)

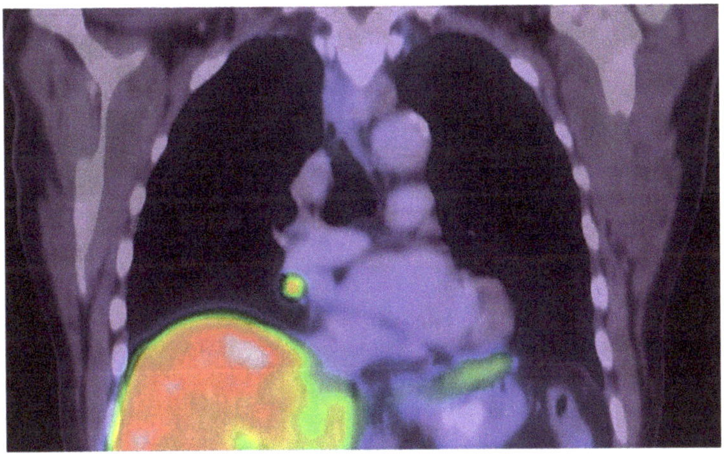

Figure 3. (a–c) Case study of a patient with evidence of a prostate-specific membrane antigen (PSMA)-avid prostatic finding in the initial staging (a) (with an initial prostate-specific antigen of 5.0 ng/mL) concordant with the histopathologically confirmed aggressive prostate carcinoma (PC) with a Gleason Score of 8 (4 + 4). The [^{18}F]PSMA-1007 positron emission tomography/computed tomography showed no locoregional lymph node metastases or skeletal metastases, but three mediastinal lymph nodes ((a): blue arrows) of normal size, located infracarinally (b) and bilaterally hilar ((c): hilar right), carrying intensive tracer uptake (the highest maximum standardized uptake value of 11.4), which were histopathologically confirmed as metastatic PC.

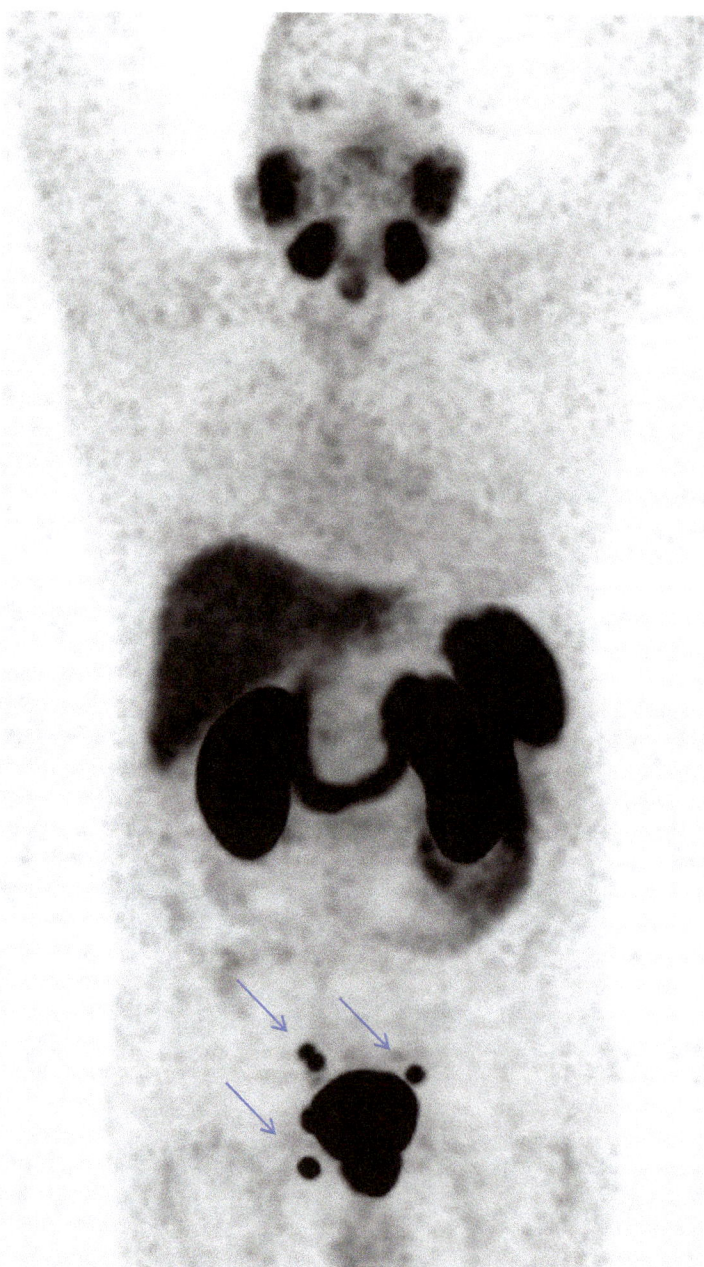

Figure 4. Case study of a patient with evidence of a prostate-specific membrane antigen (PSMA)-avid prostatic finding in the initial staging with an initial prostate-specific antigen of 13.0 ng/mL, concordant with the histopathologically confirmed aggressive prostate carcinoma (PC) with a Gleason Score of 8 (4 + 4). The [^{68}Ga]Ga-PSMA-11 positron emission tomography/computed tomography showed five locoregional lymph node metastases (blue arrows) carrying intensive tracer uptake (the highest maximum standardized uptake value of 19.4), which were histopathologically confirmed as metastatic PC.

4. Discussion

The EAU-EANM-ESTRO-ESUR-ISUP–SIOG Guidelines 2022 explicitly emphasize that most published studies on the primary staging of PC were based on ^{68}Ga-labeling for PSMA PET imaging, and few studies were based on ^{18}F labeling [2,7]. According to these guidelines, there are currently no conclusive data comparing ^{68}Ga-PSMA with ^{18}F-PSMA imaging in primary PC staging. In this context, the present study can possibly make a valuable contribution to the comparison of the two methods, ^{68}Ga-PSMA and ^{18}F-PSMA, in the clinical staging of PC.

In this comparative study of ^{68}Ga-PSMA vs. ^{18}F-PSMA in patients with newly diagnosed PC, we analyzed the PSMA-positive lesions that were determined to be malignant. PSMA-avid prostatic foci in concordance with histopathologically proven PC were found in all 52 study patients in the ^{18}F-PSMA cohort, while ^{68}Ga-PSMA showed them in 97.2% of the cohort (35/36). The imaging data for prostatic lesions were compared with histopathologic prostate biopsy results expressed as GS. Our results showed concordant findings with both tracers, which is in line with other studies comparing ^{18}F-PSMA and ^{68}Ga-PSMA in primary staging [8–10]. Kuten et al. reported in a head-to-head comparison that the identification of all intermediate- and high-risk PC lesions was comparable by both methods [8]. Hoberück et al. described, in a retrospective intraindividual comparison, that ^{18}F- as well as ^{68}Ga-PSMA appeared largely interchangeable, with neither tracer significantly outperforming the other [9]. The authors described that no significant difference considering SUV$_{max}$ of tumor lesions was shown [9]. A prospective intraindividual comparative study on ^{18}F-PSMA and ^{68}Ga-PSMA for PC staging, evaluation at biochemical recurrence and assessment of metastatic disease, by Pattison et al. demonstrated a high concordance of 92% for TNM stage [10]. Further studies confirmed similar findings in PSMA PET/CT imaging with the two radiopharmaceuticals in the setting of restaging PC patients, too [11,12]. Rauscher et al. showed similar detection rates in patients with biochemical recurrence after radical prostatectomy. However, five times as many positive findings of benign origin were found in ^{18}F-PSMA compared with ^{68}Ga-PSMA [11]. The side-by-side evaluation specifically requested by the authors for the ^{18}F-PSMA diagnosis of PET and CT images as well as intensive reader training on well-known pitfalls (for example, non-specific tracer uptake in the ganglia) in the clinical context [11] was implemented in a quality-assured manner by the diagnostic specialists in our present study. In a further restaging study by Hoffmann et al., both methods (^{18}F-PSMA and ^{68}Ga-PSMA) showed comparable overall findings [12]. Exceptions to this, however, were a clearer distinction between positive and negative results in the ^{18}F-PSMA imaging considering a PSA threshold, determined in the study, in biochemical recurrent patients after radical prostatectomy [12]. However, Rahbar et al. described on the basis of patient images that ^{18}F-PSMA offers an advantage over imaging with ^{68}Ga-PSMA for the detection of local recurrence after primary local therapy due to the later renal tracer excretion. The authors related this advantage to case constellations with unclear lesions near the ureter or the urinary bladder [13]. Renal excretion of ^{68}Ga-PSMA and radioactive bladder filling obscures local recurrence in the situation of biochemical recurrence but is of less relevance in initial tumor staging as in our study. Considering the comparison of ^{68}Ga-PSMA and the PET/CT with another ^{18}F-labeled radiotracer, named [^{18}F]rhPSMA-7 (^{18}F-rhPSMA-7), a study by Kroenke et al. showed similar tumor positivity rates and SUV$_{max}$ values for primary PC and biochemical recurrence of PC [7,14]. Giesel conducted a comparative study considering different ^{18}F-labeled PSMA PET ligands. The comparison of [^{18}F]DCFPyl PET/CT (^{18}F-DCFPyl) with ^{18}F-PSMA also showed no significant differences in the detection of carcinoma foci or their SUV$_{max}$ values [6].

In order to improve underdetection of high-grade PC and overdetection of low-grade PC [2,4], it makes sense to define a separation sharpness for the clinical setting. The cancer patients who would not benefit from a therapy should be considered separately from the patients with expected therapy success. The EAU-EANM-ESTRO-ESUR-ISUP–SIOG Guidelines 2022 do not specify how the term csPC should be defined exactly [2]. The guidelines report that studies mostly define GS 7 tumors and upwards or GS 7b tumors and upwards as clinically significant and that authors should decide for themselves and explain this in the study design [2]. In our study, we defined in one patient subgroup csPCa as any ISUP grade group ≥ 3 malignancy (patients with the high–intermediate or intermediate-unfavorable PC risk of GS 7b and above) and in a second patient subgroup csPCb as any ISUP grade group ≥ 4 malignancy (patients with the high PC risk of GS 8 and above), in order to then be able to compare both groups. Our study mainly focused on analyzing the best SUV_{max} cut-off value to identify the clinically significant PC foci and to compare the results of both methods. PSMA-avid lesions were defined as suspicious of malignancy when the uptake of the tracer was significantly higher than the surrounding benign tissue, when the tracer uptake appeared focal in character, and when the lesions were classified as primarily malignant (in the opinion of experts based on their extensive experience in the interpretation of PSMA PET/CT scans). Experience has shown that suspicious PET lesions with a SUV_{max} of 2.5 or higher were mostly associated with compatible and duplicatable visual evidence of PC foci and, therefore, this value was initially used as a cut-off to distinguish between PET positivity and negativity for both radiopharmaceuticals. Because the tumor-to-background ratio for the malignant lesions compared with the benign tissue in the PSMA PET/CT is very high according to previous studies (e.g., in comparison to FDG PET/CT, [15]) and the difference in the detected lesions was clearly shown in the present study, we did not list the SUV_{mean} values separately, as this would have no added value.

First, choosing a routinely used SUV_{max} of 2.5 as the cut-off value between csPC and clinically insignificant PC, the findings of both methods demonstrated similar concordance in our study. ^{18}F-PSMA revealed 25% (13/52) of PC prostatic lesions with histopathology of low- and intermediate-favorable risk PC (GS $\leq$ 7a) vs. 75% (39/52) with histopathology of intermediate-unfavorable and high-risk PC (GS $\geq$ 7b) with a sensitivity of 100%, a PPV of 76%, and an accuracy of 76% considering a SUV_{max} of 2.5. For ^{68}Ga-PSMA, the results were 31.4% (11/35) vs. 68.6% (24/35) with a sensitivity of 97%, a PPV of 75%, and an accuracy of 77% with the uptake of the radiotracer above a SUV_{max} of 2.5. In the present study, because the specificity of both methods was extremely low (10% vs. 27%) using a SUV_{max} threshold of 2.5, an optimal SUV_{max} cut-off value was determined for ^{18}F-PSMA and for ^{68}Ga-PSMA by Youden index calculation. The reasons for reduced specificity in PSMA imaging are well known and include neovascularization and PSMA overexpression in non-prostatic tissue, e.g., benign neoplasms, i.e., thyroid and parathyroid adenomas, and in non-prostatic malignancies such as breast cancer, thyroid cancer, gliomas, lung cancer, neuroendocrine tumors, lymphoma, and renal cell carcinoma. There are fewer false positives if the PSMA images are interpreted by experts who are aware of the various pitfalls [16].

Subsequently, ROC curves were used to characterize the diagnostic performance. By considering the PSMA-avid prostatic lesions and the corresponding classification in the GS based on the biopsy, a SUV_{max} of 8.95 was analyzed by ROC analysis ($p = 0.007$) to differentiate between csPC and clinically insignificant PC (subgroup: csPCa) for ^{18}F-PMSA with a sensitivity of 62%, a specificity of 85%, a PPV of 92%, and an accuracy of 67%. ^{68}Ga-PSMA gave similar findings for a SUV_{max} of 8.7 ($p = 0.003$) with a sensitivity of 54%, a specificity of 91%, a PPV of 93%, and an accuracy of 66%, respectively. However, our data show a higher (but also moderate) specificity and a higher PPV for ^{18}F-PSMA (52% and 61% based on a SUV_{max} of 4.75) in comparison with ^{68}Ga-PSMA (33% and 43% based on a SUV_{max} of 6.2), when differentiating between low- and intermediate-risk PC vs. high-risk PC (subgroup: csPCb), with comparable sensitivity (90% vs. 89%) and accuracy (63% both). But these data did not show statistical significance (SUV_{max} of 4.75, $p = 0.26$ and SUV_{max} of 6.2, $p = 0.055$). Kuten et al. calculated ROC curves to distinguish pathological from non-pathological components of the prostate, for which both methods proved to be suitable [8]. A comparison of the results with our calculated values is not possible because the comparison groups differ. Additionally, due to the lack of statistical significance, no optimal SUV_{max} values could be calculated in the study by Kuten et al. [8].

The results of diagnostic PSMA imaging as part of the staging of PC offer the possibility of guiding biopsy and therapy management to detect the targeted PC lesions with the most aggressive tumor foci (csPC) [17,18]. A mpMRI in combination with a PSMA hybrid imaging fusion biopsy could increase the accuracy of directed biopsy [18]. Pepe et al. demonstrated a lower false positive rate and a better negative predictive value compared with mpMRI. In 80% of the cases, a biopsy could have been omitted based on the PSMA PET/CT results [18]. As part of individual therapy management, hybrid imaging with PSMA PET/CT enables optimal patient selection as well as personalized monitoring [17]. In this regard, our calculated SUV_{max} cut-offs can be used to differentiate between low- and intermediate-favorable from intermediate-unfavorable and high-risk PC lesions. The more we know about diagnostic imaging (such as the correlation between PSMA receptor density and GS as well as PSMA imaging with different radiopharmaceuticals and their physiological expression in non-prostatic benign tissue and non-prostatic tumors, both benign and malignant) and can optimize it, the better therapy decisions can be made [17]. Because present EAU Guidelines state that there is currently no conclusive data comparing ^{68}Ga-PSMA vs. ^{18}F-PSMA imaging in primary PC staging [2], we investigated this. The comparison could not show any clear advantage for one of the methods in our study, which is also an important statement for clinical application. In all 52 study patients in the ^{18}F-PSMA cohort and in 97.2% (35/36) of the patients in the ^{68}Ga-PSMA cohort, PSMA-avid prostate lesions were detected concordant with histopathologically proven PC. PSMA-positive metastases were shown in 5.8% (3/52) in the intermediate-favorable risk ^{18}F-PSMA cohort vs. in 30.8% (16/52) in the intermediate-unfavorable risk group, but no PSMA-avid metastases (0/35) were seen in the ^{68}Ga-PSMA intermediate-favorable risk cohort vs. 25.7% (9/35) with GS $\geq$ 7b. In view of the nearly similar results and the good performance of ^{18}F- as well as ^{68}Ga-labeled compounds, the challenge for the use of the appropriate radiopharmaceutical could potentially be made depending on availability [12]. Nevertheless, further studies are needed to assess the position of routinely established ^{68}Ga- and ^{18}F-labeled compounds in PSMA imaging and their actual clinical utility. These will be carried out on the different radiotracers in order to shed light on new aspects, the overall impact on survival, and the clinical impact of PSMA-based diagnostics such as PSMA-targeted biopsies [7,18]. In this context, a randomized study that would perform a combined PSMA imaging with a mpMRI as a guide for prostate biopsy in the initial stage with a high suspicion of csPC and would consider different radiotracers might be useful [19–22]. Limitations of the present study include the retrospective nature of the analysis, the small number of patients, and the lack of an intraindividual comparison of the patients. To confirm and expand our results we recommend further studies, ideally prospective with larger patient cohorts.

5. Conclusions

^{18}F-PSMA and ^{68}Ga-PSMA both show promising results in the detection of newly diagnosed PC with comparable correlation of PSMA-avid lesions with GS. Neither method showed an outstanding superior advantage. Studies reporting ^{18}F-PSMA and ^{68}Ga-PSMA are equally relevant for the staging of patients with PC. With regard to both methods, the importance of PSMA imaging for the detection of metastases is also clear in primary staging, especially in patients with high-risk and intermediate-unfavorable risk PC. Our calculated thresholds for the SUV_{max} value may represent valuable parameters in clinical use for the discrimination of csPC from non-csPC and may also serve to guide prostate biopsies and support the identification of aggressive PC foci.

Author Contributions: Conceptualization, M.A.H., J.M.-H., F.R., N.F. and M.S.; methodology, M.A.H., J.M.-H., F.R., N.F. and M.S.; software, M.A.H., J.M.-H., N.F. and H.-G.B.; validation, M.A.H., J.M.-H., F.R., N.F., H.-G.B., H.J.W. and M.S.; formal analysis, M.A.H., F.R., N.F., F.E.v.E., H.-G.B. and H.J.W.; investigation, M.A.H., J.M.-H., F.R. and H.J.W.; resources, M.A.H., J.M.-H., H.-G.B. and H.J.W.; data curation, J.M.-H., F.R., H.J.W. and M.S.; writing—original draft preparation, M.A.H., J.M.-H., F.R., N.F., H.-G.B. and M.S.; writing—review and editing, F.E.v.E., H.J.W. and M.S.; visualization, M.A.H.,

J.M.-H., H.-G.B. and M.S.; supervision, H.J.W. and M.S.; project administration, M.A.H., J.M.-H., F.R., N.F., H.J.W. and M.S. All authors have read and agreed to the published version of the manuscript.

Funding: This research received no external funding.

Institutional Review Board Statement: The study was conducted in accordance with the Declaration of Helsinki and the German Medicinal Products Act, § 13.2b. The Ethics Committee of the Medical Association North Rhine (Aekno) (protocol code 41/2019, approval date: 22 February 2019) approved the study.

Informed Consent Statement: Informed consent was obtained from all subjects involved in the study. All patients signed an informed consent (including evaluation and publication of their anonymized data).

Data Availability Statement: The datasets analyzed during the current study are available from the Practice of Radiology and Nuclear Medicine in Cologne/Germany, named "Praxis im KölnTriangle" upon reasonable request.

Acknowledgments: The authors wish to express their gratitude to Ed Michaelson, of Fort Lauderdale, Florida, USA, for language revision.

Conflicts of Interest: The authors declare no conflict of interest.

References

1. Carioli, G.; Bertuccio, P.; Boffetta, P.; Levi, F.; La Vecchia, C.; Negri, E.; Malvezzi, M. European cancer mortality predictions for the year 2020 with a focus on prostate cancer. *Ann. Oncol.* **2020**, *31*, 650–658. [CrossRef] [PubMed]
2. *EAU Guidelines*; Edn. Presented at the EAU Annual Congress Amsterdam 2022; European Association of Urology (EAU) Guidelines Office: Arnhem, The Netherlands; 2022. ISBN 978-94-92671-16-5. Available online: https://uroweb.org/guidelines/compilations-of-all-guidelines/ (accessed on 16 July 2022).
3. Hofman, M.S.; Lawrentschuk, N.; Francis, R.J.; Tang, C.; Vela, I.; Thomas, P.; Rutherford, N.; Martin, J.M.; Frydenberg, M.; Shakher, R.; et al. Prostate-specific membrane antigen PET-CT in patients with high-risk prostate cancer before curative-intent surgery or radiotherapy (proPSMA): A prospective, randomised, multicentre study. *Lancet* **2020**, *395*, 1208–1216. [CrossRef]
4. Hoffmann, M.A.; Wieler, H.J.; Baues, C.; Kuntz, N.J.; Richardsen, I.; Schreckenberger, M. The Impact of 68Ga-PSMA PET/CT and PET/MRI on the Management of Prostate Cancer. *Urology* **2019**, *130*, 1–12. [CrossRef] [PubMed]
5. Coenen, H.H.; Gee, A.D.; Adam, M.; Antoni, G.; Cutler, C.S.; Fujibayashi, Y.; Jeong, J.M.; Mach, R.H.; Mindt, T.L.; Pike, V.W.; et al. Open letter to journal editors on: International Consensus Radiochemistry Nomenclature Guidelines. *EJNMMI Radiopharm. Chem.* **2019**, *4*, 7. [CrossRef] [PubMed]
6. Giesel, F.L.; Will, L.; Lawal, I.; Lengana, T.; Kratochwil, C.; Vorster, M.; Neels, O.; Reyneke, F.; Haberkorn, U.; Kopka, K.; et al. Intraindividual Comparison of ^{18}F-PSMA-1007 and ^{18}F-DCFPyL PET/CT in the Prospective Evaluation of Patients with Newly Diagnosed Prostate Carcinoma: A Pilot Study. *J. Nucl. Med.* **2018**, *59*, 1076–1080. [CrossRef]
7. Werner, R.A.; Derlin, T.; Lapa, C.; Sheikbahaei, S.; Higuchi, T.; Giesel, F.L.; Behr, S.; Drzezga, A.; Kimura, H.; Buck, A.K.; et al. ^{18}F-Labeled, PSMA-Targeted Radiotracers: Leveraging the Advantages of Radiofluorination for Prostate Cancer Molecular Imaging. *Theranostics* **2020**, *10*, 1–16. [CrossRef]
8. Kuten, J.; Fahoum, I.; Savin, Z.; Shamni, O.; Gitstein, G.; Hershkovitz, D.; Mabjeesh, N.J.; Yossepowitch, O.; Mishani, E.; Even-Sapir, E. Head-to-Head Comparison of ^{68}Ga-PSMA-11 with ^{18}F-PSMA-1007 PET/CT in Staging Prostate Cancer Using Histopathology and Immunohistochemical Analysis as a Reference Standard. *J. Nucl. Med.* **2020**, *61*, 527–532. [CrossRef]
9. Hoberück, S.; Löck, S.; Borkowetz, A.; Sommer, U.; Winzer, R.; Zöphel, K.; Fedders, D.; Michler, E.; Kotzerke, J.; Kopka, K.; et al. Intraindividual comparison of [^{68}Ga]-Ga-PSMA-11 and [^{18}F]-F-PSMA-1007 in prostate cancer patients: A retrospective single-center analysis. *EJNMMI Res.* **2021**, *11*, 109. [CrossRef]
10. Pattison, D.A.; Debowski, M.; Gulhane, B.; Arnfield, E.G.; Pelecanos, A.M.; Garcia, P.L.; Latter, M.J.; Lin, C.Y.; Roberts, M.J.; Ramsay, S.C.; et al. Prospective intra-individual blinded comparison of [^{18}F]PSMA-1007 and [^{68}Ga]Ga-PSMA-11 PET/CT imaging in patients with confirmed prostate cancer. *Eur. J. Nucl. Med. Mol. Imaging.* **2022**, *49*, 763–776. [CrossRef]
11. Rauscher, I.; Krönke, M.; König, M.; Gafita, A.; Maurer, T.; Horn, T.; Schiller, K.; Weber, W.; Eiber, M. Matched-Pair Comparison of ^{68}Ga-PSMA-11 PET/CT and ^{18}F-PSMA-1007 PET/CT: Frequency of Pitfalls and Detection Efficacy in Biochemical Recurrence After Radical Prostatectomy. *J. Nucl. Med.* **2020**, *61*, 51–57. [CrossRef]
12. Hoffmann, M.A.; von Eyben, F.E.; Fischer, N.; Rosar, F.; Müller-Hübenthal, J.; Buchholz, H.G.; Wieler, H.J.; Schreckenberger, M. Comparison of [^{18}F]PSMA-1007 with [^{68}Ga]Ga-PSMA-11 PET/CT in Restaging of Prostate Cancer Patients with PSA Relapse. *Cancers* **2022**, *14*, 1479. [CrossRef] [PubMed]
13. Rahbar, K.; Weckesser, M.; Ahmadzadehfar, H.; Schäfers, M.; Stegger, L.; Bögemann, M. Advantage of ^{18}F-PSMA-1007 over ^{68}Ga-PSMA-11 PET imaging for differentiation of local recurrence vs. urinary tracer excretion. *Eur. J. Nucl. Med. Mol. Imaging.* **2018**, *45*, 1076–1077. [CrossRef] [PubMed]

14. Kroenke, M.; Mirzoyan, L.; Horn, T.; Peeken, J.C.; Wurzer, A.; Wester, H.-J.; Makowski, M.; Weber, W.A.; Eiber, M.; Rauscher, I. Matched-Pair Comparison of ^{68}Ga-PSMA-11 and ^{18}F-rhPSMA-7 PET/CT in Patients with Primary and Biochemical Recurrence of Prostate Cancer: Frequency of Non-Tumor-Related Uptake and Tumor Positivity. *J. Nucl. Med.* **2021**, *62*, 1082–1088. [CrossRef] [PubMed]
15. Zhou, X.; Li, Y.; Jiang, X.; Wang, X.; Chen, S.; Shen, T.; You, J.; Lu, H.; Liao, H.; Li, Z.; et al. Intra-Individual Comparison of ^{18}F-PSMA-1007 and ^{18}F-FDG PET/CT in the Evaluation of Patients with Prostate Cancer. *Front. Oncol.* **2021**, *10*, 585213. [CrossRef] [PubMed]
16. Malan, N.; Vangu, M.-d.-T. Normal Variants, Pitfalls, and Artifacts in Ga-68 Prostate Specific Membrane Antigen (PSMA) PET/CT Imaging. *Front. Nucl. Med.* **2022**, *2*, 825512. [CrossRef]
17. Kaewput, C.; Vinjamuri, S. Update of PSMA Theranostics in Prostate Cancer: Current Applications and Future Trends. *J. Clin. Med.* **2022**, *11*, 2738. [CrossRef]
18. Pepe, P.; Roscigno, M.; Pepe, L.; Panella, P.; Tamburo, M.; Marletta, G.; Savoca, F.; Candiano, G.; Cosentino, S.; Ippolito, M.; et al. Could 68Ga-PSMA PET/CT Evaluation Reduce the Number of Scheduled Prostate Biopsies in Men Enrolled in Active Surveillance Protocols? *J. Clin. Med.* **2022**, *11*, 3473. [CrossRef]
19. Emmett, L.; Buteau, J.; Papa, N.; Moon, D.; Thompson, J.; Roberts, M.J.; Rasiah, K.; Pattison, D.A.; Yaxley, J.; Thomas, P.; et al. The Additive Diagnostic Value of Prostate-specific Membrane Antigen Positron Emission Tomography Computed Tomography to Multiparametric Magnetic Resonance Imaging Triage in the Diagnosis of Prostate Cancer (PRIMARY): A Prospective Multicentre Study. *Eur. Urol.* **2021**, *80*, 682–689. [CrossRef]
20. Kesch, C.; Vinsensia, M.; Radtke, J.P.; Schlemmer, H.P.; Heller, M.; Ellert, E.; Holland-Letz, T.; Duensing, S.; Grabe, N.; Afshar-Oromieh, A.; et al. Intraindividual Comparison of ^{18}F-PSMA-1007 PET/CT, Multiparametric MRI, and Radical Prostatectomy Specimens in Patients with Primary Prostate Cancer: A Retrospective, Proof-of-Concept Study. *J. Nucl. Med.* **2017**, *58*, 1805–1810. [CrossRef]
21. Wang, X.; Wen, Q.; Zhang, H.; Ji, B. Head-to-Head Comparison of ^{68}Ga-PSMA-11 PET/CT and Multiparametric MRI for Pelvic Lymph Node Staging Prior to Radical Prostatectomy in Patients with Intermediate to High-Risk Prostate Cancer: A Meta-Analysis. *Front. Oncol.* **2021**, *11*, 737989. [CrossRef]
22. Ling, S.W.; de Jong, A.C.; Schoots, I.G.; Nasserinejad, K.; Busstra, M.B.; van der Veldt, A.; Brabander, T. Comparison of ^{68}Ga-labeled Prostate-specific Membrane Antigen Ligand Positron Emission Tomography/Magnetic Resonance Imaging and Positron Emission Tomography/Computed Tomography for Primary Staging of Prostate Cancer: A Systematic Review and Meta-analysis. *Eur. Urol. Open Sci.* **2021**, *33*, 61–71. [CrossRef] [PubMed]

Article

Functional Investigation of the Tumoural Heterogeneity of Intrahepatic Cholangiocarcinoma by In Vivo PET-CT Navigation: A Proof-of-Concept Study

Luca Viganò [1,2,*,†], Egesta Lopci [3,†], Luca Di Tommaso [2,4], Annarita Destro [4], Alessio Aghemo [2,5], Lorenza Rimassa [2,6], Luigi Solbiati [2,7], Arturo Chiti [2,5], Guido Torzilli [2,8] and Francesco Fiz [3,9]

1. Hepatobiliary Unit, Department of Minimally Invasive General & Oncologic Surgery, Humanitas Gavazzeni University Hospital, Viale M. Gavazzeni 21, 24125 Bergamo, Italy
2. Department of Biomedical Sciences, Humanitas University, Viale Rita Levi Montalcini 4, 20090 Milan, Italy
3. Department of Nuclear Medicine, Humanitas Research Hospital—IRCCS, 20089 Milan, Italy
4. Pathology Unit, Humanitas Research Hospital—IRCCS, 20089 Milan, Italy
5. Department of Internal Medicine, Division of Internal Medicine and Hepatology, Humanitas Research Hospital—IRCCS, 20089 Milan, Italy
6. Medical Oncology and Hematology Unit, Humanitas Research Hospital—IRCCS, 20089 Milan, Italy
7. Department of Radiology, Humanitas Research Hospital—IRCCS, 20089 Milan, Italy
8. Department of Surgery, Division of Hepatobiliary and General Surgery, Humanitas Research Hospital—IRCCS, 20089 Milan, Italy
9. Department of Nuclear Medicine and Clinical Molecular Imaging, University Hospital, 72076 Tübingen, Germany

* Correspondence: luca.vigano@hunimed.eu; Tel.: +39-035-4204326; Fax: +39-035-4204944
† These authors contributed equally to this work.

Abstract: Intra-tumoural heterogeneity (IH) is a major determinant of resistance to therapy and outcomes but remains poorly translated into clinical practice. Intrahepatic cholangiocarcinoma (ICC) often presents as large heterogeneous masses at imaging. The present study proposed an innovative in vivo technique to functionally assess the IH of ICC. Preoperative 18F-FDG PET-CT and intraoperative ultrasonography were merged to perform the intraoperative navigation of functional tumour heterogeneity. The tumour areas with the highest and the lowest metabolism (SUV) at PET-CT were selected, identified during surgery, and sampled. Three consecutive patients underwent the procedure. The areas with the highest uptake at PET-CT had higher proliferation index (KI67) values and higher immune infiltration compared to areas with the lowest uptake. One of the patients showed a heterogeneous presence of FGFR2 translocation within the samples. Tumour heterogeneity at PET-CT may drive biopsy to sample the most informative ICC areas. Even more relevant, these preliminary data show the possibility of achieving a non-invasive evaluation of IH in ICC, paving the way for an imaging-based precision-medicine approach.

Keywords: intra-tumoural heterogeneity; intrahepatic cholangiocarcinoma; positron emission tomography–computed tomography; immunology; FGFR2 translocation; imaging fusion; navigation technology

1. Introduction

Intra-tumoural heterogeneity (IH) is regarded as a major determinant of resistance to therapy and patients' prognosis but remains poorly translated into clinical practice [1–3]. The evaluation of IH has been mostly determined from the laboratory analyses of resected specimens, while, more recently, much of the research has been concentrated on imaging. The possibility of achieving a non-invasive mapping of IH is extremely appealing, because it would allow a better characterisation of the tumour (IH-based biopsies), a more precise prediction of prognosis, and a more effective treatment (IH-based therapies). Progress in medical imaging modalities open new opportunities for the investigation of IH. Positron emission tomography–computed tomography (PET-CT) offers unique functional imaging of liver tumours [4–6]. Navigation technology systems [7,8] may merge different imaging modalities (morphologic and functional ones) to optimise the identification of the different tumour areas.

Among liver tumours, intrahepatic cholangiocellular carcinoma (ICC) is probably the most adequate to study IH. It is often diagnosed at an advanced stage and presents as large heterogeneous masses with a non-homogeneous uptake at PET-CT [9]. This presentation at imaging corresponds to a major genetic IH [10,11], even if the two have never been associated.

The present study depicts an innovative in vivo technique to functionally study the IH of ICC. Preoperative 18F-fluorodeoxyglucose (FDG) PET-CT images were merged with ultrasonography ones to navigate the tumour and to precisely explore the association between IH at imaging and IH at pathology. In this proof-of-concept study, we tested the procedure during surgery to unequivocally evaluate its reliability and accuracy.

2. Materials and Methods

All consecutive patients affected by ICC and undergoing surgery were considered. Inclusion criteria were (a) aged $\geq$18 years; (b) ICC size >50 mm; (c) preoperative PET-CT with evidence of tumour areas having a heterogeneous uptake. Exclusion criteria were: (a) diagnosis of mixed hepato-cholangiocarcinoma at the final pathology; (b) preoperative chemotherapy or any preoperative loco-regional treatment, including thermal ablation, chemoembolisation, or radioembolisation; (c) uncontrolled diabetes or any metabolic alteration preventing an accurate SUV evaluation. The standard preoperative imaging included thoracoabdominal CT and hepatic magnetic resonance imaging (MRI). A multidisciplinary team discussed the management of every patient. Informed consent was signed by all the participants. The local ethics committee approved the study (approval number: 146/20 on 20 February 2020).

2.1. PET-CT Imaging

FDG PET-CT were performed on General Electric Discovery 690 (General Electric Healthcare, Waukesha, WI, USA) according to standard procedures. Reconstructed images were examined and interpreted by an experienced nuclear medicine physician (EL). The tumour areas with different metabolic activities at PET-CT were preoperatively identified. In each ICC, we considered sampling only the spots with the highest and with the lowest standardised uptake value (SUVmax and SUVmin, respectively) within the tumour. The low-uptake areas corresponding to necrosis at morphologic imaging (CT and MRI) were not considered.

2.2. IOUS and Intraoperative Navigation

At the point of laparotomy, intraoperative ultrasonography (IOUS) was performed using an Esaote Twice ultrasound system (Esaote, Genoa, Italy), equipped with an intraoperative T-shaped probe (IOT332 probe, Esaote, Genoa, Italy), working at 3–11 MHz frequency.

The two imaging modalities (PET-CT and IOUS) were synchronised by a semi-automatic system in the following steps. The images of PET-CT were uploaded to the ultrasound machine and then projected onto the screen beside the standard IOUS images. Some intrahepatic anatomic landmarks identified on the PET-CT (e.g., umbilical portion, first-order bifurcation of the right portal branch, hepato-caval confluence) were manually identified at IOUS. Once a landmark was visualised at IOUS, the axial image of PET-CT with the same landmark was identified and selected, and a mark was placed on the anatomical structure in the two imaging modalities. After the identification and selection of two landmarks, the machine provided an automatic synchronisation of the two imaging modalities. The correct synchronisation between the two imaging modalities was then verified by scanning all the liver. If any discordance was observed, some additional anatomic landmarks were selected to refine the process until a perfect overlapping of all intrahepatic anatomical structures was achieved. Once the process was completed, the overlapping of the full liver was obtained, and the PET-CT navigation was possible (Figure 1). The SUVmax and the SUVmin tumour areas selected at PET-CT were identified and sampled using a 16-gauge Trucut needle (Figure 2); the needle trajectory was selected to be fully included within the resected portion of the liver to avoid any risk of tumour-seeding in the future liver remnant. At least two biopsies were taken from each area. At the end of the resection, the same targeted areas were again identified, and a macrobiopsy was performed. Only samples with an adequate cellular composition were retained for the analyses (through a quick histologic check after sampling).

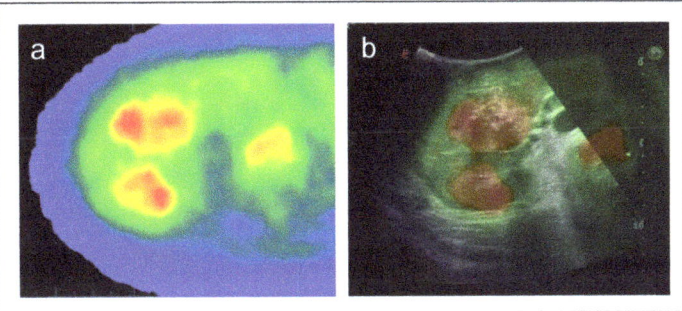

Figure 1. Navigation technology with the intraoperative fusion of preoperative PET-CT and IOUS. The tumour areas having different uptake at PET-CT are identified in vivo during surgery. (**a**) PET axial view of ICC; (**b**) Intraoperative fusion of PET-CT and IOUS images.

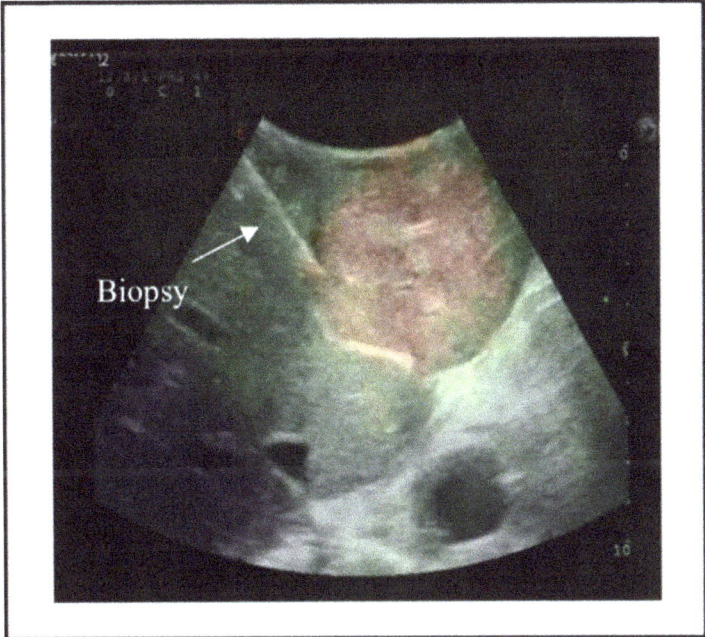

Figure 2. IOUS-guided biopsy of the tumour areas having different uptake at PET-CT.

2.3. Pathology Analyses

The specimens were fixed in formalin, paraffin-embedded, and stained with haematoxylin-eosin. Each sample had a standard morphological evaluation. Immunohistochemistry (IHC) was used to analyse the following parameters: the expression of CK7 and CK19; immune infiltrate (CD3+, T-lymphocyte marker; CD4+, helper/inducer T-lymphocyte marker; CD8+, suppressor/cytotoxic T-lymphocyte marker; CD68+, macrophage marker; and CD163+, M2 macrophage marker); the expression of programmed cell death protein 1 (PD1), its ligand (PD-L1), and tumour protein p53; proliferation index (Ki67); and metabolic enzymes glucose-6-phosphate dehydrogenase (G6PD) and citrate synthase (CS). We analysed the presence of FGFR2 translocations and the presence of microsatellite instability, and the loss of heterozygosity (1p36) using fluorescence in situ hybridisation. For PD1, PD-L1, p53, Ki67, G6PD, and CS, data were expressed as the percentage of immunoreactive cells compared to the total number of neoplastic cells. For the immune infiltrate (CD3, CD4, CD8, CD68, CD163), data were expressed as the percentage of immunoreactive cells compared to the total number of immune cells.

The specimens from SUVmax and SUVmin areas were separately analysed, and their data were compared. Both IOUS-guided tumour biopsies before resection and macroscopical biopsies at the end of resection were analysed. The concordance between samples from the same area was assessed.

3. Results

We enrolled three consecutive patients with a diagnosis of ICC confirmed at pathology. Table 1 summarises the patients' characteristics. The mean tumour size was 92 mm (range 60–120). At PET-CT, the mean SUVmax was 11.2 (8.9–14.7), the mean SUVmin was 5.3 (5.1–5.5), and the mean difference between the two was 5.8 (3.5–9.6). The synchronisation of PET-CT with IOUS and its navigation was successful in all patients.

Table 1. Clinical characteristics of the patients.

	Patient #1	Patient #2	Patient #3
Age	76	60	71
Sex	Male	Male	Male
Tumour size, mm	120	60	97
Number of tumours	1	1	1
Grading	G2	G2	G3
Surgical margin, mm	3	10	1
Microscopic vascular invasion	Y	N	Y
Perineural infiltration	N	N	Y

Table 2 summarises the pathology data. The IH of ICC was evident in different analyses. One patient had a lower tumour grading in the SUVmin area than in the SUVmax one (G1 vs. G2). One patient had a phenotypic IH, i.e., variable CK19 positivity in areas with a different uptake. One patient had a molecular IH: FGFR2 translocation was evident in the high-uptake area, while it was not in the low-uptake one. PET-CT uptake was also associated with the proliferative index in two patients (70% in the SUVmax area vs. 10% in the SUVmin area of one patient; 70 vs. 20%, respectively, in one). Finally, IH on PET-CT corresponded to heterogeneous immune infiltration: SUVmax areas had a higher CD8+ infiltrate in all patients (a mean of 15 vs. 8%), and a higher CD4+ (30 vs. 10%), CD68+ (25 vs. 10%), and CD163+ (30 vs. 12%) infiltrate in two patients. Metabolic indexes, PD1, PD-L1, and p53 expression were similar between areas.

Table 2. Summary of the pathology results.

	Patient #1		Patient #2		Patient #3	
	Area SUV Min	Area SUV Max	Area SUV Min	Area SUV Max	Area SUV Min	Area SUV Max
SUV	5.1	14.7	5.5	9.9	5.4	8.9
Morphology	stroma < cells	cells > stroma	cells = stroma	cells = stroma	cells = stroma	cells = stroma
Phenotype	CK7$^+$ CK19$^{-/+}$	CK7$^+$ CK19$^{-/+}$	CK7$^+$ CK19$^{/+}$	CK7$^+$ CK19$^{-/+}$	CK7$^+$ CK19$^{-/+}$	CK7$^+$ CK19$^-$
Grading	G1	G2	G2	G2	G3	G3
Proliferation index (KI67)	15%	15%	10%	70%	20%	70%
P53	20%	10%	30%	30%	60%	60%
PDL-1	Neg	Neg	Neg	Neg	Neg	Neg
PD1	5%	Neg	5%	10%	5%	Neg
FGFR2	WT	WT	WT	Translocated	WT	WT
1p36	LOH	LOH	Conserved	Conserved	Conserved	Conserved
Immune infiltrate						
CD3	10%	10%	10%	10%	10%	20%
CD4	10%	20%	10%	40%	20%	20%
CD8	5%	10%	10%	20%	5%	15%
CD68	10%	20%	10%	30%	20%	20%
CD163	20%	20%	20%	50%	5%	10%
Metabolic indexes						
G6PD	80%	80%	40%	100%	50%	50%
CS	100%	60%	80%	100%	20%	20%

CD163, marker of M2 macrophages; CD3 (cluster of differentiation 3), marker of T-lymphocytes; CD4, marker of helper/inducer T-lymphocyte; CD68, pan-macrophage or M1 marker; CD8, marker of suppressor/cytotoxic T-lymphocyte; CK19, cytokeratin 19; CK7, cytokeratin 7; CS, citrate synthase; FGFR2, fibroblast growth factor receptor 2; G6PD, glucose-6-phosphate dehydrogenase; Ki67, proliferation index; LOH, loss of heterozygosity; Neg, negative; p53, tumour suppressor protein; PD-1, programmed cell death protein 1; PD-L1, programmed death ligand 1; SUV, (standardised uptake value) semiquantitative parameter of FDG uptake; WT, wild type.

The pathology data of IOUS-guided biopsies and macrobiopsies after resection obtained from the same area were concordant.

4. Discussion

ICC is an aggressive malignancy with a poor prognosis. Standard chemotherapy has scarce disease control [12], but targeted therapies and immunotherapy could change this scenario. Some of the commonest ICC mutations concern the p53 pathway, Ras/Raf/MEK/ERK pathway, metabolic pathway (IDH1/IDH2), FGFR2, and 1p36 [10,11,13]. To date, targeted therapies for FGFR2 rearrangements and IDH1 mutations have been approved, and some other drugs have had tissue-agnostic approval [14,15]. However, the effectiveness of systemic therapies is limited by profound tumour genetic heterogeneity [10,11]. Walter et al. depicted varying expression patterns of MSH6 (mismatch repair protein) in peripheral and central areas of ICC [16]. Goyal et al. reported intra-tumoural clonal heterogeneity, in terms of acquired resistance to FGFR inhibition, in patients with FGFR2-fusion-positive tumours [17]. The possibility of predicting IH with non-invasive imaging is of major interest but has not been demonstrated yet.

ICC malignant cells have increased their expression of glucose transporters and a high activity of hexokinase, which leads to augmented glucose metabolism [4]. It corresponds to an increased FDG accumulation at PET-CT, especially in moderately and poorly differentiated ICCs [5]. High glucose metabolism in ICC is expected to be associated with increased tumour aggressiveness. Indeed, Seo et al. reported a high SUV as an independent predictor of postoperative recurrence [6].

We investigated the association between the heterogeneous uptake of ICC at PET-CT and IH. Among liver tumours, ICC is the most adequate for this analysis: it is usually diagnosed at an advanced stage (large masses); FDG PET-CT uptake is often non-homogeneous; and resectable patients do not receive preoperative chemotherapy, which could compromise PET-CT findings. Navigation technology provided a fundamental contribution. It is commonly used to guide the percutaneous interstitial treatment of tumours not visible on ultrasound [7]. In liver surgery, navigation technology merges preoperative and intraoperative imaging to identify the anatomy and the correct plane [8]. We used the fusion of preoperative PET-CT with IOUS to have an accurate identification of tumour areas with a different uptake at PET-CT. The intraoperative analysis allowed us to maximise the precision of the biopsy and unequivocally ascertain the capability of PET-driven biopsies to detect IH.

In the present series, PET-CT effectively caught IH. FDG uptake was associated with proliferative index (Ki67) and tumour grading: the areas with the highest SUV were the most aggressive parts of ICC. We also observed interesting results concerning genetic mutations and immune infiltration. In one patient, PET-CT identified a heterogeneous mutational status of FGFR2 (a wild-type in the SUVmin area and translocated in the SUVmax one). The remaining two patients had a wild-type status of FGFR2 in all biopsies. Considering immune infiltration, tumour areas with a higher FDG uptake had higher levels of T-lymphocytes (CD3+ and CD4+/CD8+) and macrophages (CD68+/CD163+) compared to areas with a lower uptake. Those data are clinically relevant: FGFR2 mutations are the target of approved drugs [14,18,19], and the immune infiltrate is a major determinant of prognosis in ICC patients [20,21]. A further result deserves consideration. In general, the key enzymes of anaerobic glycolysis and mitochondrial respiration (G6PD and CS, respectively) did not show a clear association with the SUV. Even if FDG PET-CT detects an augmented glucose metabolism [22], the different uptake did not always correspond to a heterogeneous metabolic pattern. Due to the study design (three patients), we can formulate some hypotheses about the mechanisms underlying the heterogeneous FDG uptake, also considering that they can vary among patients. In one patient, the expression of citrate synthase, which is used in oxygen-dependent ATP production, dropped in the high-SUV area. This finding is consistent with the concept of increased glucose consumption in the hypoxic areas of the tumours, which are forced to switch to the energy-inefficient anaerobic glycolysis and thus require many times more substrate for the same ATP output [23]. In the remaining two patients, the high-uptake areas were probably related to a major increase in the proliferative index (of both patients) and an FGFR2 translocation (in one). Investigations on the link between the latter gene and glucose metabolism are thus far limited, but the FGF/FGFR pathway involves anti-apoptosis signalling, proliferation, and angiogenesis [24].

The present study is in line with modern oncological research. Advanced imaging and analyses achieved excellent results for ICC, being able to provide a non-invasive prediction of tumour pathology data and prognosis [25,26]. Focusing on PET-CT, Yugawa et al. demonstrated that FDG uptake is associated with immune infiltration [27]. Fiz et al. reported that the radiomic analysis of the ICC and peritumoral tissue accurately predicts tumour grading, microvascular invasion, and survival [28]. Our preliminary data are coherent with such literature but represent a major step forward, thanks to IH mapping.

The proposed approach is clinically relevant for at least two reasons. First, the fusion of two different imaging modalities—morphological (ultrasound) and functional (PET)—provided a non-invasive depiction of ICC heterogeneity and detection of the most significant tumour portions. Even if our data are preliminary, the concordance of these results among multiple samplings from the same area strengthens the reliability and the reproducibility of the present technique. PET-driven biopsies could become a new standard in ICC patients: to catch the most relevant and aggressive areas of the tumour, have a more precise prediction of prognosis, and schedule a more effective patient-tailored treatment. Theoretically, the same approach could be applied to other liver tumours (primary or metastatic) and tracers. Liver metastases from colorectal cancers have both an intense FDG uptake with heterogeneous areas and a proven intralesional heterogeneity that correlates with prognosis [29–31]. Metastatic neuroendocrine tumours have a known inter-lesional heterogeneous DOTA peptides uptake, which can bear relevance for treatment strategies [32]. The tracers of the PSMA molecules can visualise the heterogeneity of prostate cancer metastases and, more recently, primary hepatic malignancies [33,34]. The uptake can depict variations in vascularity across the tumoural volume [34].

Second, the present technique was the first one that reliably associates the different FDG-uptake areas with tumour heterogeneity at a phenotypic, molecular, and genetic level and with immune infiltration. Our experience only provides a preliminary exploration of the concept but could be the basis for a better understanding of IH, a precision-medicine approach, and the identification of new biomarkers and therapeutic targets. By analysing a larger population, we could identify the SUV values and patterns which are able to non-invasively predict tumour characteristics.

5. Conclusions

The present study demonstrates that the fusion of morphological and functional imaging modalities may allow an in vivo and reliable evaluation of tumour heterogeneity. Discrepant intra-tumoural phenotypic, molecular, and genetic patterns were identified, as well as heterogeneous immune infiltrations. The proposed approach could increase the efficacy of percutaneous biopsies and could be the basis for a better understanding of IH.

Author Contributions: Conceptualisation, L.V., E.L., F.F., L.D.T., A.A., L.R., L.S., A.C. and G.T.; methodology, L.V., E.L., F.F., A.D. and L.S.; software, E.L. and L.S.; formal analysis, L.D.T. and A.D.; investigation, L.V., E.L., L.D.T., A.D., L.S., A.C. and G.T.; data curation, A.A., F.F. and L.R.; writing—original draft preparation, L.V., E.L., F.F. and A.D.; writing—review and editing, L.D.T., A.A., L.R., L.S., A.C. and G.T.; supervision, L.V., A.A., L.R., L.S., A.C. and G.T. All authors have read and agreed to the published version of the manuscript.

Funding: This research received no external funding.

Institutional Review Board Statement: The study was conducted in accordance with the Declaration of Helsinki and was approved by the Institutional Review Board (or Ethics Committee) of Humanitas Clinical & Research Hospital (protocol code 146/20 on 20 February 2020).

Informed Consent Statement: Informed consent was obtained from all subjects involved in the study.

Data Availability Statement: The data presented in this study are available from the corresponding author on reasonable request.

Conflicts of Interest: The authors declare no conflict of interest pertinent to the present manuscript. Considering the conflicts of interest in general, we state that: (1) L.V. received speaker's honoraria from Johnson & Johnson. (2) A.C. received speaker's honoraria from Advanced Accelerator Applications, General Electric Healthcare, Sirtex Medical Europe and AmGen Europe; received travel grants form General Electric Healthcare and Sirtex Medical Europe; he is a member of Blue Earth Diagnostics' and Advanced Accelerator Applications' advisory boards; received scientific support, in terms of a three-year Ph.D. fellowship, from the Sanofi Genzyme. (3) L.R. reports receiving consulting fees from Amgen, ArQule, AstraZeneca, Basilea, Bayer, BMS, Celgene, Eisai, Exelixis, Genenta, Hengrui, Incyte, Ipsen, IQVIA, Lilly, MSD, Nerviano Medical Sciences, Roche, Sanofi, Servier, Taiho Oncology, Zymeworks; lecture fees from AbbVie, Amgen, Bayer, Eisai, Gilead, Incyte, Ipsen, Lilly, Merck Serono, Roche, Sanofi; travel expenses from AstraZeneca; and institutional research funding from Agios, ARMO BioSciences, AstraZeneca, BeiGene, Eisai, Exelixis, Fibrogen, Incyte, Ipsen, Lilly, MSD, Nerviano Medical Sciences, Roche, Zymeworks. All other authors have no relevant disclosures.

References

1. Gerlinger, M.; Rowan, A.J.; Horswell, S.; Math, M.; Larkin, J.; Endesfelder, D.; Gronroos, E.; Martinez, P.; Matthews, N.; Stewart, A.; et al. Intratumor heterogeneity and branched evolution revealed by multiregion sequencing. *N. Engl. J. Med.* **2012**, *366*, 883–892. [CrossRef]
2. Kreso, A.; O'Brien, C.A.; van Galen, P.; Gan, O.I.; Notta, F.; Brown, A.M.; Ng, K.; Ma, J.; Wienholds, E.; Dunant, C.; et al. Variable clonal repopulation dynamics influence chemotherapy response in colorectal cancer. *Science* **2013**, *339*, 543–548. [CrossRef]
3. Laurent-Puig, P.; Pekin, D.; Normand, C.; Kotsopoulos, S.K.; Nizard, P.; Perez-Toralla, K.; Rowell, R.; Olson, J.; Srinivasan, P.; Le Corre, D.; et al. Clinical relevance of KRAS-mutated subclones detected with picodroplet digital PCR in advanced colorectal cancer treated with anti-EGFR therapy. *Clin. Cancer Res.* **2015**, *21*, 1087–1097. [CrossRef]

4. Haberkorn, U.; Ziegler, S.I.; Oberdorfer, F.; Trojan, H.; Haag, D.; Peschke, P.; Berger, M.R.; Altmann, A.; van Kaick, G. FDG uptake, tumor proliferation and expression of glycolysis associated genes in animal tumor models. *Nucl. Med. Biol.* **1994**, *21*, 827–834. [CrossRef]
5. Paudyal, B.; Oriuchi, N.; Paudyal, P.; Higuchi, T.; Nakajima, T.; Endo, K. Expression of glucose transporters and hexokinase II in cholangiocellular carcinoma compared using [18F]-2-fluro-2-deoxy-D-glucose positron emission tomography. *Cancer Sci.* **2008**, *99*, 260–266. [CrossRef]
6. Seo, S.; Hatano, E.; Higashi, T.; Nakajima, A.; Nakamoto, Y.; Tada, M.; Tamaki, N.; Iwaisako, K.; Mori, A.; Doi, R.; et al. Fluorine-18 fluorodeoxyglucose positron emission tomography predicts lymph node metastasis, P-glycoprotein expression, and recurrence after resection in mass-forming intrahepatic cholangiocarcinoma. *Surgery* **2008**, *143*, 769–777. [CrossRef]
7. Mauri, G.; Gennaro, N.; De Beni, S.; Ierace, T.; Goldberg, S.N.; Rodari, M.; Solbiati, L.A. Real-Time US-(18)FDG-PET/CT Image Fusion for Guidance of Thermal Ablation of (18)FDG-PET-Positive Liver Metastases: The Added Value of Contrast Enhancement. *Cardiovasc. Interv. Radiol.* **2019**, *42*, 60–68. [CrossRef]
8. Hallet, J.; Gayet, B.; Tsung, A.; Wakabayashi, G.; Pessaux, P.; 2nd International Consensus Conference on Laparoscopic Liver Resection group. Systematic review of the use of pre-operative simulation and navigation for hepatectomy: Current status and future perspectives. *J. Hepatobiliary Pancreat Sci.* **2015**, *22*, 353–362. [CrossRef]
9. Banales, J.M.; Cardinale, V.; Carpino, G.; Marzioni, M.; Andersen, J.B.; Invernizzi, P.; Lind, G.E.; Folseraas, T.; Forbes, S.J.; Fouassier, L.; et al. Expert consensus document: Cholangiocarcinoma: Current knowledge and future perspectives consensus statement from the European Network for the Study of Cholangiocarcinoma (ENS-CCA). *Nat. Rev. Gastroenterol. Hepatol.* **2016**, *13*, 261–280. [CrossRef]
10. Brandi, G.; Farioli, A.; Astolfi, A.; Biasco, G.; Tavolari, S. Genetic heterogeneity in cholangiocarcinoma: A major challenge for targeted therapies. *Oncotarget* **2015**, *6*, 14744–14753. [CrossRef]
11. Putra, J.; de Abreu, F.B.; Peterson, J.D.; Pipas, J.M.; Mody, K.; Amos, C.I.; Tsongalis, G.J.; Suriawinata, A.A. Molecular profiling of intrahepatic and extrahepatic cholangiocarcinoma using next generation sequencing. *Exp. Mol. Pathol.* **2015**, *99*, 240–244. [CrossRef]
12. Valle, J.; Wasan, H.; Palmer, D.H.; Cunningham, D.; Anthoney, A.; Maraveyas, A.; Madhusudan, S.; Iveson, T.; Hughes, S.; Pereira, S.P.; et al. Cisplatin plus gemcitabine versus gemcitabine for biliary tract cancer. *N. Engl. J. Med.* **2010**, *362*, 1273–1281. [CrossRef]
13. Limpaiboon, T.; Tapdara, S.; Jearanaikoon, P.; Sripa, B.; Bhudhisawasdi, V. Prognostic significance of microsatellite alterations at 1p36 in cholangiocarcinoma. *World J. Gastroenterol.* **2006**, *12*, 4377–4382. [CrossRef]
14. Kam, A.E.; Masood, A.; Shroff, R.T. Current and emerging therapies for advanced biliary tract cancers. *Lancet Gastroenterol. Hepatol.* **2021**, *6*, 956–969. [CrossRef]
15. Search Results for "Cholangiocarcinoma" on the FDA Search Tool. Available online: https://www.fda.gov/search?s=cholangiocarcinoma (accessed on 27 August 2022).
16. Walter, D.; Doring, C.; Feldhahn, M.; Battke, F.; Hartmann, S.; Winkelmann, R.; Schneider, M.; Bankov, K.; Schnitzbauer, A.; Zeuzem, S.; et al. Intratumoral heterogeneity of intrahepatic cholangiocarcinoma. *Oncotarget* **2017**, *8*, 14957–14968. [CrossRef]
17. Goyal, L.; Saha, S.K.; Liu, L.Y.; Siravegna, G.; Leshchiner, I.; Ahronian, L.G.; Lennerz, J.K.; Vu, P.; Deshpande, V.; Kambadakone, A.; et al. Polyclonal Secondary FGFR2 Mutations Drive Acquired Resistance to FGFR Inhibition in Patients with FGFR2 Fusion-Positive Cholangiocarcinoma. *Cancer Dis.* **2017**, *7*, 252–263. [CrossRef]
18. Borad, M.J.; Champion, M.D.; Egan, J.B.; Liang, W.S.; Fonseca, R.; Bryce, A.H.; McCullough, A.E.; Barrett, M.T.; Hunt, K.; Patel, M.D.; et al. Integrated genomic characterization reveals novel, therapeutically relevant drug targets in FGFR and EGFR pathways in sporadic intrahepatic cholangiocarcinoma. *PLoS Genet.* **2014**, *10*, e1004135. [CrossRef]
19. Mazzaferro, V.; El-Rayes, B.F.; Droz Dit Busset, M.; Cotsoglou, C.; Harris, W.P.; Damjanov, N.; Masi, G.; Rimassa, L.; Personeni, N.; Braiteh, F.; et al. Derazantinib (ARQ 087) in advanced or inoperable FGFR2 gene fusion-positive intrahepatic cholangiocarcinoma. *Br. J. Cancer* **2019**, *120*, 165–171. [CrossRef]
20. Vigano, L.; Soldani, C.; Franceschini, B.; Cimino, M.; Lleo, A.; Donadon, M.; Roncalli, M.; Aghemo, A.; Di Tommaso, L.; Torzilli, G. Tumor-Infiltrating Lymphocytes and Macrophages in Intrahepatic Cholangiocellular Carcinoma. Impact on Prognosis after Complete Surgery. *J. Gastrointest Surg.* **2019**, *23*, 2216–2224. [CrossRef]
21. Asukai, K.; Kawamoto, K.; Eguchi, H.; Konno, M.; Nishida, N.; Koseki, J.; Noguchi, K.; Hasegawa, S.; Ogawa, H.; Yamada, D.; et al. Prognostic Impact of Peritumoral IL-17-Positive Cells and IL-17 Axis in Patients with Intrahepatic Cholangiocarcinoma. *Ann. Surg. Oncol.* **2015**, *22* (Suppl. S3), S1524–S1531. [CrossRef]
22. Kowalik, M.A.; Guzzo, G.; Morandi, A.; Perra, A.; Menegon, S.; Masgras, I.; Trevisan, E.; Angioni, M.M.; Fornari, F.; Quagliata, L.; et al. Metabolic reprogramming identifies the most aggressive lesions at early phases of hepatic carcinogenesis. *Oncotarget* **2016**, *7*, 32375–32393. [CrossRef]
23. Liberti, M.V.; Locasale, J.W. The Warburg Effect: How Does it Benefit Cancer Cells? *Trends Biochem. Sci.* **2016**, *41*, 211–218. [CrossRef]
24. Katoh, M.; Nakagama, H. FGF receptors: Cancer biology and therapeutics. *Med. Res. Rev.* **2014**, *34*, 280–300. [CrossRef]
25. King, M.J.; Hectors, S.; Lee, K.M.; Omidele, O.; Babb, J.S.; Schwartz, M.; Tabrizian, P.; Taouli, B.; Lewis, S. Outcomes assessment in intrahepatic cholangiocarcinoma using qualitative and quantitative imaging features. *Cancer Imaging* **2020**, *20*, 43. [CrossRef]
26. Fiz, F.; Jayakody Arachchige, V.S.; Gionso, M.; Pecorella, I.; Selvam, A.; Wheeler, D.R.; Sollini, M.; Viganò, L. Radiomics of Biliary Tumors: A Systematic Review of Current Evidence. *Diagnostics* **2022**, *12*, 826. [CrossRef]

27. Yugawa, K.; Itoh, S.; Iseda, N.; Kurihara, T.; Kitamura, Y.; Toshima, T.; Harada, N.; Kohashi, K.; Baba, S.; Ishigami, K.; et al. Obesity is a risk factor for intrahepatic cholangiocarcinoma progression associated with alterations of metabolic activity and immune status. *Sci. Rep.* **2021**, *11*, 5845. [CrossRef]
28. Fiz, F.; Masci, C.; Costa, G.; Sollini, M.; Chiti, A.; Ieva, F.; Torzilli, G.; Viganò, L. PET/CT-based radiomics of mass-forming intrahepatic cholangiocarcinoma improves prediction of pathology data and survival. *Eur. J. Nucl. Med. Mol. Imaging* **2022**, *49*, 3387–3400. [CrossRef]
29. Watanabe, A.; Harimoto, N.; Yokobori, T.; Araki, K.; Kubo, N.; Igarashi, T.; Tsukagoshi, M.; Ishii, N.; Yamanaka, T.; Handa, T.; et al. FDG-PET reflects tumor viability on SUV in colorectal cancer liver metastasis. *Int. J. Clin. Oncol.* **2020**, *25*, 322–329. [CrossRef]
30. Goasguen, N.; de Chaisemartin, C.; Brouquet, A.; Julié, C.; Prevost, G.P.; Laurent-Puig, P.; Penna, C. Evidence of heterogeneity within colorectal liver metastases for allelic losses, mRNA level expression and in vitro response to chemotherapeutic agents. *Int. J. Cancer* **2010**, *127*, 1028–1037. [CrossRef] [PubMed]
31. Menck, K.; Wlochowitz, D.; Wachter, A.; Conradi, L.C.; Wolff, A.; Scheel, A.H.; Korf, U.; Wiemann, S.; Schildhaus, H.U.; Bohnenberger, H.; et al. High-Throughput Profiling of Colorectal Cancer Liver Metastases Reveals Intra- and Inter-Patient Heterogeneity in the EGFR and WNT Pathways Associated with Clinical Outcome. *Cancers* **2022**, *14*, 2084. [CrossRef]
32. Graf, J.; Pape, U.F.; Jann, H.; Denecke, T.; Arsenic, R.; Brenner, W.; Pavel, M.; Prasad, V. Prognostic Significance of Somatostatin Receptor Heterogeneity in Progressive Neuroendocrine Tumor Treated with Lu-177 DOTATOC or Lu-177 DOTATATE. *Eur. J. Nucl. Med. Mol. Imaging* **2020**, *47*, 881–894. [CrossRef] [PubMed]
33. Damjanovic, J.; Janssen, J.C.; Prasad, V.; Diederichs, G.; Walter, T.; Brenner, W.; Makowski, M.R. (68)Ga-PSMA-PET/CT for the evaluation of liver metastases in patients with prostate cancer. *Cancer Imaging* **2019**, *19*, 37. [CrossRef] [PubMed]
34. Chen, W.; Lee, Z.; Awadallah, A.; Zhou, L.; Xin, W. Peritumoral/vascular expression of PSMA as a diagnostic marker in hepatic lesions. *Diagn. Pathol.* **2020**, *15*, 92. [CrossRef] [PubMed]

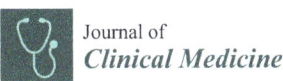

Review

Assessment of Response to Immunotherapy in Patients with Hodgkin Lymphoma: Towards Quantifying Changes in Tumor Burden Using FDG-PET/CT

Francesca Tutino [1], Elisabetta Giovannini [1], Silvia Chiola [2], Giampiero Giovacchini [1] and Andrea Ciarmiello [1,*]

1. Nuclear Medicine Unit, Ospedale Civile Sant'Andrea, Via Vittorio Veneto 170, 19124 La Spezia, Italy
2. Nuclear Medicine Unit, IRCCS Ospedale Policlinico San Martino, 16132 Genoa, Italy
* Correspondence: andrea.ciarmiello@asl5.liguria.it

Abstract: Immune checkpoint inhibitors are currently the standard of care for many advanced solid tumors, and they have been recently approved for the treatment of relapsed/refractory Hodgkin lymphoma and primary mediastinal B cell lymphoma. Assessments of the response to immunotherapy may be complicated by the occurrence of the flare/pseudoprogression phenomenon, consisting of initial tumor enlargement and even the appearance of new lesions, followed by a response, which may initially be indistinguishable from true progression. There have been efforts to characterize and capture the new patterns of response observed during immunotherapy, namely, pseudoprogression and delayed response, and several immune-related response criteria have been proposed. Confirming progression on a subsequent scan and measuring the total tumor burden are both common in immune-related criteria. Due to the peculiarity of hematologic malignancies, lymphoma-specific immune-related criteria have been developed (LYRIC), and they have been evaluated in research studies in comparison to the Lugano Classification. In this review work, we illustrate the evolution of the response criteria in lymphomas from the first CT-based criteria to the development of the PET-based Lugano Classification, further refined to take into account the flare phenomenon encountered during immunotherapy. We also describe the additional contribution of PET-derived volumetric parameters to the interpretation of responses during immunotherapy.

Keywords: immunotherapy; Hodgkin lymphoma; FDG-PET; pseudoprogression; LYRIC; MTV

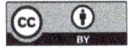

1. Introduction

In the last decade, novel biological agents with an immune mechanism have entered the clinical world; the newest agents are immune checkpoint inhibitors. Nowadays, immune checkpoint inhibitors represent the standard of care for advanced melanoma, non-small-cell lung cancer, renal carcinoma and head and neck tumors [1–3]. In the last decade, the impressive results of phase I and II studies exploring the effectiveness and safety of PD-1 inhibitors in Hodgkin lymphoma (HL) [4,5] and primary mediastinal B cell lymphoma (PMBCL) [6] granted the accelerated approval of anti-PD-1 by the FDA without a confirmatory phase III study. In 2016, nivolumab was approved by the FDA for the treatment of relapsed/refractory classical HL (cHL) after autologous stem cell transplantation and brentuximab vedotin as the first hematologic indication. Pembrolizumab was approved for relapsed/refractory cHL after at least three lines of therapy in 2017 and for relapsed PMBCL after the failure of two or more lines of therapy in 2018 (Keynote 013 study).

The impact of immune checkpoint inhibitors on the treatment of HL is related to the unique property of HL of being constituted only by a minority of malignant cells (Reed–Stemberg cells) embedded in an abundant microenvironment, whose cells overexpress PD1-PDL1 due to a genetic aberration in the 9p23-24 locus. Immune checkpoint inhibitors are of minor importance in non-Hodgkin lymphoma (NHL); no immune checkpoint inhibitor approval exists for NHL. However, for relapsed/refractory NHL, the option of chimeric antigen receptor T (CAR-T) cell therapy is gaining ground. CAR-T therapy was recently approved by the FDA and EMA for the treatment of relapsed/refractory diffuse large B cell lymphoma.

Immune checkpoint inhibitors, working with an immune mechanism, may cause a transient increase in tumor burden due to inflammation, named pseudoprogression, and they may alter tumor metabolism, yielding false positive and false negative results on FDG-PET/TC. In recent years, novel response criteria were designed in an attempt to capture these additional response patterns beyond those observed in conventional chemotherapy.

In this review work, we examine the evolution of response criteria from the first efforts to describe the effects of conventional chemotherapy on tumor growth to the development of lymphoma-specific criteria and their refinement to be suitable to capture the benefit provided by immunotherapy. We also describe the contribution of additional FDG-PET/CT quantitative parameters, such as metabolic tumor volume (MTV) and total lesion glycolysis (TLG), to assessing changes in tumor burden in the course of immunotherapy.

2. Immunobiology of Immune Checkpoints

Tumor cell growth is promoted by the ability of tumor cells to "escape" from the immune system and to be immunotolerant. Tumor cells lose their immunogenic antigens and manipulate the microenvironment dysregulating immune checkpoints to express inhibitory signals [7–9]. The rationale of immunotherapy is to restore a florid T-cell cytotoxic response directed against the tumor, and this can be achieved either by activating stimulatory checkpoints or by inhibiting inhibitory checkpoints [10].

The most relevant inhibitory checkpoints are programmed death cell receptor 1 (PD1) and cytotoxic T-lymphocyte-associated protein 4 (CTLA-4), both being receptors expressed on the T-cell surface inducing T-cell anergy. PD1, through the interaction with its ligand, programmed death cell ligand 1 (PDL1), expressed in antigen-presenting cells (APCs), activated T cells and tumor cells, inhibits the T-cell cytotoxic response [11]. CTLA-4 inhibits T-cell proliferation by blocking the costimulatory molecules of the B7-CD28 superfamily expressed on APCs [12].

The knowledge about the expression of immune inhibitory checkpoints in hematologic malignancies has been illustrated in a recent review work by Witkowska and Smolewsky [13]. HL widely overexpresses PD1/PDL1 due to a widespread genetic alteration in the locus 9p23-24 and the subsequent activation of Janus kinase 2 [14]. PMBCL shows a high expression of PD1 ligands, especially the EBV-positive subtype, probably mediated by virus latent proteins [15,16]. Follicular lymphoma (FL), originating from B germinal centers similarly to HL and PMBCL, may express PD1 ligands [17]. CTLA-4 expression, of which little is known about, might be observed in T-cell lymphomas and Sezary syndrome [18].

3. Review of PET-Based Criteria for Response Assessment

3.1. Background and Assessment of Response to Conventional Chemotherapy

The first effort towards the standardization of assessments of the response to cancer treatment was a handbook published in 1979 promoted by the World Health Organization (WHO) [19]. The WHO criteria stated the concept of the tumor bidimensional measurement of tumor burden as a sum of the products of lesion diameters before and after therapy and established the four response categories still currently in use: complete response, partial response, stable disease and progressive disease.

The first guidelines to incorporate the metabolic data provided by FDG-PET/CT in response assessment were the European Organization for Research and Treatment of Cancer (EORTC) criteria, released in 1999 [20]. The reference region for complete metabolic response was the background adjacent to lesions. The main goal of the EORTC criteria was to evaluate the viability of residual masses: based on metabolic activity, it was feasible to discriminate fibrotic/necrotic changes from residual tumors.

A new set of joint EORTC/National Cancer Institute CT-based guidelines for response assessment, the Response Evaluation Criteria in Solid Tumors (RECIST), was first published in 2000 [21] and then revised and updated in 2009 (RECIST 1.1) [22]. In contrast to the bidimensional assessment of the WHO criteria, being laborious and time consuming, the RECIST criteria rely on a unidimensional assessment of the largest axial diameters of the tumors [23]. Moreover, RECIST introduced the concept of target lesions.

In the same year, 2009, on the heels of RECIST, Wahl et al. published the PET Response Criteria in Solid Tumors (PERCIST) [24]. Similarly to RECIST, the PERCIST criteria rely on the assessment of residual metabolic activity in target lesions (hottest lesions). The remarkable innovations of PERCIST are the introduction of SUV lean (SUL, SUV normalized for lean body mass) and SUL peak and the definition of the minimum measurable activity as 1.5 times hepatic activity.

Due to the peculiarity of hematologic malignancies, specialized criteria for response assessment in lymphomas were developed. The first effort to design response criteria specific for lymphomas was the International Working Group (IWG) criteria [25], sponsored by the National Institute of Health, published in 1998. The IWG criteria were CT-based criteria, and they introduced a fifth response category, namely, complete response/unconfirmed (CRu), defined as the persistence of residual nodal masses despite a reduction greater than 75% in the sum of the product of diameters. CRu reflects the difficulty of assessing the origin of residual masses based purely on radiological data.

In the early 2000s as the fast growth of PET began and as PET/CT tomographs were developed, the gain in accuracy provided by PET, able to assess the viability of residual masses, was recognized, leading to the proposal of the so-called IWG+PET criteria by Juweid et al. in 2005 [26]. Soon after in 2007, in the context of a project promoted by the German Study Group, the International Harmonization Project, two publications by Cheson et al. [27] and by Juweid et al. [28] updated the IWG criteria, embodying PET in the response evaluation. These modified criteria were based on an integrated evaluation of CT and PET. The PET evaluation was qualitative and provided a positive or negative classification based on a comparison of activity in residuals with activity in reference regions (mediastinal blood pool for residual masses greater than 2 cm and adjacent background for smaller lesions). The assessment of viability in residual tumors enabled by PET/TC led to the elimination of the ambiguous CRu category.

In 2009, an International workshop held in Deauville (France) formulated novel response criteria, the Deauville Score (DS) [29,30]. DS is a five-point scale based on a visual comparison of activity in residual tumors with activity in reference regions (mediastinal blood pool and liver). In 2013, at the 12th International Conference on Malignant Lymphomas, the Lugano Classification was developed [31], a body of consensus recommendations for staging and response assessment in lymphomas. According to the Lugano guidelines, both contrast CT and PET have to be performed in the setting of response assessment. Separate sets of response criteria for CT and PET evaluations were published. For PET interpretation, DS was adopted. DS, being simple and easy to implement, had widespread diffusion and underwent a process of standardization across centers, becoming the gold standard for response assessment in lymphomas.

In the case of uncertainty of DS attribution, research groups active in the field recommend confirming visual evaluations with the SUV ratio between residual tumors and reference regions [32]. Recently, quantitative extensions of DS were also developed, particularly qPET [33,34], but these methods have not yet been prospectively validated and need standardization.

The evolution of the response criteria in oncology and hematology over time is presented in Figure 1.

3.2. Pseudoprogression and Hyperprogression

The Lugano Classification was designed to assess the response to traditional chemotherapy or conventional chemo-immunotherapeutic regimens, including rituximab. The patterns of response to immunotherapy differ from the patterns observed in conventional treatments. Usually, response occurs early after immunotherapy, and, consequently, an early response evaluation after two–three cycles of therapy is advisable. Response assessment may be confounded by the phenomena of delayed response and flare/pseudoprogression. Delayed response consists of a late objective response in the course of treatment, after initial tumor growth and apparent progression of the disease. Flare/pseudoprogression was first described in lymphomas and chronic lymphocytic leukemia receiving lenalinomide as a rapid increase in the size of lymph nodes, often painful, accompanied by fever and lymphocytosis [35–37]. Flare/pseudoprogression is defined as an increase in the size of baseline lesions and even the appearance of new lesions when the patient is clinically improving. It represents an apparent progression on imaging, in the absence of clinical deterioration of the patient, and it is followed by a response. Pseudoprogression usually occurs early during treatment. The increase in the size of baseline lesions is an inflammatory phenomenon due to T-cell recruitment, NK activation and a massive release of cytokines [38]. It is crucial to recognize pseudoprogression and to not discontinue treatment before achieving clinical benefit.

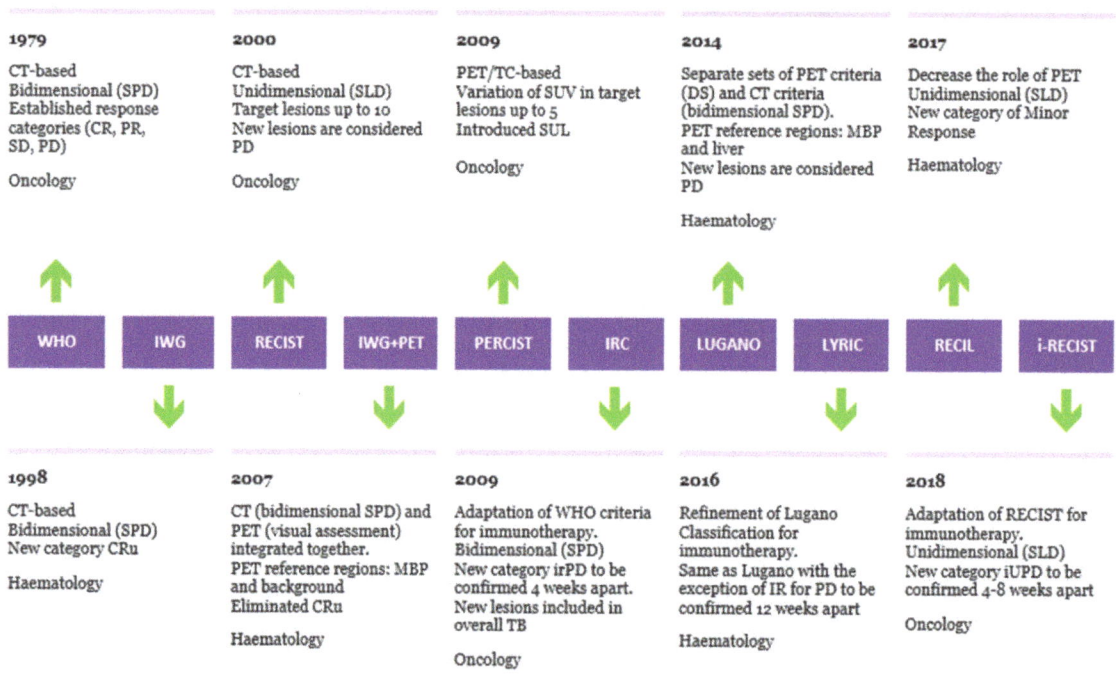

Figure 1. Evolution of criteria for response to cancer treatment. Timeline illustrating the evolution of response criteria over time in oncology and hematology, outlining the differences in method of tumor measurement, PET interpretation and assessment of progression of disease. SPD: sum of products of diameters. SLD: sum of longest axial diameters. MBP: mediastinal blood pool. SUL: standardized uptake lean mass. DS: Deauville Score. Cru: unconfirmed complete response. irPD: immune-related progression of disease. IR: indeterminate response. iUPD: immune-unconfirmed progression of disease.

Hyperprogression, defined as a rapid acceleration of tumor growth, is a new aggressive pattern reported in a fraction of lung cancer, melanoma, renal carcinoma [39] and head and neck carcinoma [40] cases treated with anti-PD-1/PD-L1. Compared to pseudoprogression described above, hyperprogression is a disruptive phenomenon, and it is not prone to uncertainty in interpretation.

3.3. Assessment of Response to Immunotherapy

Atypical responses encountered in patients under immune checkpoint blockade, due to delayed responses and pseudoprogression, and additional response patterns beyond those of conventional chemotherapy classified by the WHO and RECIST criteria were shown to be associated with survival benefit comparable to typical responses [41] and needed to be taken into account in response assessment. There have been efforts to characterize these phenomena and to incorporate them into novel response criteria.

In 2009, a publication by Wholchok et al. proposed the Immune-Related Response Criteria (IRC) [41], novel CT-based immune therapy response criteria adapted from the WHO criteria, based on the experience of community workshops using data from patients with advanced melanoma treated with ipilimumab. Across this cohort of patients, four patterns of response to ipilimumab were reported. Two patterns were captured by conventional response criteria: (1) a shrinkage in baseline lesions without new lesions and (2) "stable" disease, eventually followed by a slow steady decline of tumor burden (TB). The other two were new and were beyond conventional response assessment: (3) response after an initial increase in TB and (4) a reduction in overall TB concomitantly with the appearance of new lesions.

The main statements of the IRC can be resumed as follows:

1. Immune-related progression (irPD) of disease needs to be confirmed in a subsequent scan at least 4 weeks later in the absence of clinical deterioration and the worsening of laboratory parameters, aimed to uncover delayed response and pseudoprogression phenomena. PD confirmation is required before withdrawing treatment.
2. Stable disease is considered a therapeutic effect and a surrogate end-point for clinical benefit in contrast to assessment of the response to conventional cytotoxic therapy.
3. Overall, TB has to be measured, even when new lesions appear. The threshold for SD and partial response (PR) are the same as that in the WHO criteria, but new lesions are included in TB assessment.

The IRC have been implemented into clinical trials evaluating immune checkpoint inhibitors in solid tumors.

In 2013, the IRC were adapted to the unidimensional RECIST criteria and called Immune-Related RECIST (irRECIST) [42]. In 2017, the RECIST working group adapted the RECIST 1.1 criteria to the new body of knowledge about the patterns of response to immunotherapy in solid tumors and developed the so-called Immune-RECIST (i-RECIST) [43]. i-RECIST have a new response category of "immune unconfirmed progression" that requires confirmation on a subsequent scan within 6–8 weeks, accounting for the occurrence of pseudoprogression and delayed response.

In the studies on the immune checkpoint blockade in LH and N, a similar incidence of delayed response and flare/pseudoprogression, and response patterns similar to those reported in solid tumors have been observed. However, merely translating the IRC in the setting of response assessment in lymphomas was not considered totally appropriate for the following reasons: First, over time, there was an independent evolution of the response criteria for solid tumors and lymphomas. Response in solid tumors is assessed using morphologic unidimensional criteria, the RECIST criteria, whereas response in lymphomas is evaluated using the Lugano Classification based on PET/TC and on a bidimensional assessment of lymph node size on CT. Second, progression is defined by the WHO criteria as an increase in size >25% of the sum of the product of the diameters of solid tumors, whereas in lymphomas, an increase in the size of a single lymph node accompanied by PET positivity is adequate to discern progression. Third, response assessment in solid tumors is based on a dimensional evaluation of masses, always considered abnormal, whereas in the setting of lymphomas, residual masses do not have just an interpretation, since they can represent fibrotic/necrotic changes, according to metabolic activity.

To address these issues, in 2016, the LYRIC criteria (Lymphoma Response to Immunomodulatory Therapy Criteria) [44] were developed as a refinement of the Lugano Classification accounting for features specific of immunotherapy. In the LYRIC criteria, a CT-based size assessment and a PET/TC evaluation are integrated together. LYRIC introduced the novel category of indeterminate response (IR) to account for flare/pseudoprogression and delayed response, requiring a confirmatory study, either a biopsy or subsequent imaging within 12 weeks. Three types of IR were identified:

- IR(1): Progression (defined as >50% increase in overall TB) in the first 12 weeks of therapy without clinical deterioration.
- IR(2): Appearance of new lesions in the context of overall TB stability (Figure 2).
- IR(3): Increase in the uptake of existing lesions without a concomitant increase in lesion size and number (Figure 3).

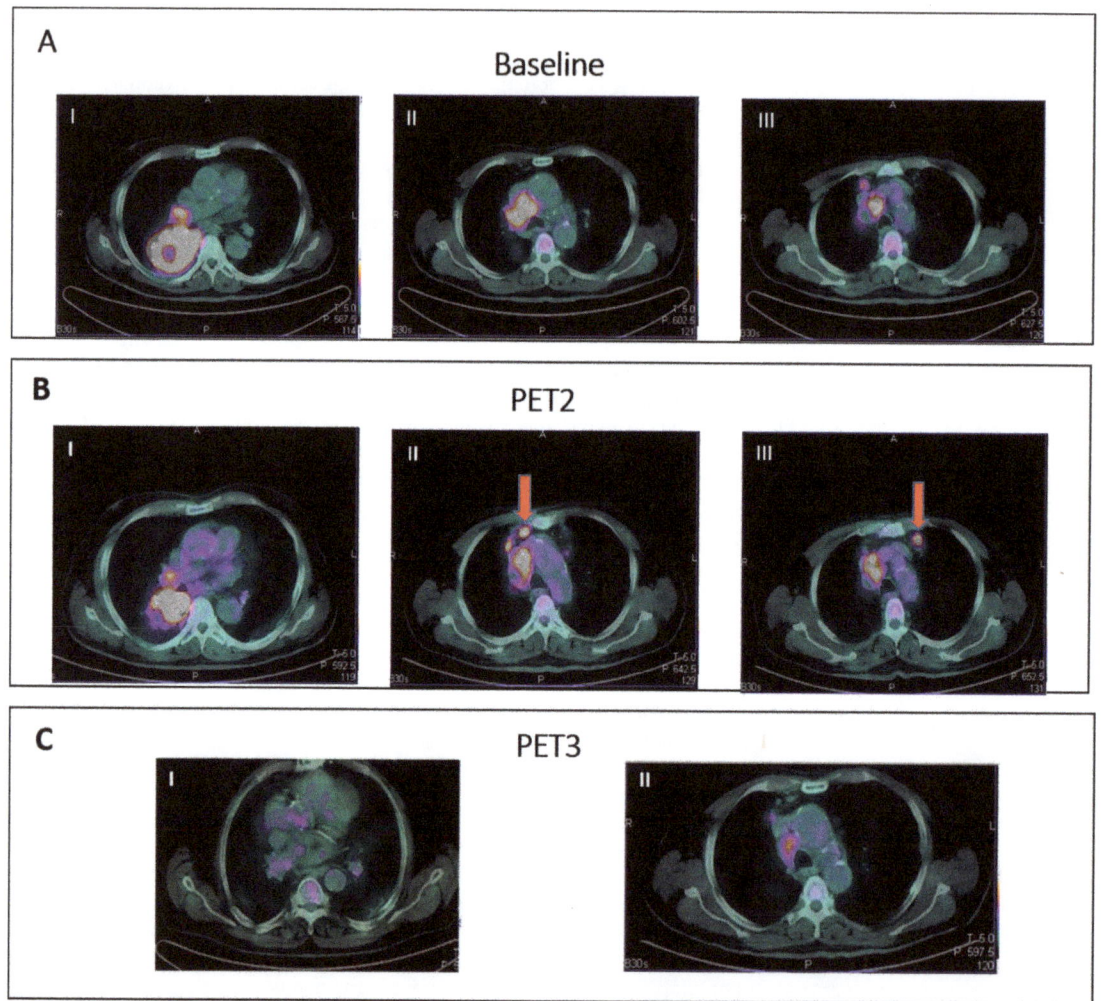

Figure 2. IR (2): Pseudoprogression in a patient on nivolumab for Hodgkin lymphoma. Panel (**A**) shows baseline disease. Panel (**B**) (II–III) shows the appearance of new nodal lesions (red arrows) in early PET evaluation after four cycles of immunotherapy. PET/TC evaluation at a later time point (**C**) demonstrates regression of the nodal flares and metabolic response.

The LYRIC criteria were applied in studies assessing the response to immunotherapy in lymphomas and were compared with the Lugano Classification.

In 2017, with the aim of unifying the response criteria in lymphoma with the response criteria in solid tumors in the context of clinical trials evaluating new therapeutic agents in a mixed population of patients with lymphoma and patients with solid tumors, an international working group developed the Response Evaluation Criteria in Lymphoma (RECIL) [45]. RECIL looks at the RECIST criteria, proposing a unidimensional evaluation of the sum of the longest axial diameters in a maximum of three target lesions, instead of the sum of the product of diameters in up to six target lesions as suggested by the Lugano criteria. Based on the hypothesis that new therapeutic agents can alter a tumor's metabolism and, thus, have the potential to increase false-positive and false-negative FDG-PET results, RECIL decreased the role of PET in response assessment in lymphomas. Although in the Lugano Classification, complete response (CR) was represented by PET negativity (DS 1–3) regardless of lesion size, in RECIL, the CR response category requires a shrinkage >30% of lesions besides PET negativity. The PR category was also modified to capture the mixed responses encountered with novel treatments. In the Lugano Classification, the increase in size >50% of a single lesion is sufficient to discern PD, even if other lesions concomitantly decrease in size. In contrast, in RECIL, similarly to the IRC and LYRIC seen above, the overall tumor burden is considered, and this case may discern PR, defined as a decrease in size >30% of overall TB accompanied by PET positivity (DS 4 or 5). RECIL introduced a novel provisional category of minor response, defined as a shrinkage of lesions >10% and <29% accompanied by any PET status, aiming to account for a response that does not fulfill the criteria for traditional response categories but may be associated with survival benefit. A comparison of the Lugano Classification, LYRIC and RECIL 2017 is presented in Table 1.

Table 1. Comparison between Lugano lymphoma classification, LYRIC and RECIL 2017.

	Lugano	LYRIC	RECIL 2017
Number of target lesions	Up to 6	Up to 6	Up to 3
Measurement method	Bidimensional: perpendicular diameters	Bidimensional: perpendicular diameters	Unidimensional: long diameter of any target lesion
Complete response (CR)	PET negativity (DS 1–3) with or without a residual mass	Same as Lugano	PET negativity (DS 1–3) plus reduction in SLD > 30%
Minor response (MR)	No	Same as Lugano	Yes: reduction in SLD between $\geq$10% and <30%
Partial response (PR)	Reduced FDG-PET uptake (DS 4–5) Decrease SPD $\geq$ 50%	Same as Lugano	Reduction in SLD $\geq$ 30% not meeting criteria for CR New lesions are included in overall TB
Stable disease (SD)	Stable FDG-PET uptake (DS 4–5) Decrease SPD < 50%	Same as Lugano	Decrease <10% to increase $\leq$20% in SLD
Progression of disease (PD)	Increased FDG-PET uptake (DS 4–5) Increase SPD $\geq$ 50% New lesions	As with Lugano, with the exception of IR IR(1): $\geq$50% increase in SPD in first 12 weeks IR(2): <50% increase in SPD with new lesion(s), or $\geq$50% increase in PPD of a lesion or set of lesions IR(3): increase in FDG uptake without a concomitant increase in lesion size	Increase in SLD by 20%. For relapse from CR, at least one lesion should measure 2 cm in the long axis with or without PET activity

SPD: sum of product of perpendicular diameters of target lesions. SLD: sum of the longest diameters of target lesions. IR: indeterminate response.

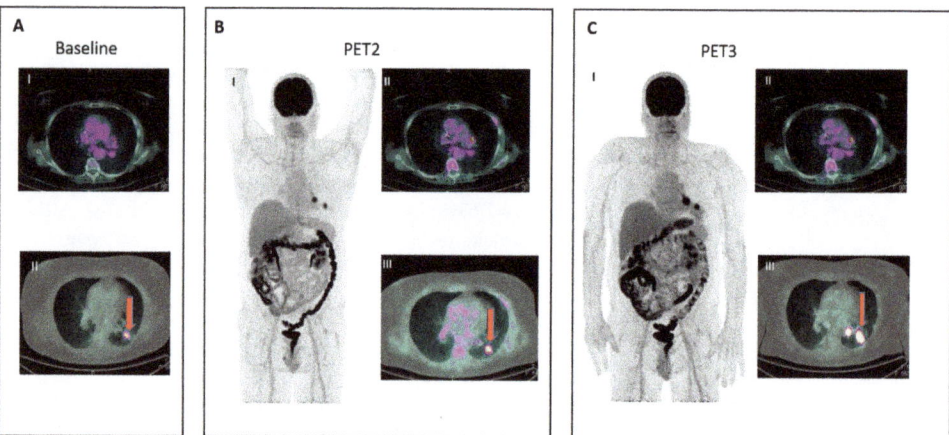

Figure 3. IR (3): Panel (**A**) shows baseline lesions (red arrow). Early PET evaluation (**B**) during nivolumab for Hodgkin lymphoma shows increase in FDG uptake (red arrow) in baseline lesions without concomitant increase in size. At subsequent PET evaluation (**C**), there is a concordant increment in size (red arrow), and criteria for true progression are met.

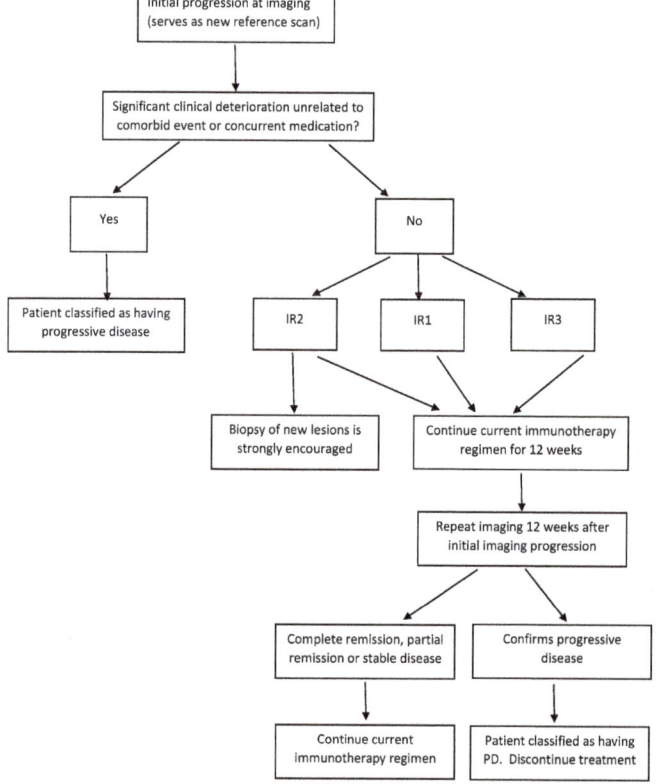

Figure 4. Flowchart of assessment of response to immunotherapy in lymphoma.

For an assessment of the response to immunotherapy in lymphomas, FDG-PET should be performed at baseline and repeated after three–four cycles (at 9–12 weeks). Immune checkpoint inhibitors induce inflammation that can translate into increased FDG uptake and even into the appearance of new lesions in the absence of true progression. In the assessment of patients with lymphoma during the course of immunotherapy, collaboration between clinicians, radiologists and PET readers in the context of a multidisciplinary approach is advisable in equivocal and challenging cases to discriminate treatment-induced inflammation/pseudoprogression from true progression. Decisions must be based on a repeated scan taken 12 weeks later. A re-biopsy, when feasible, might be necessary in cases of persistent FDG uptake, and it is encouraged in cases with the appearance of new lesions of indeterminate origin. We illustrate a possible algorithmic approach to patients with HL on immunotherapy in Figure 4.

4. Contribution of PET/CT-Derived Volumetric Parameters to Response Assessment

The morphologic CT-based criteria most widely adopted, the RECIST criteria, rely on a unidimensional assessment of target lesions, with up to five (two per organ maximum) intended to represent a sample of the total TB. Indeed, the assessment of the entire TB using CT in an individual patient is time consuming and complex. In contrast, by using PET/CT, exploiting the quantitative potential of parametric images, foci that accumulate FDG can be outlined by grouping together pixels with SUV above a chosen threshold (typically 41% of the maximum), quantified and summed up, with the aid of semiautomatic software for segmentation and with minimal manual intervention [46]. It is feasible to measure the total TB as metabolically active volume (MTV). Consequently, it is possible to easily assess the variations in TB between baseline and after therapy. Total lesion glycolysis, defined as MTV multiplied by SUVmean, can also be assessed using semiautomatic software, combining volumetric data with metabolic parameters.

EANM guidelines for the use of PET/CT to evaluate the response to immunotherapy recommend performing the computation of volumetric parameters at baseline to study their modifications later during treatment [47].

The additional contribution of PET-derived volumetric parameters has been evaluated in recent research studies (Table 2). Two single-center, retrospective studies [48,49] suggested that the SUV metric is suitable to evaluate the response to immunotherapy in relapsed/refractory HL. They outlined a significantly greater MTV (ΔMTV) and TLG reduction (ΔTLG) in responders (CR and PR according to DS) than in non-responders. A study by Castello [49] and colleagues also showed that, in the majority of responders (29/31), tumor burden shrinkage was greater than 50%. In this study, the variation in the tumor burden metrics at an early evaluation (8 weeks) correlated with variation at later time points and accurately predicted the long-term outcomes of the patients.

Table 2. Contribution of MTV to assessment of response to immunotherapy.

Study	Patients	Treatment	Time Points	Response Criteria	SUV Metrics	Results
Savas et al. (2018) [50]	13 I-IV HL Newly diagnosed	PEM	3 cycles	Lugano	MTV	Mean ΔMTV-90% CR 50%
Dercle et al. (2018) [48]	16 R/R HL	Nivolumab/ PEM	3 mth	Lugano LYRIC	SUVmax SUVmean MTV TLG	ΔMTV-90% in responders (PR+CR) ΔMTV < 50% in refractory (SD+PD)
Castello et al. (2019) [49]	43 R/R HL	Nivolumab/ PEM	Early (8 wks) Interim (17 wks)	Lugano LYRIC	SUVmax SUVmean MTV TLG	ΔMTV > 50% in 29/31 responders (PR+CR) Median MTV-95% CR 60%
Voltin et al. (2020) [51]	53 IIb HL therapy naïve	Nivolumab	4 cycles (16 wks)	Lugano	MTV TLG	Average ΔMTV-91% CR 46.4%

R/R: relapsed/refractory. PEM: pembrolizumab.

The feasibility of response assessment using PET-derived volumetric parameters has been evaluated in small cohorts of naïve patients receiving HL therapy. A study by Savas et al. [50] in 13 patients with newly diagnosed HL assessed ΔMTV and ΔTLG after 3 sequential cycles of pembrolizumab. Based on the analysis of the response rates at the end of treatment, this study suggested that the response to pembrolizumab is better captured by the dramatic decline in TB at an early assessment compared to conventional criteria, namely, DS and SPD. Similarly, a study by Voltin [51] in 53 patients with early unfavorable HL (stage II) treated with nivolumab showed an early near-complete MTV reduction (ΔMTV 91%), despite there being lower rates of CR assessed with conventional criteria. Based on the outcome analysis on a follow-up period of 12 months, the authors suggested that conventional criteria could underestimate the response in this cohort of stage II HL.

Recently, considering tumor heterogeneity and differences in therapy response, artificial intelligence (AI) approaches, radiomics and machine learning algorithms, have emerged as non-invasive technologies using medical imaging analyses. AI can extract significant quantitative data from patients' medical images and correlate image features with diagnostic and therapeutic outcomes [52,53]. Radiomics has been applied in lymphomas to examine baseline FDG-PET for differential diagnosis from other malignancies and in evaluations of bone marrow involvement and pre-treatment risk [54,55], but, currently, no data are available for radiomic analyses in the context of assessments of the response to immunotherapy in lymphomas [56,57].

As the state of the art, it is recommended to assess MTV and TLG before treatment and during treatment in scheduled PET scans to quantify changes in tumor burden, as this can orient the interpretation of the response to immunotherapy.

5. Immune-Related Adverse Events

Immune-related adverse events (irAEs) represent a major cause of treatment discontinuation and a confounding factor in response assessment at imaging. However, the side effects experienced during immunotherapy seem to be better tolerated than the side effects due to cytotoxic therapy; a lower risk of serious (grade III–IV) adverse events has been reported [58].

IrAEs are related to the recruitment of an immune infiltrate in the organs involved. From this perspective, IrAEs can be seen as an "undesirable" sign of immune activation or rather that immunotherapy is acting effectively, as suggested by some studies reporting an association between irAEs and treatment efficacy [59,60].

The first sign of immune activation is the inversion of the liver-to-spleen ratio, which may be accompanied by splenomegaly. Speen activation can be associated with a mild diffuse uptake in bone marrow. In an early phase, reactive lymph nodes may be seen in the basin of the tumor. A sarcoid-like reaction, consisting of an increased uptake in mediastinal hilar lymph nodes and pulmonary granulomatosis, can also occur. These phenomena are transient, self-limiting and require monitoring until their resolution.

IrAEs can affect any organ, particularly the endocrine system's glands (hypophysitis, thyroiditis and adrenalitis). A symmetrical enlargement of the adrenal gland with diffusely increased FDG uptake can be due to adrenalitis (Figure 5). With particular reference to nivolumab-induced thyrotoxicity, in a recent metanalysis by Barroso-Sousa and colleagues [61], incidence rates of 6.5% for hypothyroidism and of 2.5% for thyrotoxicosis are reported. Nivolumab-induced thyroid dysfunction is due to painless thyroiditis, characterized in most cases by an early-onset, transient, thyrotoxic phase, commonly followed by hypothyroidism. A research study investigated the underlying mechanism of the thyroid [62], suggesting that, since normal thyroid tissue expresses PDL1 and PDL2 mRNA and proteins, PD1 pathway blockade impairs immunotolerance and can induce autoimmune thyroiditis in the absence of TRAb positivity. The appearance of a diffusely increased FDG uptake in the thyroid gland in the course of immunotherapy (Figure 6) should be considered suggestive of incipient thyroiditis, even before clinical manifestation and obtaining laboratory findings [63].

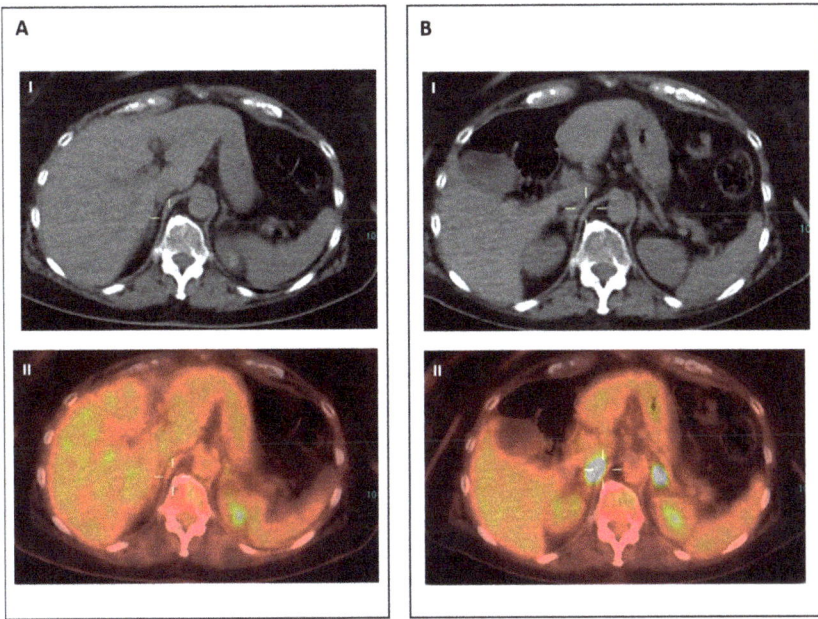

Figure 5. Adrenalitis: patient with advanced melanoma. Panel (**A**) shows CT (I) and PET/CT (II) during therapy with tyrosine kinase inhibitors; adrenal glands appear normal. Note the appearance of intense hypermetabolism in the adrenal glands (box (**B**), II) accompanied by symmetrical enlargement in CT images (box (**B**), I) during combined nivolumab plus ipilimumab treatment.

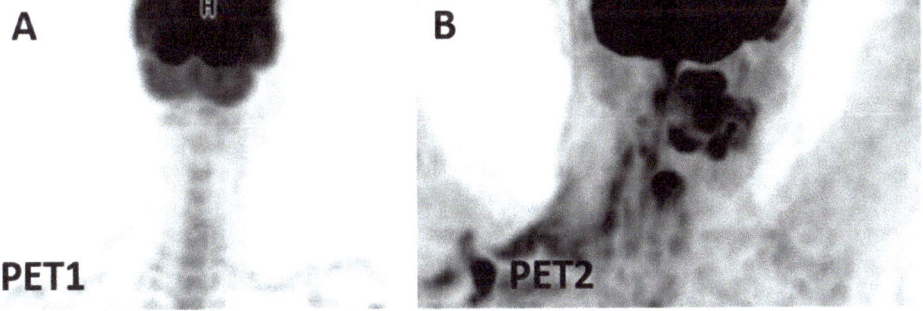

Figure 6. Nivolumab-induced thyroiditis: (**A**) no uptake in the thyroid gland at baseline. (**B**) appearance of diffuse mild uptake in the thyroid gland in a patient receiving nivolumab for Hodgkin lymphoma who developed thyroiditis.

A threatening irAE that can limit treatment cycles is checkpoint-inhibitor-related pneumonitis (CPI). An accurate diagnosis of CIP can be difficult since, during the treatment of oncological patients, other factors (infections, radiation therapy and other drugs) are often mixed. In recent years, several studies [64,65] have demonstrated the potential of CT radiomics to differentiate CIP from other conditions, such as radiation-induced pneumonitis, leading to the development of the Rad-score [66], a robust model combining 11 imaging histological features with bilateral involvement and sharp borders.

The spleen must be critically checked: spleen enlargement and the inversion of the physiological spleen-to-liver ratio can occur in the course of immunotherapy, similarly to what is observed during conventional rituximab-based regimens, and should not be mistaken for lymphoma involvement.

IrAEs can be asymptomatic; in this context, FDG-PET/CT, being sensitive to foci of active inflammation, including those due to immune activation, has the unique ability to detect irAEs before clinical manifestation.

6. Future Perspectives

The selection of patients suitable to receive immunotherapy relies on several biomarkers (PD-L1 immunohistochemistry, immunohistochemistry for mismatch repair proteins, PCR-based assays for microsatellite instability and sequencing for tumor mutational burden on biopsy); however, they are not perfect and cannot accurately predict patient outcome. Furthermore, the current approach to assessing PD1 status cannot detect heterogeneity over time and across lesions due to the dedifferentiation of tumor clones, which may occur during therapy. To address these limitations, novel PET tracers, designed as antibodies or fragments of antibodies for specific immunotargets (immune-PET), were developed in the past few years. Immuno-PET offers the possibility to non-invasively image in vivo the whole body biodistribution of immune checkpoints and hold the potential to guide treatment decision making.

The first human PD-L1 PET study was conducted with ^{89}Zr -atezolizumab in 22 patients with metastatic non-small-cell lung cancer (NSCLC), bladder cancer and triple-negative breast cancer [67]. The patients were imaged before starting immunotherapy. The study demonstrated a high tracer uptake in normal lymphoid tissue and sites of inflammation. Tumor lesions showed a generally high tumor uptake, with great intra-patient and inter-patient heterogeneity. [89Zr]Zr-atezolizumab uptake in tumor lesions correlated with the response to therapy, PFS and OS and outperformed immunohistochemistry on a fresh biopsy in the prediction of clinical response.

CD8 cells play an essential role in the cytotoxic response to tumors boosted by immunotherapy. The results of a clinical study evaluating the CD8 PET tracer 89ZED88082A, a zirconium-89-labeled one-armed antibody in solid tumors, have recently been published [68]. In this study, PET imaging was performed before and during immunotherapy. The pre-treatment biodistribution of the tracer showed specific CD8 targeting, with a high tracer uptake in normal lymphoid tissue. The tracer uptake in tumor lesions was variable within and between patients. The tumor uptake was higher in patients with mismatch-repair-deficient tumors and was correlated with CD8 cell density in tumors stained immunohistochemically. A higher SUVmax in tumor lesions at baseline showed a trend with improved OS. The results of serial 89ZED88082A imaging during immunotherapy showed a great spatial and temporal heterogeneity of the behavior of lesions in responders, providing an insight into the complex dynamic tumor microenvironment. A phase II trial investigating the efficacy of atezolizumab consolidation therapy in high-risk DLBCL is ongoing (HOVON 151) (NCT03850028) (https://clinicaltrials.gov last update posted 18 June 2019, accessed on 25 April 2023). In this study, patients are evaluated with sequential ^{89}Zr-atezolizumab imaging before and after R-CHOP induction therapy, during atezolizumab consolidation therapy and at the time of suspected relapse. The HOVON 151 trial reflects the application of immune-PET in the clinical setting and may widen therapeutic options in lymphomas.

In the future, the promising field of immuno-PET may hopefully improve patient selection for immunotherapy and response assessment, and it may guide the development of new agents.

7. Conclusions

The criteria for response assessment in lymphoma have deeply evolved in the last decade, assigning an outstanding role to FDG-PET/CT. This path starts from the first lymphoma-specific CT-based criteria and leads towards the PET-based Lugano Classification, which, nowadays, represents the gold standard. The LYRIC criteria, the recent refinement of the

Lugano Classification, were conceived to capture the new patterns of response observed during treatment with novel immunotherapy agents that have entered the clinic. In this context, PET/CT has the unique ability to assess response and uncover immune-related adverse events. PET/CT quantitative parameters, such as MTV and TLG, assessing changes in tumor burden may be useful tools in interpreting the response to immunotherapy.

Author Contributions: Conception and design, F.T. and A.C.; literature search, F.T., E.G. and S.C.; writing-original draft preparation, F.T., E.G. and G.G.; writing—review and editing, G.G., A.C.; visualization, S.C.; supervision, G.G. and A.C.; project administration, A.C. All authors have read and agreed to the published version of the manuscript.

Funding: This research received no external funding.

Conflicts of Interest: The authors declare no conflict of interest.

References

1. Schadendorf, D.; Hodi, F.S.; Robert, C.; Weber, J.S.; Margolin, K.; Hamid, O.; Patt, D.; Chen, T.T.; Berman, D.M. Pooled Analysis of Long-Term Survival Data From Phase II and Phase III Trials of Ipilimumab in Unresectable or Metastatic Melanoma. *J. Clin. Oncol.* **2015**, *33*, 1889–1894. [CrossRef] [PubMed]
2. Robert, C.; Ribas, A.; Wolchok, J.D.; Hodi, F.S.; Hamid, O.; Kefford, R.; Weber, J.S.; Joshua, A.M.; Hwu, W.J.; Gangadhar, T.C.; et al. Anti-programmed-death-receptor-1 treatment with pembrolizumab in ipilimumab-refractory advanced melanoma: A randomised dose-comparison cohort of a phase 1 trial. *Lancet* **2014**, *384*, 1109–1117. [CrossRef] [PubMed]
3. Larkin, J.; Chiarion-Sileni, V.; Gonzalez, R.; Grob, J.J.; Cowey, C.L.; Lao, C.D.; Schadendorf, D.; Dummer, R.; Smylie, M.; Rutkowski, P.; et al. Combined Nivolumab and Ipilimumab or Monotherapy in Untreated Melanoma. *N. Engl. J. Med.* **2015**, *373*, 23–34. [CrossRef] [PubMed]
4. Ansell, S.M.; Lesokhin, A.M.; Borrello, I.; Halwani, A.; Scott, E.C.; Gutierrez, M.; Schuster, S.J.; Millenson, M.M.; Cattry, D.; Freeman, G.J.; et al. PD-1 blockade with nivolumab in relapsed or refractory Hodgkin's lymphoma. *N. Engl. J. Med.* **2015**, *372*, 311–319. [CrossRef] [PubMed]
5. Younes, A.; Santoro, A.; Shipp, M.; Zinzani, P.L.; Timmerman, J.M.; Ansell, S.; Armand, P.; Fanale, M.; Ratanatharathorn, V.; Kuruvilla, J.; et al. Nivolumab for classical Hodgkin's lymphoma after failure of both autologous stem-cell transplantation and brentuximab vedotin: A multicentre, multicohort, single-arm phase 2 trial. *Lancet Oncol.* **2016**, *17*, 1283–1294. [CrossRef]
6. Armand, P.; Rodig, S.; Melnichenko, V.; Thieblemont, C.; Bouabdallah, K.; Tumyan, G.; Ozcan, M.; Portino, S.; Fogliatto, L.; Caballero, M.D.; et al. Pembrolizumab in Relapsed or Refractory Primary Mediastinal Large B-Cell Lymphoma. *J. Clin. Oncol.* **2019**, *37*, 3291–3299. [CrossRef]
7. Porta, C.; Sica, A.; Riboldi, E. Tumor-associated myeloid cells: New understandings on their metabolic regulation and their influence in cancer immunotherapy. *FEBS J.* **2018**, *285*, 717–733. [CrossRef]
8. Zhu, Y.; Knolhoff, B.L.; Meyer, M.A.; Nywening, T.M.; West, B.L.; Luo, J.; Wang-Gillam, A.; Goedegebuure, S.P.; Linehan, D.C.; DeNardo, D.G. CSF1/CSF1R blockade reprograms tumor-infiltrating macrophages and improves response to T-cell checkpoint immunotherapy in pancreatic cancer models. *Cancer Res.* **2014**, *74*, 5057–5069. [CrossRef]
9. Waniczek, D.; Lorenc, Z.; Snietura, M.; Wesecki, M.; Kopec, A.; Muc-Wierzgon, M. Tumor-Associated Macrophages and Regulatory T Cells Infiltration and the Clinical Outcome in Colorectal Cancer. *Arch. Immunol. Ther. Exp.* **2017**, *65*, 445–454. [CrossRef]
10. Pardoll, D.M. The blockade of immune checkpoints in cancer immunotherapy. *Nat. Rev. Cancer* **2012**, *12*, 252–264. [CrossRef]
11. Bochtler, P.; Kroger, A.; Schirmbeck, R.; Reimann, J. Type I IFN-induced, NKT cell-mediated negative control of CD8 T cell priming by dendritic cells. *J. Immunol.* **2008**, *181*, 1633–1643. [CrossRef] [PubMed]
12. Kolar, P.; Knieke, K.; Hegel, J.K.; Quandt, D.; Burmester, G.R.; Hoff, H.; Brunner-Weinzierl, M.C. CTLA-4 (CD152) controls homeostasis and suppressive capacity of regulatory T cells in mice. *Arthritis Rheum.* **2009**, *60*, 123–132. [CrossRef] [PubMed]
13. Witkowska, M.; Smolewski, P. Immune Checkpoint Inhibitors to Treat Malignant Lymphomas. *J. Immunol. Res.* **2018**, *2018*, 1982423. [CrossRef] [PubMed]
14. Green, M.R.; Monti, S.; Rodig, S.J.; Juszczynski, P.; Currie, T.; O'Donnell, E.; Chapuy, B.; Takeyama, K.; Neuberg, D.; Golub, T.R.; et al. Integrative analysis reveals selective 9p24.1 amplification, increased PD-1 ligand expression, and further induction via JAK2 in nodular sclerosing Hodgkin lymphoma and primary mediastinal large B-cell lymphoma. *Blood* **2010**, *116*, 3268–3277. [CrossRef]
15. Green, M.R.; Rodig, S.; Juszczynski, P.; Ouyang, J.; Sinha, P.; O'Donnell, E.; Neuberg, D.; Shipp, M.A. Constitutive AP-1 activity and EBV infection induce PD-L1 in Hodgkin lymphomas and posttransplant lymphoproliferative disorders: Implications for targeted therapy. *Clin. Cancer Res.* **2012**, *18*, 1611–1618. [CrossRef] [PubMed]
16. Shi, M.; Roemer, M.G.; Chapuy, B.; Liao, X.; Sun, H.; Pinkus, G.S.; Shipp, M.A.; Freeman, G.J.; Rodig, S.J. Expression of programmed cell death 1 ligand 2 (PD-L2) is a distinguishing feature of primary mediastinal (thymic) large B-cell lymphoma and associated with PDCD1LG2 copy gain. *Am. J. Surg. Pathol.* **2014**, *38*, 1715–1723. [CrossRef] [PubMed]

17. Nam-Cha, S.H.; Roncador, G.; Sanchez-Verde, L.; Montes-Moreno, S.; Acevedo, A.; Dominguez-Franjo, P.; Piris, M.A. PD-1, a follicular T-cell marker useful for recognizing nodular lymphocyte-predominant Hodgkin lymphoma. *Am. J. Surg. Pathol.* **2008**, *32*, 1252–1257. [CrossRef]
18. Sekulic, A.; Liang, W.S.; Tembe, W.; Izatt, T.; Kruglyak, S.; Kiefer, J.A.; Cuyugan, L.; Zismann, V.; Legendre, C.; Pittelkow, M.R.; et al. Personalized treatment of Sezary syndrome by targeting a novel CTLA4:CD28 fusion. *Mol Genet. Genom. Med.* **2015**, *3*, 130–136. [CrossRef]
19. Miller, A.B.; Hoogstraten, B.; Staquet, M.; Winkler, A. Reporting results of cancer treatment. *Cancer* **1981**, *47*, 207–214. [CrossRef]
20. Young, H.; Baum, R.; Cremerius, U.; Herholz, K.; Hoekstra, O.; Lammertsma, A.A.; Pruim, J.; Price, P. Measurement of clinical and subclinical tumour response using [18F]-fluorodeoxyglucose and positron emission tomography: Review and 1999 EORTC recommendations. European Organization for Research and Treatment of Cancer (EORTC) PET Study Group. *Eur. J. Cancer* **1999**, *35*, 1773–1782. [CrossRef]
21. Therasse, P.; Arbuck, S.G.; Eisenhauer, E.A.; Wanders, J.; Kaplan, R.S.; Rubinstein, L.; Verweij, J.; Van Glabbeke, M.; van Oosterom, A.T.; Christian, M.C.; et al. New guidelines to evaluate the response to treatment in solid tumors. European Organization for Research and Treatment of Cancer, National Cancer Institute of the United States, National Cancer Institute of Canada. *J. Natl. Cancer Inst.* **2000**, *92*, 205–216. [CrossRef] [PubMed]
22. Eisenhauer, E.A.; Therasse, P.; Bogaerts, J.; Schwartz, L.H.; Sargent, D.; Ford, R.; Dancey, J.; Arbuck, S.; Gwyther, S.; Mooney, M.; et al. New response evaluation criteria in solid tumours: Revised RECIST guideline (version 1.1). *Eur. J. Cancer* **2009**, *45*, 228–247. [CrossRef] [PubMed]
23. James, K.; Eisenhauer, E.; Christian, M.; Terenziani, M.; Vena, D.; Muldal, A.; Therasse, P. Measuring response in solid tumors: Unidimensional versus bidimensional measurement. *J. Natl. Cancer Inst.* **1999**, *91*, 523–528. [CrossRef] [PubMed]
24. Wahl, R.L.; Jacene, H.; Kasamon, Y.; Lodge, M.A. From RECIST to PERCIST: Evolving Considerations for PET response criteria in solid tumors. *J. Nucl. Med.* **2009**, *50*, 122S–150S. [CrossRef]
25. Cheson, B.D.; Horning, S.J.; Coiffier, B.; Shipp, M.A.; Fisher, R.I.; Connors, J.M.; Lister, T.A.; Vose, J.; Grillo-Lopez, A.; Hagenbeek, A.; et al. Report of an international workshop to standardize response criteria for non-Hodgkin's lymphomas. NCI Sponsored International Working Group. *J. Clin. Oncol.* **1999**, *17*, 1244. [CrossRef]
26. Juweid, M.E.; Wiseman, G.A.; Vose, J.M.; Ritchie, J.M.; Menda, Y.; Wooldridge, J.E.; Mottaghy, F.M.; Rohren, E.M.; Blumstein, N.M.; Stolpen, A.; et al. Response assessment of aggressive non-Hodgkin's lymphoma by integrated International Workshop Criteria and fluorine-18-fluorodeoxyglucose positron emission tomography. *J. Clin. Oncol.* **2005**, *23*, 4652–4661. [CrossRef]
27. Cheson, B.D. The International Harmonization Project for response criteria in lymphoma clinical trials. *Hematol. Oncol. Clin. N. Am.* **2007**, *21*, 841–854. [CrossRef]
28. Juweid, M.E.; Stroobants, S.; Hoekstra, O.S.; Mottaghy, F.M.; Dietlein, M.; Guermazi, A.; Wiseman, G.A.; Kostakoglu, L.; Scheidhauer, K.; Buck, A.; et al. Use of positron emission tomography for response assessment of lymphoma: Consensus of the Imaging Subcommittee of International Harmonization Project in Lymphoma. *J. Clin. Oncol.* **2007**, *25*, 571–578. [CrossRef]
29. Meignan, M.; Gallamini, A.; Haioun, C.; Polliack, A. Report on the Second International Workshop on interim positron emission tomography in lymphoma held in Menton, France, 8–9 April 2010. *Leuk. Lymphoma* **2010**, *51*, 2171–2180. [CrossRef]
30. Meignan, M.; Gallamini, A.; Itti, E.; Barrington, S.; Haioun, C.; Polliack, A. Report on the Third International Workshop on Interim Positron Emission Tomography in Lymphoma held in Menton, France, 26–27 September 2011 and Menton 2011 consensus. *Leuk. Lymphoma* **2012**, *53*, 1876–1881. [CrossRef]
31. Barrington, S.F.; Mikhaeel, N.G.; Kostakoglu, L.; Meignan, M.; Hutchings, M.; Mueller, S.P.; Schwartz, L.H.; Zucca, E.; Fisher, R.I.; Trotman, J.; et al. Role of imaging in the staging and response assessment of lymphoma: Consensus of the International Conference on Malignant Lymphomas Imaging Working Group. *J. Clin. Oncol.* **2014**, *32*, 3048–3058. [CrossRef] [PubMed]
32. Annunziata, S.; Cuccaro, A.; Calcagni, M.L.; Hohaus, S.; Giordano, A.; Rufini, V. Interim FDG-PET/CT in Hodgkin lymphoma: The prognostic role of the ratio between target lesion and liver SUVmax (rPET). *Ann. Nucl. Med.* **2016**, *30*, 588–592. [CrossRef] [PubMed]
33. Hasenclever, D.; Kurch, L.; Mauz-Korholz, C.; Elsner, A.; Georgi, T.; Wallace, H.; Landman-Parker, J.; Moryl-Bujakowska, A.; Cepelova, M.; Karlen, J.; et al. qPET—A quantitative extension of the Deauville scale to assess response in interim FDG-PET scans in lymphoma. *Eur. J. Nucl. Med. Mol. Imaging* **2014**, *41*, 1301–1308. [CrossRef] [PubMed]
34. Georgi, T.W.; Kurch, L.; Hasenclever, D.; Warbey, V.S.; Pike, L.; Radford, J.; Sabri, O.; Kluge, R.; Barrington, S.F. Quantitative assessment of interim PET in Hodgkin lymphoma: An evaluation of the qPET method in adult patients in the RAPID trial. *PLoS ONE* **2020**, *15*, e0231027. [CrossRef]
35. Chanan-Khan, A.; Miller, K.C.; Musial, L.; Lawrence, D.; Padmanabhan, S.; Takeshita, K.; Porter, C.W.; Goodrich, D.W.; Bernstein, Z.P.; Wallace, P.; et al. Clinical efficacy of lenalidomide in patients with relapsed or refractory chronic lymphocytic leukemia: Results of a phase II study. *J. Clin. Oncol.* **2006**, *24*, 5343–5349. [CrossRef]
36. Eve, H.E.; Rule, S.A. Lenalidomide-induced tumour flare reaction in mantle cell lymphoma. *Br. J. Haematol.* **2010**, *151*, 410–412. [CrossRef]
37. Corazzelli, G.; De Filippi, R.; Capobianco, G.; Frigeri, F.; De Rosa, V.; Iaccarino, G.; Russo, F.; Arcamone, M.; Becchimanzi, C.; Crisci, S.; et al. Tumor flare reactions and response to lenalidomide in patients with refractory classic Hodgkin lymphoma. *Am. J. Hematol.* **2010**, *85*, 87–90. [CrossRef]

38. Chanan-Khan, A.A.; Chitta, K.; Ersing, N.; Paulus, A.; Masood, A.; Sher, T.; Swaika, A.; Wallace, P.K.; Mashtare, T.L.; Wilding, G., Jr.; et al. Biological effects and clinical significance of lenalidomide-induced tumour flare reaction in patients with chronic lymphocytic leukaemia: In vivo evidence of immune activation and antitumour response. *Br. J. Haematol.* **2011**, *155*, 457–467. [CrossRef]
39. Champiat, S.; Dercle, L.; Ammari, S.; Massard, C.; Hollebecque, A.; Postel-Vinay, S.; Chaput, N.; Eggermont, A.; Marabelle, A.; Soria, J.C.; et al. Hyperprogressive Disease Is a New Pattern of Progression in Cancer Patients Treated by Anti-PD-1/PD-L1. *Clin. Cancer Res.* **2017**, *23*, 1920–1928. [CrossRef]
40. Saada-Bouzid, E.; Defaucheux, C.; Karabajakian, A.; Coloma, V.P.; Servois, V.; Paoletti, X.; Even, C.; Fayette, J.; Guigay, J.; Loirat, D.; et al. Hyperprogression during anti-PD-1/PD-L1 therapy in patients with recurrent and/or metastatic head and neck squamous cell carcinoma. *Ann. Oncol.* **2017**, *28*, 1605–1611. [CrossRef]
41. Wolchok, J.D.; Hoos, A.; O'Day, S.; Weber, J.S.; Hamid, O.; Lebbe, C.; Maio, M.; Binder, M.; Bohnsack, O.; Nichol, G.; et al. Guidelines for the evaluation of immune therapy activity in solid tumors: Immune-related response criteria. *Clin. Cancer Res.* **2009**, *15*, 7412–7420. [CrossRef] [PubMed]
42. Nishino, M.; Giobbie-Hurder, A.; Gargano, M.; Suda, M.; Ramaiya, N.H.; Hodi, F.S. Developing a common language for tumor response to immunotherapy: Immune-related response criteria using unidimensional measurements. *Clin. Cancer Res.* **2013**, *19*, 3936–3943. [CrossRef] [PubMed]
43. Seymour, L.; Bogaerts, J.; Perrone, A.; Ford, R.; Schwartz, L.H.; Mandrekar, S.; Lin, N.U.; Litiere, S.; Dancey, J.; Chen, A.; et al. iRECIST: Guidelines for response criteria for use in trials testing immunotherapeutics. *Lancet Oncol.* **2017**, *18*, e143–e152. [CrossRef] [PubMed]
44. Cheson, B.D.; Ansell, S.; Schwartz, L.; Gordon, L.I.; Advani, R.; Jacene, H.A.; Hoos, A.; Barrington, S.F.; Armand, P. Refinement of the Lugano Classification lymphoma response criteria in the era of immunomodulatory therapy. *Blood* **2016**, *128*, 2489–2496. [CrossRef]
45. Younes, A.; Hilden, P.; Coiffier, B.; Hagenbeek, A.; Salles, G.; Wilson, W.; Seymour, J.F.; Kelly, K.; Gribben, J.; Pfreundschuh, M.; et al. International Working Group consensus response evaluation criteria in lymphoma (RECIL 2017). *Ann. Oncol.* **2017**, *28*, 1436–1447. [CrossRef]
46. Boellaard, R.; Delgado-Bolton, R.; Oyen, W.J.; Giammarile, F.; Tatsch, K.; Eschner, W.; Verzijlbergen, F.J.; Barrington, S.F.; Pike, L.C.; Weber, W.A.; et al. FDG PET/CT: EANM procedure guidelines for tumour imaging: Version 2.0. *Eur. J. Nucl. Med. Mol. Imaging* **2015**, *42*, 328–354. [CrossRef]
47. Lopci, E.; Hicks, R.J.; Dimitrakopoulou-Strauss, A.; Dercle, L.; Iravani, A.; Seban, R.D.; Sachpekidis, C.; Humbert, O.; Gheysens, O.; Glaudemans, A.; et al. Joint EANM/SNMMI/ANZSNM practice guidelines/procedure standards on recommended use of [(18)F]FDG PET/CT imaging during immunomodulatory treatments in patients with solid tumors version 1.0. *Eur. J. Nucl. Med. Mol. Imaging* **2022**, *49*, 2323–2341. [CrossRef]
48. Dercle, L.; Seban, R.D.; Lazarovici, J.; Schwartz, L.H.; Houot, R.; Ammari, S.; Danu, A.; Edeline, V.; Marabelle, A.; Ribrag, V.; et al. (18)F-FDG PET and CT Scans Detect New Imaging Patterns of Response and Progression in Patients with Hodgkin Lymphoma Treated by Anti-Programmed Death 1 Immune Checkpoint Inhibitor. *J. Nucl. Med.* **2018**, *59*, 15–24.
49. Castello, A.; Grizzi, F.; Qehajaj, D.; Rahal, D.; Lutman, F.; Lopci, E. (18)F-FDG PET/CT for response assessment in Hodgkin lymphoma undergoing immunotherapy with checkpoint inhibitors. *Leuk Lymphoma* **2019**, *60*, 367–375. [CrossRef]
50. Allen, P.B.; Karmali, R.; Pro, B.; Evens, A.M.; Dillehay, G.; Rademaker, A.; Palmer, B.; Advani, R.; Gordon, L.I.; Winter, J.N. A Phase II Study of Sequential Pembrolizumab (PEM) Followed by AVD for Frontline Treatment of Classical Hodgkin Lymphoma (CHL): Quantifying Response Following PEM Monotherapy with FDG-PET-Derived Metabolic Tumor Volume and Total Lesion Glycolysis. *Blood* **2018**, *2*, 42. [CrossRef]
51. Voltin, C.A.; Mettler, J.; van Heek, L.; Goergen, H.; Muller, H.; Baues, C.; Keller, U.; Meissner, J.; Trautmann-Grill, K.; Kerkhoff, A.; et al. Early Response to First-Line Anti-PD-1 Treatment in Hodgkin Lymphoma: A PET-Based Analysis from the Prospective, Randomized Phase II NIVAHL Trial. *Clin. Cancer Res.* **2021**, *27*, 402–407. [CrossRef] [PubMed]
52. Kim, N.; Lee, E.S.; Won, S.E.; Yang, M.; Lee, A.J.; Shin, Y.; Ko, Y.; Pyo, J.; Park, H.J.; Kim, K.W. Evolution of Radiological Treatment Response Assessments for Cancer Immunotherapy: From iRECIST to Radiomics and Artificial Intelligence. *Korean J. Radiol.* **2022**, *23*, 1089–1101. [CrossRef] [PubMed]
53. Oriuchi, N.; Endoh, H.; Kaira, K. Monitoring of Current Cancer Therapy by Positron Emission Tomography and Possible Role of Radiomics Assessment. *Int. J. Mol. Sci.* **2022**, *23*, 9394. [CrossRef] [PubMed]
54. Jiang, H.; Li, A.; Ji, Z.; Tian, M.; Zhang, H. Role of Radiomics-Based Baseline PET/CT Imaging in Lymphoma: Diagnosis, Prognosis, and Response Assessment. *Mol. Imaging Biol.* **2022**, *24*, 537–549. [CrossRef]
55. Cottereau, A.S.; Meignan, M.; Nioche, C.; Clerc, J.; Chartier, L.; Vercellino, L.; Casasnovas, O.; Thieblemont, C.; Buvat, I. New Approaches in Characterization of Lesions Dissemination in DLBCL Patients on Baseline PET/CT. *Cancers* **2021**, *13*, 3998. [CrossRef]
56. Lopci, E. Immunotherapy Monitoring with Immune Checkpoint Inhibitors Based on [(18)F]FDG PET/CT in Metastatic Melanomas and Lung Cancer. *J. Clin. Med.* **2021**, *10*, 5160. [CrossRef]
57. Kiamanesh, Z.; Ayati, N.; Sadeghi, R.; Hawkes, E.; Lee, S.T.; Scott, A.M. The value of FDG PET/CT imaging in outcome prediction and response assessment of lymphoma patients treated with immunotherapy: A meta-analysis and systematic review. *Eur. J. Nucl. Med. Mol. Imaging* **2022**, *49*, 4661–4676. [CrossRef]

58. Nishijima, T.F.; Shachar, S.S.; Nyrop, K.A.; Muss, H.B. Safety and Tolerability of PD-1/PD-L1 Inhibitors Compared with Chemotherapy in Patients with Advanced Cancer: A Meta-Analysis. *Oncologist* **2017**, *22*, 470–479. [CrossRef]
59. Haratani, K.; Hayashi, H.; Nakagawa, K. Association of immune-related adverse events with immune checkpoint inhibitor efficacy: Real or imaginary? *BMC Med.* **2020**, *18*, 111. [CrossRef]
60. Nobashi, T.; Baratto, L.; Reddy, S.A.; Srinivas, S.; Toriihara, A.; Hatami, N.; Yohannan, T.K.; Mittra, E. Predicting Response to Immunotherapy by Evaluating Tumors, Lymphoid Cell-Rich Organs, and Immune-Related Adverse Events Using FDG-PET/CT. *Clin. Nucl. Med.* **2019**, *44*, e272–e279. [CrossRef]
61. Barroso-Sousa, R.; Barry, W.T.; Garrido-Castro, A.C.; Hodi, F.S.; Min, L.; Krop, I.E.; Tolaney, S.M. Incidence of Endocrine Dysfunction Following the Use of Different Immune Checkpoint Inhibitor Regimens: A Systematic Review and Meta-analysis. *JAMA Oncol.* **2018**, *4*, 173–182. [CrossRef] [PubMed]
62. Yamauchi, I.; Sakane, Y.; Fukuda, Y.; Fujii, T.; Taura, D.; Hirata, M.; Hirota, K.; Ueda, Y.; Kanai, Y.; Yamashita, Y.; et al. Clinical Features of Nivolumab-Induced Thyroiditis: A Case Series Study. *Thyroid* **2017**, *27*, 894–901. [CrossRef]
63. Eshghi, N.; Garland, L.L.; Nia, E.; Betancourt, R.; Krupinski, E.; Kuo, P.H. (18)F-FDG PET/CT Can Predict Development of Thyroiditis Due to Immunotherapy for Lung Cancer. *J. Nucl. Med. Technol.* **2018**, *46*, 260–264. [CrossRef]
64. Chen, X.; Sheikh, K.; Nakajima, E.; Lin, C.T.; Lee, J.; Hu, C.; Hales, R.K.; Forde, P.M.; Naidoo, J.; Voong, K.R. Radiation versus immune checkpoint inhibitor associated pneumonitis: Distinct radiologic morphologies. *Oncologist* **2021**, *26*, e1822–e1832. [CrossRef] [PubMed]
65. Cheng, J.; Pan, Y.; Huang, W.; Wang, L.; Ni, D.; Tan, P. Differentiation between immune checkpoint inhibitor-related and radiation pneumonitis in lung cancer by CT radiomics and machine learning. *Med. Phys.* **2022**, *49*, 1547–1558. [CrossRef] [PubMed]
66. Qiu, Q.; Xing, L.; Wang, Y.; Feng, A.; Wen, Q. Development and validation of a radiomics nomogram using computed tomography for differentiating immune checkpoint inhibitor-related pneumonitis from radiation pneumonitis for patients with non-small cell lung cancer. *Front. Immunol.* **2022**, *13*, 870842. [CrossRef] [PubMed]
67. Bensch, F.; van der Veen, E.L.; Lub-de Hooge, M.N.; Jorritsma-Smit, A.; Boellaard, R.; Kok, I.C.; Oosting, S.F.; Schröder, C.P.; Hiltermann, T.J.N.; van der Wekken, A.J.; et al. ^{89}Zr-atezolizumab imaging as a non-invasive approach to assess clinical response to PD-L1 blockade in cancer. *Nat. Med.* **2018**, *24*, 1852–1858. [CrossRef]
68. Kist de Ruijter, L.; van de Donk, P.P.; Hooiveld-Noeken, J.S.; Giesen, D.; Elias, S.G.; Lub-de Hooge, M.N.; Oosting, S.F.; Jalving, M.; Timens, W.; Brouwers, A.H.; et al. Whole-body CD8$^+$ T cell visualization before and during cancer immunotherapy: A phase 1/2 trial. *Nat. Med.* **2022**, *28*, 2601–2610. [CrossRef] [PubMed]

Disclaimer/Publisher's Note: The statements, opinions and data contained in all publications are solely those of the individual author(s) and contributor(s) and not of MDPI and/or the editor(s). MDPI and/or the editor(s) disclaim responsibility for any injury to people or property resulting from any ideas, methods, instructions or products referred to in the content.

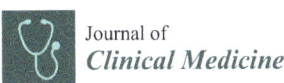

Article

Diagnostic Performance of Dynamic Whole-Body Patlak [^{18}F]FDG-PET/CT in Patients with Indeterminate Lung Lesions and Lymph Nodes

Matthias Weissinger [1,2], Max Atmanspacher [1], Werner Spengler [3], Ferdinand Seith [2], Sebastian Von Beschwitz [1], Helmut Dittmann [1], Lars Zender [3], Anne M. Smith [4], Michael E. Casey [4], Konstantin Nikolaou [2,5,6], Salvador Castaneda-Vega [1,7,*] and Christian la Fougère [1,5,6]

[1] Department of Nuclear Medicine and Clinical Molecular Imaging, University Hospital Tuebingen, 72076 Tuebingen, Germany; max.atmanspacher@student.uni-tuebingen.de (M.A.)
[2] Department of Diagnostic and Interventional Radiology, University Hospital Tuebingen, 72076 Tuebingen, Germany
[3] Department for Internal Medicine VIII, University Hospital Tuebingen, 72076 Tuebingen, Germany
[4] Siemens Medical Solutions USA, Inc., Molecular Imaging, Knoxville, TN 37932, USA
[5] iFIT-Cluster of Excellence, Eberhard Karls University Tuebingen, 72076 Tuebingen, Germany
[6] German Cancer Consortium (DKTK), Partner Site Tuebingen, 72076 Tuebingen, Germany
[7] Werner Siemens Imaging Center, Department of Preclinical Imaging and Radiopharmacy, Eberhard Karls University Tuebingen, 72076 Tuebingen, Germany
* Correspondence: salvador.castaneda@med.uni-tuebingen.de

Abstract: Background: Static [^{18}F]FDG-PET/CT is the imaging method of choice for the evaluation of indeterminate lung lesions and NSCLC staging; however, histological confirmation of PET-positive lesions is needed in most cases due to its limited specificity. Therefore, we aimed to evaluate the diagnostic performance of additional dynamic whole-body PET. Methods: A total of 34 consecutive patients with indeterminate pulmonary lesions were enrolled in this prospective trial. All patients underwent static (60 min p.i.) and dynamic (0–60 min p.i.) whole-body [^{18}F]FDG-PET/CT (300 MBq) using the multi-bed-multi-timepoint technique (Siemens mCT FlowMotion). Histology and follow-up served as ground truth. Kinetic modeling factors were calculated using a two-compartment linear Patlak model (FDG influx rate constant = Ki, metabolic rate = MR-FDG, distribution volume = DV-FDG) and compared to SUV using ROC analysis. Results: MR-FDG$_{mean}$ provided the best discriminatory power between benign and malignant lung lesions with an AUC of 0.887. The AUC of DV-FDG$_{mean}$ (0.818) and SUV$_{mean}$ (0.827) was non-significantly lower. For LNM, the AUCs for MR-FDG$_{mean}$ (0.987) and SUV$_{mean}$ (0.993) were comparable. Moreover, the DV-FDG$_{mean}$ in liver metastases was three times higher than in bone or lung metastases. Conclusions: Metabolic rate quantification was shown to be a reliable method to detect malignant lung tumors, LNM, and distant metastases at least as accurately as the established SUV or dual-time-point PET scans.

Keywords: whole-body; dynamic PET; parametric FDG; Patlak; FDG; PET/CT

Citation: Weissinger, M.; Atmanspacher, M.; Spengler, W.; Seith, F.; Von Beschwitz, S.; Dittmann, H.; Zender, L.; Smith, A.M.; Casey, M.E.; Nikolaou, K.; et al. Diagnostic Performance of Dynamic Whole-Body Patlak [^{18}F]FDG-PET/CT in Patients with Indeterminate Lung Lesions and Lymph Nodes. *J. Clin. Med.* **2023**, *12*, 3942. https://doi.org/10.3390/jcm12123942

Academic Editors: Arutselvan Natarajan and Filippo Lococo

Received: 5 April 2023
Revised: 22 May 2023
Accepted: 30 May 2023
Published: 9 June 2023

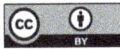

Copyright: © 2023 by the authors. Licensee MDPI, Basel, Switzerland. This article is an open access article distributed under the terms and conditions of the Creative Commons Attribution (CC BY) license (https:// creativecommons.org/licenses/by/ 4.0/).

1. Introduction

Lung cancer continues to be the tumor disease with the leading number of cancer deaths worldwide [1]. Precise staging is essential for the initiation of adequate therapy [2]. PET/CT with the glucose analog [^{18}F]Fluorodeoxyglucose ([^{18}F]FDG) assumes a central function for staging lung cancer, according to international guidelines [3,4]. [^{18}F]FDG-PET is generally performed as a static scan, at a defined uptake time of 60 to 90 min after intravenous (i.v.) tracer application. However, due to increased [^{18}F]FDG affinity in inflammatory tissue, [^{18}F]FDG-PET is known to have limited specificity for an accurate evaluation of thoracic lymph nodes, especially in the presence of frequently associated tumor inflammatory pulmonary disease. Thus, [^{18}F]FDG-avid lymph nodes must be biopsied before surgery or radiotherapy to rule out malignancy histologically [3,4]. However, such an intervention is often difficult and risky in clinical practice due to the often-limited cardiopulmonary reserve. Furthermore, the evaluation of indeterminate lung lesions, which cannot be biopsied due to their location or unfavorable risk–benefit to the patient, is also an indication for PET [3,4].

One way to generate complementary PET information is to quantify the tracer distribution over time. Until recently, this was typically feasible using two workflows with significant limitations. The first option is a dynamic acquisition, where the tracer distribution is continuously measured in a defined but limited anatomical region. Using this method, the axial field of view of current well-established PET scanners (generally between 15 and 30 cm) limits the anatomical coverage, which in turn restricts the dynamic acquisition of whole-body data [5,6]. A second option is a dual-/multi-time-point PET: this technique combines two or more static PET examinations and calculates the difference in [^{18}F]FDG uptake [7–9]. Whereas traditional dynamic PET is not suitable for whole-body staging due to the limited FOV of the PET scanner, dual-time-point imaging has already shown significantly increased accuracy for the assessment of mediastinal lymph node metastases (LNM) in a large meta-analysis of 654 patients with non-small cell lung cancer (NSCLC) [7].

Dynamic whole-body PET data can be produced using an innovative combination of dynamic acquisition at the start of the scan followed by multiple subsequent whole-body scans either in the "step-and-shoot" or in the "continuous-bed-motion" technique. This form of dynamic data acquisition can be used for Patlak kinetic modeling, which enables the assessment of [^{18}F]FDG distribution in different compartments separately for each organ and tissue in the body [10–13]. However, the clinical benefit of this technique and of dynamic information on tumor staging has not been completely elucidated.

Therefore, the aim of this prospective study was to assess the feasibility of dynamic whole-body PET acquisition in a clinical setting and to evaluate the diagnostic performance of parametric imaging in the classification of indeterminate lung lesions and lymph nodes.

2. Materials and Methods

2.1. Study Design

Thirty-three consecutive patients with indeterminate pulmonary lesions and a clinical indication for [^{18}F]FDG-PET/CT were enrolled into this prospective unicentric trial between June 2019 and April 2022, as shown in detail in the Consolidated Standards of Reporting Trials (CONSORT) flow diagram (Figure 1). This prospective trial was approved by the Institutional Review Board (registry No. 333/2019BO2) and is listed in the German Clinical Trial Register (DRKS-ID: DRKS00017717). All patients signed an informed consent.

2.2. PET/CT Examination Protocol

Patients were asked to fast for at least 6 h prior to examination. Weight, size, and blood sugar level were measured before i.v. tracer administration. Blood glucose level was below 140 mg/dL in all patients without the administration of insulin 8 h prior to tracer application. [^{18}F]FDG dosing was weight-based using 4.0 ± 0.6 MBq/kg. All patients were positioned with arms up on a vacuum mattress on the PET/CT (Biograph mCT, Siemens Healthineers) table to reduce motion artifacts and were asked to breathe as calmly and steadily as possible.

Before PET, a full diagnostic CT with adaptable tube voltage and tube current (CARE KV 120–140 kV, CARE Dose 4D 40–280 mAs) was performed. An iodinated contrast agent (80–100 mL Ultravist® 370, Bayer Vital GmbH, Leverkusen, Germany) was administered to all patients except for contraindications.

The dynamic PET acquisition started simultaneously with the i.v. injection of [^{18}F]FDG and lasted a total of 80 min. The initial table position was centered over the cardiac region (BI $\approx$ 6 min) to acquire the individual input function followed by whole-body (WB) dynamic PET of skull to mid-thigh (WB $\approx$ 74 min) using continuous-bed-motion as described in detail by Karakatsanis et al. and Rahmim et al. [10–12].

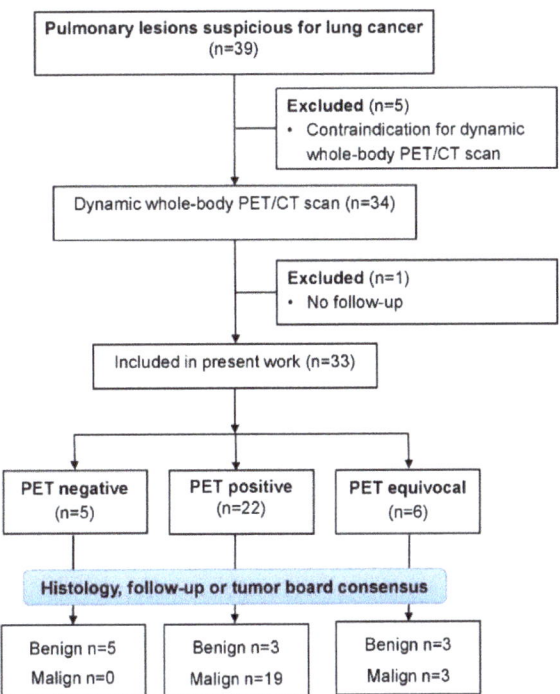

Figure 1. CONSORT flow diagram for patient enrolment. PET = Positron Emission Tomography; CT = Computer Tomography.

Image data were subdivided into 43 time frames (12 × 5 s, 6 × 10 s, 8 × 30 s, 7 × 180 s, and 10 × 300 s.) The time activity curve (TAC) was derived by an automatically generated cylindric volume of interest (VOI: 10 mm diameter and 20 mm long) centered in the descending aorta with acquired CT images using ALPHA (automated learning and parsing of human anatomy) as implemented in the vendor's software (VG70A, Siemens Healthcare GmbH, Erlangen, Germany).

2.3. Reconstruction and Postprocessing

Dynamic PET data (cardiac region and WB) were reconstructed with OSEM 3D reconstruction applying point-spread-function (PSF) and time-of-flight (TOF)—using two iterations, 21 subsets, a 200 × 200 matrix, and a 5 mm Gaussian filter. The reconstructed passes 12–17 of the WB and the resulting TAC were used to perform the Patlak reconstructions with two iterations, 21 subsets, a 200 × 200 matrix, and a Gaussian 5 mm filter as implemented in the vendor's software (VG70A, Siemens Healthcare GmbH).

A standard of care static whole-body image was reconstructed by using passes 15–17 of the WB, with ultraHD-PET (PSF + TOF), two iterations, 21 subsets, and a 400 × 400 matrix with a Gaussian 2 mm filter.

[^{18}F]FDG kinetics were modeled using a two-compartment model based on linear Patlak analysis [14,15], as described in detail by A. M. Smith et al. [16], resulting in the generation of whole-body Patlak slope and Patlak intercept parametric images. Patlak slope, which represents the constant influx rate of [^{18}F]FDG (Ki_{mean}, given in mL/(min × 100 mL) = 0.01 × min^{-1}), was multiplied by the blood glucose level to calculate the metabolic rate of [^{18}F]FDG (MR-FDG$_{mean}$) and is expressed as μmol/(min × 100 mL). Patlak intercept is expressed in percent and represents the distribution volume of free [^{18}F]FDG (DV-FDG$_{mean}$) in the reversible compartments and fractional blood volume [13]. Semiquantitative measurements were performed in static images using SUV_{max}, SUV_{mean} (50% isocontour), and SUV_{peak} (1 mL sphere).

2.4. Image Evaluation and Segmentation

Parametric images were produced and quantified using syngo.via® 8.2 (Siemens Healthineers, Erlangen, Germany). Volumes of interest (VOIs) were manually delineated in the fused PET/CT images and validated by a certified expert in nuclear medicine with more than five years of experience in PET/CT. VOIs were overlaid on the Ki dataset, DV-FDG, and on the static PET images for data extraction. If necessary, manual coregistration was performed to assure adequate realignment.

2.5. Ground Truth

The final diagnosis was provided by histology, long-time follow-up, and/or as a consensus decision of the institutional interdisciplinary tumor board.

2.6. Statistical Analysis

Differences in the mean values of two groups, features, or methods were tested for significance using the two-sided Student's t-test. Levene's test was performed to assess the equality of variance before the t-tests.

One-way ANOVA was performed to compare the dignity (inflammation, benign, or malign) of the different groups for the studied metrics (e.g., DV-FDGmean, MR-FDGmean). An alpha level of 0.05 was used for analysis. Subsequent multiple comparison correction was performed using Tukey's honestly significant difference procedure. Results of the ANOVA are shown with p values in the main manuscript. Correlation coefficients were calculated according to Pearson and a Pearson correlation coefficient of $r > 0.7$ was defined as strong, 0.7–0.3 as moderate, and <0.3 as a weak linear correlation. A p-value < 0.05 was considered statistically significant.

The intersection of the false-negative and false-positive rates was defined as the optimal cut-off value. Statistical analysis was performed with SPSS Statistics 28.0 software (IBM Inc., Armonk, NY, USA), MATLAB v. R2022b (The MathWorks, Inc., Natick, MA, USA), and MS Excel 2019 v.2206 (Microsoft corporation, Redmond, WA, USA).

3. Results

3.1. Patient Cohort

Thirty-nine patients met the inclusion criteria for this prospective study between October 2019 and April 2022, of whom 34 consented to study-related dynamic PET acquisition. One patient received further treatment abroad and dropped out of the analysis. Consequently, 33 patients with complete datasets were included in the analysis. Gender distribution was 42% women (14/33) and 58% men (19/33). Male patients were significantly older (68 ± 9 yrs vs. 60 ± 10 yrs, respectively, $p = 0.032$) and taller (178 ± 9 cm vs. 161 ± 9 cm, respectively, $p < 0.001$) than female patients with comparable weight (78 ± 22 kg vs. 70 ± 10 kg, respectively, $p = 0.053$) and BMI (26 ± 6 vs. 27 ± 4, respectively, $p = 0.475$). The blood glucose level before tracer administration did not differ between the sexes and was 5.44 ± 0.94 mmol/L.

3.2. Pulmonary Lesions

Detailed pulmonary lesion analysis is shown in Table 1 with 66.7% (22/33) classified as malignant and 33.3% as benign. In one patient, the lung lesion had completely regressed between external CT-scan and PET/CT, so that no lung lesion measurements could be obtained. The final diagnosis was confirmed histologically in 64.6% of the patients (21/33), by follow-up in 21.2% (7/33), and as a consensus decision of the interdisciplinary tumor board in 15.2% (5/33).

Table 1. Patients' characteristics and diagnosis.

Study-ID	Sex	Age at PET	Final Diagnosis of Lung Lesion	Diagnosis Confirmation	Tumor Stage T	N	M
1	f	54	Inflammation	Follow-up			
2	m	81	CLL	Biopsy			
3	f	56	Benign	Follow-up			
4	m	75	NSCLC	Surgery	T4	N2	M1a
5	m	61	Hematoma	Follow-up			
6	m	58	NSCLC	Surgery	pT3	pN0	cM0
7	m	64	Inflammation	Follow-up			
8	m	78	NSCLC	Biopsy	cT3	cN2	cM0
9	f	50	NSCLC	Biopsy	cT4	cN3	cM1
10	m	82	Benign	Follow-up			
11	m	66	NSCLC	Biopsy	pT2a	N0	M0
12	m	79	Inflammatory myofibroblastic tumor	Surgery			
13	m	69	SCLC	Biopsy	cT4	cN3	cM1c
14	f	71	NSCLC	Surgery	pT2a	pN0	cM0
15	f	73	NSCLC	Surgery	pT1b	pN0	cM0
16	m	77	Malign	Interdisciplinary Tumor board	cT1b	N0	M0
17	f	76	NET	Surgery	pT2a	pN0	pM0
18	f	41	Benign	Interdisciplinary Tumor board			
20	m	69	NSCLC	Surgery	pT1b	pN0	pM0
21	f	57	NSCLC	Surgery	pT1c	pN0	pM0
22	f	56	Hamartoma	Follow-up			
23	f	56	Sarcoidosis	Biopsy			
24	f	73	Regredient Lesion	Interdisciplinary Tumor board			
25	f	57	NSCLC	Biopsy	cT3c	cN1	pM1a
26	m	52	Inflammation	Follow-up			
28	m	61	Primary Lung Tumor	Interdisciplinary Tumor board	cT1b	cN0	cM0
29	m	66	Primary Lung Tumor	Interdisciplinary Tumor board	cT4	cN2	cM1b
30	f	69	NSCLC	Biopsy	cT4	cN0	cM0
31	m	59	NSCLC	Surgery	pT2b	pN0	cM0
32	f	54	NSCLC	Surgery	pT2a / pT1a	pN1 / pN0	pMx / pMx
33	m	73	NSCLC	Biopsy	T2b	Nx	M1
35	m	54	Inflammation	Biopsy			
36	m	65	NSCLC	Biopsy	cT2a	cN2	cM0

CLL = Chronic Lymphatic Leukemia; NET = Neuroendocrine Tumor; NSCLC = Non-Small Cell Lung Cancer; SCLC = Small Cell Lung Cancer.

3.3. Feasibility of Patlak-PET Data Acquisition

All patients tolerated the complete scheduled acquisition time. No examination had to be discontinued or repeated due to technical difficulties. A representative multiparametric scan is presented in Figure 2.

3.4. Effect of Quantification Method on Diagnostic Accuracy

Each semiquantitative PET measurement was performed using three different quantification methods: max, mean (50% isocontour), and peak (1 mL sphere). The quantification method showed no significant effect on the AUC, neither for the lung lesions nor for the lymph nodes, as detailed in Supplementary Tables S1 and S2. For clarity, only the "mean" value is reported in the results.

Malignant lung lesions revealed a significantly higher tumor volume, SUV_{mean}, Patlak Ki_{mean}, $MR-FDG_{mean}$, and $DV-FDG_{mean}$ compared with benign lung lesions, as detailed in Table 2 and Figure 3. Benign pulmonary nodules were markedly smaller than inflammatory sites, however, this difference was not significant in this cohort ($p = 0.057$).

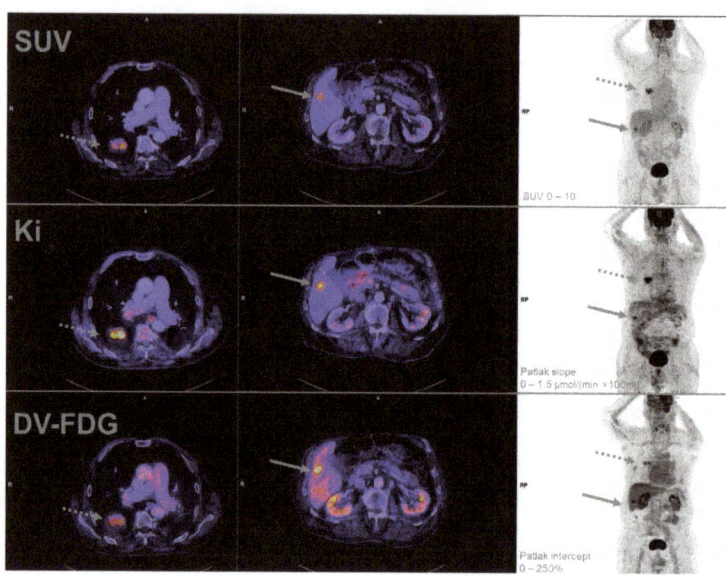

Figure 2. Representative example of multiparametric [^{18}F]FDG PET-imaging of a patient (Study-ID 33) suffering from an adenocarcinoma of the lung (dotted arrow). A single liver metastasis was detected with PET and was histologically confirmed (solid arrow). Of note is the high DV-FDG of the liver metastasis compared to the lung tumor in combination with homogeneous imaging of the surrounding tumor-free liver parenchyma. DV-FDG = Distribution Volume of FDG; FDG = Fluorodeoxyglucose; Ki = Influx Rate Constant; PET = Positron Emission Tomography; SUV = Standardized Uptake Value.

Table 2. Measurements of lung lesions, lymph nodes, and metastases depending on their classification as benign, malignant, or inflammatory.

	Total	Malign	Benign	Inflammation
Lung lesions	n = 32	n = 21	n = 6	n = 5
Volume (mL)	33.41 ± 58.63	48.34 ± 67.09	1.85 ± 1.71 *	8.63 ± 5.80 *
Density (HU)	19.55 ± 28.93	20.78 ± 30.18	3.72 ± 23.26 *	33.40 ± 25.16
SUV$_{mean}$	6.45 ± 5.56	8.40 ± 5.89	2.05 ± 1.33 *	3.50 ± 1.89
Patlak Ki$_{mean}$ (mL/(min × 100 mL))	1.93 ± 2.1	2.67 ± 2.26	0.30 ± 0.17 *	0.78 ± 0.56
MR-FDG$_{mean}$ (µmol/(min × 100 mL))	10.82 ± 12.62	15.01 ± 13.68	1.56 ± 0.80 *	3.88 ± 3.38
DV-FDG$_{mean}$ (%)	110.35 ± 99.56	114.25 ± 106.95	31.13 ± 9.87 *	63.03 ± 26.89
Lymph nodes	n = 65	n = 6	n = 47	n = 12
Short-axis (mm)	9.38 ± 5.75	17.73 ± 8.22	7.61 ± 2.73 *	6.57 ± 0.54 *
Long-axis (mm)	15.95 ± 7.97	26.52 ± 10.35	12.32 ± 4.27 *	12.45 ± 3.93 *
Volume (mL)	2.05 ± 6.40	8.17 ± 13.63	0.65 ± 7.22	0.77 ± 0.66
SUV$_{mean}$	3.43 ± 4.60	11.09 ± 6.54	1.67 ± 0.68 *	1.86 ± 0.38 *
Patlak Ki$_{mean}$ (mL/(min × 100 mL))	0.70 ± 1.14	2.47 ± 1.80	0.28 ± 0.16 *	0.40 ± 0.69 *
MR-FDG$_{mean}$ (µmol/(min × 100 mL))	3.85 ± 6.58	14.31 ± 10.13	1.50 ± 0.83 *	1.32 ± 0.30 *
DV-FDG$_{mean}$ (%)	57.02 ± 36.00	112.69 ± 44.81	43.13 ± 17.24 *	54.50 ± 12.35 *
Metastases		n = 7		
SUV$_{mean}$		6.94 ± 4.00		
Patlak Ki$_{mean}$ (mL/(min × 100 mL))		1.47 ± 1.03		
MR-FDG$_{mean}$ (µmol/(min × 100 mL))		8.37 ± 5.82		
DV-FDG$_{mean}$ (%)		69.45 ± 49.63		

* The asterisk and bold font reflects the significant result ($p < 0.01$) of Tukey's honestly significant difference procedure for multiple comparison correction when separately comparing benign and inflammation to malign findings. One-way ANOVA was significant for main group effects in all evaluations ($p < 0.05$). HU: Hounsfield Units.

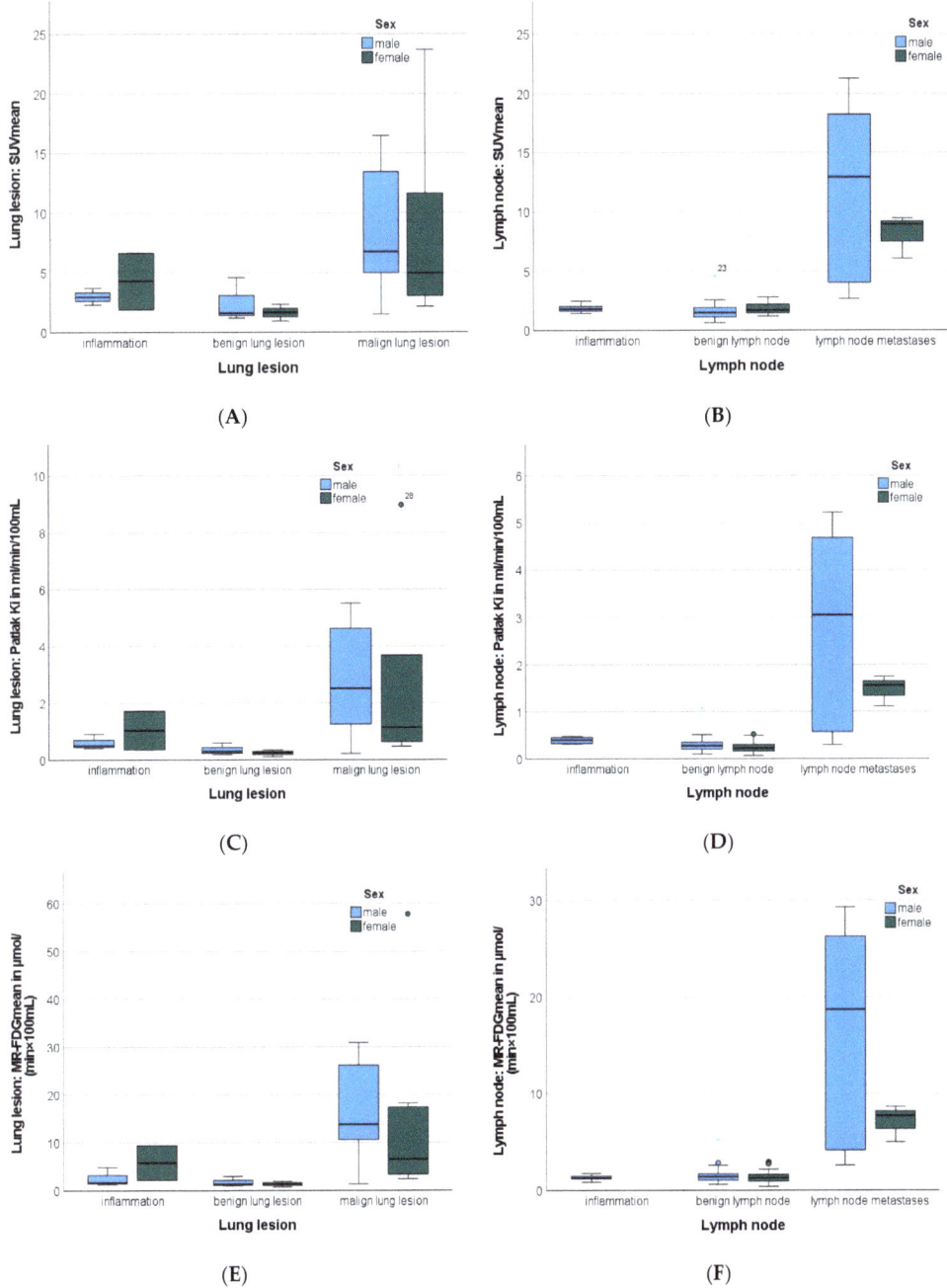

Figure 3. *Cont.*

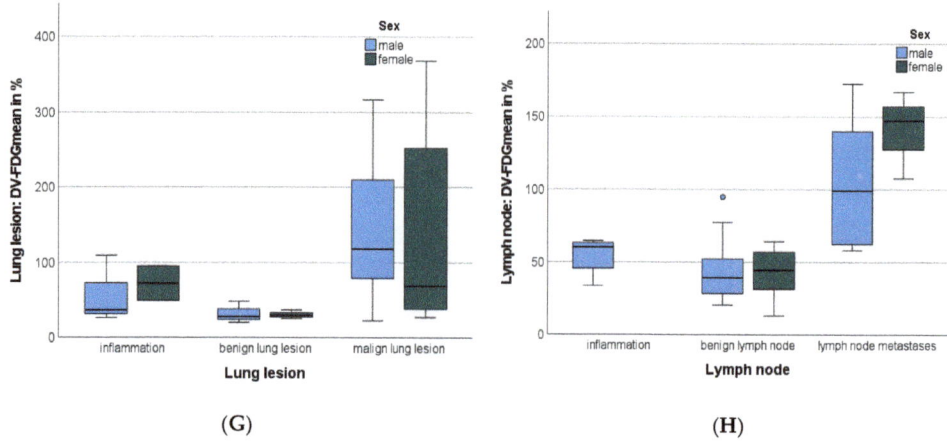

Figure 3. Boxplots illustrating gender-specific SUV$_{mean}$ (**A,B**) Patlak Ki$_{mean}$ (**C,D**) MR-FDG$_{mean}$ (**E,F**) and DV-FDG$_{mean}$ (**G,H**) measurements in the function of lung lesions (**A,C,E,G**) and lymph nodes (**B,D,F,H**). Asterisk (⋆) represents an extreme value. Circle (o) represents an outlier. DV-FDG = Distribution Volume of FDG; FDG = Fluorodeoxyglucose; Ki = Influx Rate Constant; MR = Metabolic Rate; PET = Positron Emission Tomography; SUV = Standardized Uptake Value.

3.5. Lymph Nodes Characteristics

LNM had a significantly higher SUV$_{mean}$, Patlak Ki$_{mean}$, MR-FDG$_{mean}$, and DV-FDG$_{mean}$ compared to benign and to inflammatory altered LN. Furthermore, LNM presented a significantly larger short- and long-axis diameter compared to benign and to inflammatory-altered LN, as presented in Table 2. Tumor volume was not a feature that was consistently increased in malignant lesions and could, therefore, not significantly discriminate dignity between the three groups in this cohort.

3.6. Patlak FDG-PET: Dynamic Parameter Evaluation

Liver tissue was chosen as the reference organ and measurements were performed in all patients (n = 33) in tumor-free liver tissue (SUV$_{mean}$: 2.79; MR-FDG$_{mean}$: 2.08 µmol/(min × 100 mL); Ki$_{mean}$: 0.406 mL/(min × 100 mL).

Ki$_{mean}$ and MR-FDG$_{mean}$ correlated strongly for lung lesions (r = 0.989; $p < 0.001$) and LN (r = 0.994; $p < 0.001$), so that only MR-FDG$_{mean}$ is shown in the following figures for reasons of conciseness. Quantified MR-FDG$_{mean}$ correlated strongly with SUV$_{mean}$ for lung lesions (r = 0.930; $p < 0.001$) as well as LN (r = 0.967; $p < 0.001$), as presented in Figure 4. The correlation between DV-FDG$_{mean}$ and MR-FDG$_{mean}$ was slightly lower but still strong and significant (lung lesions: 0.826, LN: 0.760, $p < 0.001$).

In distant metastases, MR-FDG$_{mean}$ quantification showed a strong correlation (r = 0.943; $p < 0.001$) with SUV$_{mean}$, regardless of the location of metastases or histology of primary tumors, as presented in the scatterplot in Figure 5A.

When only bone and lung metastases were considered, a strong correlation between SUV$_{mean}$ and Patlak intercept was observed (r = 0.891; $p = 0.017$).

In contrast, DV-FDG$_{mean}$ revealed a three-times higher value in an NSCLC liver metastasis (153.63%) compared to the other bone and lung metastases (55.54%), as shown in Figure 5B. As a result, the correlation with SUV$_{mean}$ fell below the significance level (r: 0.457, $p = 0.302$). However, considering only bone and pulmonary metastases, a strong correlation between SUV$_{mean}$ and DV-FDG$_{mean}$ r = 0.891 ($p = 0.017$) was found.

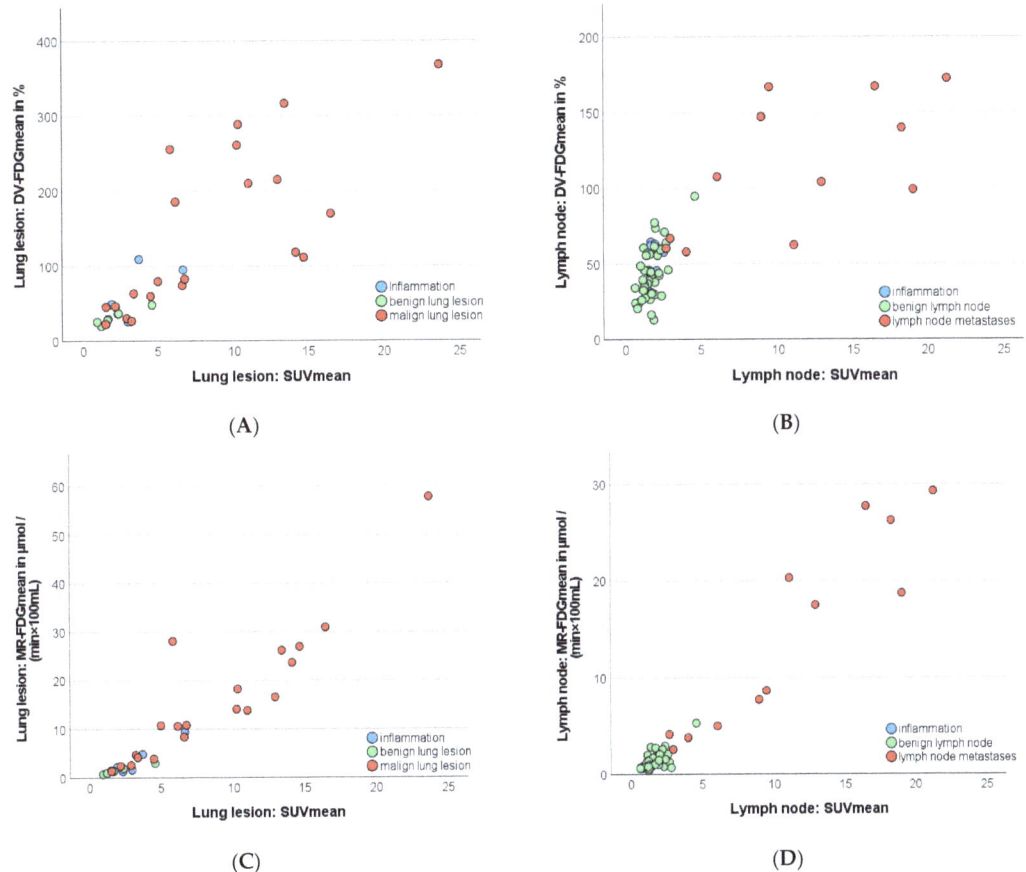

Figure 4. Scatterplots illustrating the correlation between SUV_{mean}, $MR\text{-}FDG_{mean}$, and $DV\text{-}FDG_{mean}$ of different types of lung lesions (**A**,**C**) and lymph nodes (**B**,**D**). Interestingly, $DV\text{-}FDG_{mean}$ (**B**) and $MR\text{-}FDG_{mean}$ (**D**) of the lymph nodes were proportionally half of the values of primary lesions (**A**,**C**), while the magnitude of SUV_{mean} of lymph nodes and primary lesions was found similar. DV-FDG = Distribution Volume of FDG; FDG = Fluorodeoxyglucose; Ki = Influx Rate Constant; MR = Metabolic Rate; PET = Positron Emission Tomography; SUV = Standardized Uptake Value.

3.7. Discriminatory Power between Benign and Malignant Lung Lesions

SUV_{mean} and the dynamic parameters Patlak Ki_{mean}, $MR\text{-}FDG_{mean}$, and $DV\text{-}FDG_{mean}$ revealed very good discriminatory power in the AUC-analysis between benign and malignant lung lesions even at high-significance levels ($p < 0.001$), as detailed in Figure 6 and Table 3.

Table 3. AUC values of pulmonary lesions (n = 32, prevalence: 52.4%).

	AUC	Std. Error	95% CI	*p*-Value	Cut-off Value	Sens.	Spez.
PET: SUV_{mean}	0.827	0.073	0.684–0.970	0.003	3.08	81.0%	72.7%
PET: $MR\text{-}FDG_{mean}$	0.887	0.057	0.775–1.000	<0.001	61.7 (μmol/(min × 100 mL))	81.0%	81.8%
PET: Patlak $Ki\text{-}FDG_{mean}$	0.861	0.065	0.735–0.988	0.001	0.68 (mL/(min × 100 mL))	81.0%	81.8%

Table 3. Cont.

	AUC	Std. Error	95% CI	p-Value	Cut-off Value	Sens.	Spez.
PET: DV-FDG$_{mean}$	0.818	0.075	0.671–0.965	**0.004**	54.3%	76.2%	81.8%
Ratio: SUV$_{mean}$ lesion/SUV$_{mean}$ blood pool	0.835	0.070	0.698–0.973	**0.002**	1.86	71.4%	72.7%
Ratio: SUV$_{mean}$ lesion/SUV$_{mean}$ liver tissue	0.838	0.071	0.699–0.977	**0.002**	1.38	71.4%	72.7%
CT: Lesion volume	0.797	0.078	0.643–0.950	**0.007**	5.6 mL	71.4%	72.7%
CT: Lesion density	0.550	0.109	0.335–0.764	0.648	17.0 HU	61.9%	63.6%
CT: Lesion SD density	0.677	0.103	0.475–0.880	0.104	15.1 HU	76.2%	63.2%

Significant results are highlighted in bold.

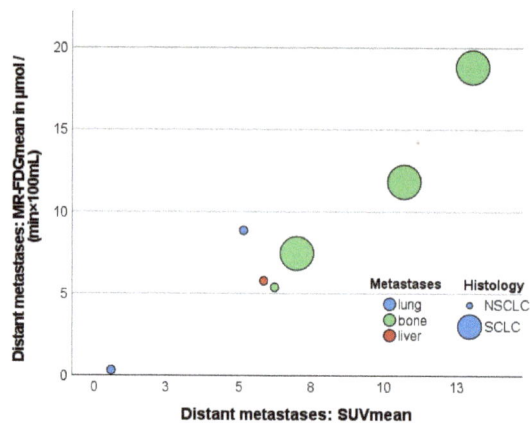

(A)

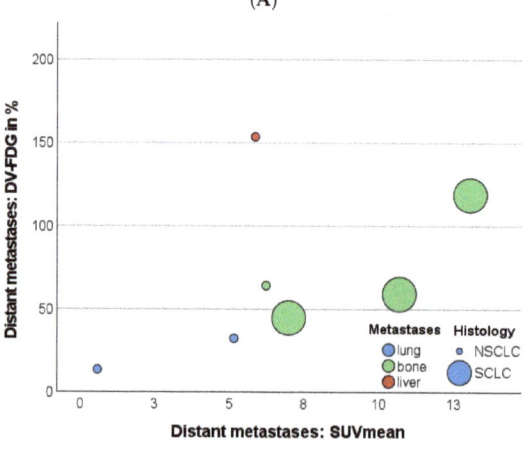

(B)

Figure 5. Scatterplots illustrating the correlation between SUV$_{mean}$ and MR-FDG$_{mean}$ (**A**); and SUV$_{mean}$ and DV-FDG$_{mean}$ (**B**) measurements in the function of the type of distant metastases and primary tumor histology. Metastases of NSCLC are coded as small circle, SCLC as large circle. DV-FDG = Distribution Volume of FDG; FDG = Fluorodeoxyglucose; MR = Metabolic Rate; NSCLC = Non Small Cell Lung Cancer; SUV = Standardized Uptake Value; SCLC = Small Cell Lung Cancer.

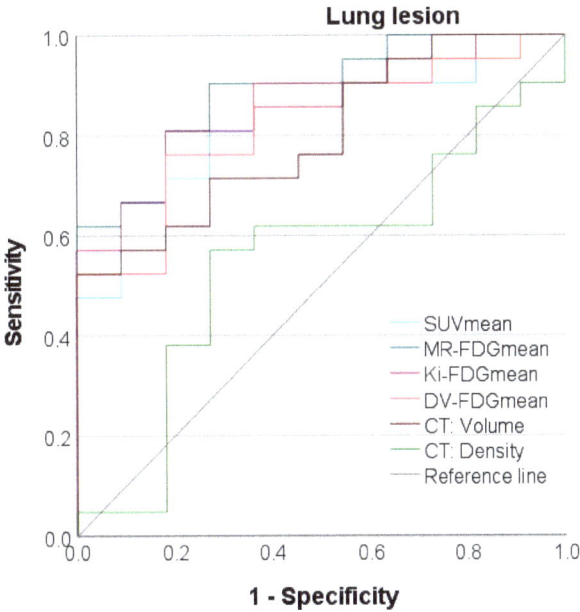

Figure 6. ROC analyses of CT morphologic, static as well as parametric, PET data to differentiate between malignant and benign lung lesions. CT = Computer Tomography; DV-FDG = Distribution Volume of FDG; FDG = Fluorodeoxyglucose; Ki = Influx Rate Constant; MR = Metabolic Rate; NSCLC = Non Small Cell Lung Cancer; SUV = Standardized Uptake Value; SCLC = Small Cell Lung Cancer.

MR-FDG$_{mean}$ provided the best discriminatory power between benign and malignant lung lesions with a high AUC of 0.887. At a somewhat lower level, the AUC of DV-FDG$_{mean}$ was 0.818 and that of the SUV$_{mean}$ was 0.827, although the difference did not reach significance in the AUC comparison in this cohort. MR-FDG$_{mean}$ was slightly more specific than SUV$_{mean}$ (81.8% vs. 72.7%, respectively) at a sensitivity of 81.0% (cut-off value of 61.7 µmol/(min × 100 mL)).

Normalizing the SUV$_{mean}$ of the lung lesions to the SUV$_{mean}$ of the blood pool in the descending aorta or the hepatic parenchyma did not result in a relevant AUC improvement, as presented in Table 3.

Regarding CT features, malignant lung lesions presented with significantly larger volume, as detailed in Table 2. Determination of the pulmonary nodule density was not able to reliably distinguish tumor foci from benign lung lesions ($p = 0.65$).

3.8. Discriminatory Power between Benign and Malignant Lymph Nodes

The parametric PET parameters MR-FDG$_{mean}$, Patlak Ki$_{mean}$, and DV-FDG$_{mean}$ provided excellent discriminatory power between LNM and benign LN. The AUC of the static PET parameter SUV$_{mean}$ (AUC 0.993) was slightly, but not significantly, higher than parametric PET parameters, as detailed in the ROC (Figure 7) and Table 4. SUV$_{mean}$ showed the highest sensitivity and specificity within all PET parameters at an optimal cut-off value of SUV 2.6.

For parametric PET, MR-FDG$_{mean}$ revealed the highest AUC of 0.987 followed by Patlak Ki$_{mean}$ and DV-FDG$_{mean}$ with non-significantly lower AUC of 0.958 and 0.948, respectively. Semiautomatic diameter measurements also reached excellent AUC with 0.969 for the short-axis and 0.947 for the long-axis diameter, as shown in Figure 7 and Table 4. The calculation of the tumor-to-liver or tumor-to-metastases ratios did not improve AUC for either Patlak Ki$_{mean}$, MR-FDG$_{mean}$, DV-FDG$_{mean}$, or SUV$_{mean}$.

Table 4. AUC values of mediastinal lymph nodes (n = 65, prevalence: 18.5%).

	AUC	Std. Error	95% CI	*p*-Value	Cut-off Value	Sens.	Spez.
PET: SUV_{mean}	**0.993**	0.007	0.979–1.000	**<0.001**	2.61	100%	94.3%
PET: MR-FDG_{mean}	**0.987**	0.011	0.966–1.000	**<0.001**	2.58 $(\mu mol/(min \times 100\ mL))$	91.7%	90.6%
PET: Patlak Ki-FDG_{mean}	**0.958**	0.034	0.891–1.000	**<0.001**	0.49 $(mL/(min \times 100\ mL))$	83.3%	92.5%
PET: DV-FDG_{mean}	**0.948**	0.028	0.893–1.000	**<0.001**	60.5 %	83.3%	81.1%
CT: short axis	**0.969**	0.020	0.929–1.000	**<0.001**	10.5 mm	91.7%	84.9%
CT: long axis	**0.947**	0.028	0.893–1.000	**<0.001**	16.1 mm	83.3%	84.9%

Significant results are highlighted in bold.

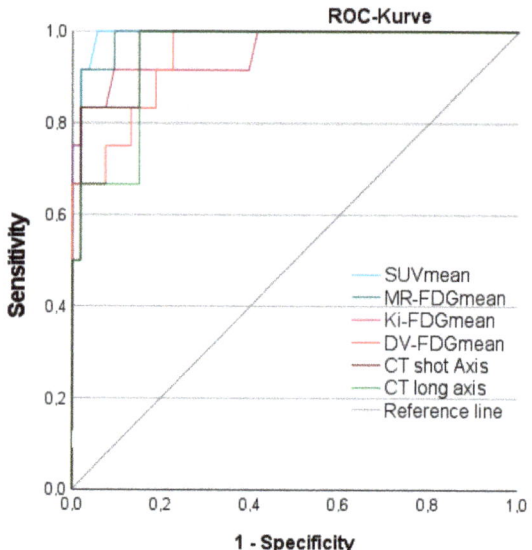

Figure 7. ROC analyses of CT morphologic, static as well as parametric, PET data to differentiate between malignant and benign lymph nodes. CT = Computer Tomography; DV-FDG = Distribution Volume of FDG; FDG = Fluorodeoxyglucose; Ki = Influx Rate Constant; MR = Metabolic Rate; NSCLC = Non Small Cell Lung Cancer; SUV = Standardized Uptake Value; SCLC = Small Cell Lung Cancer.

3.9. Effect of Distant Metastases on SUV_{mean}, Patlak Ki_{mean}, and DV-FDG_{mean} Values of Primary Tumor and LNM

A further analysis was performed to assess the differences in SUV, Patlak Ki, MR-FDG_{mean}, and DV-FDG_{mean} of lung lesions and LNM in patients with or without distant metastasis (M1, contralateral thoracic and/or extrathoracic). LNM presented with significantly higher SUV_{mean} (M1: 13.49 ± 5.65; M0: 3.89 ± 1.89 p = 0.018), Patlak Ki_{mean} (M1: 3.09 ± 1.63; M0: 0.63 ± 0.43 mL/min/100 mL, p = 0.031), and MR-FDG (M1: 17.78 ± 9.31; M0: 3.90 ± 1.22 µmol/(min × 100 mL), p = 0.032), but non significantly higher DV-FDG_{mean} (M1: 124.16% ± 44.78; M0: 78.23 ± 25.55, p = 0.129) values in patients with distant metastases (n = 5) compared to M0.

However, primary tumors showed only non-significantly higher SUV_{mean} (10.33 ± 5.37 vs. 5.73 ± 5.37%), Patlak Ki_{mean} (3.2 ± 1.85 vs. 1.69 ± 2.1 mL/min/100 mL), MR-FDG_{mean} (18.23 ± 11.01 vs. 9.45 ± 12.60 µmol/(min × 100 mL)), and DV-FDG_{mean} (143.11 ± 91.01 vs. 104.28 ± 101.48%) values in patients with M1 compared to M0.

4. Discussion

This prospective study investigates the additional diagnostic value of whole-body parametric Patlak analysis of [^{18}F]FDG PET in patients with indeterminate lung lesions in a clinical setting. Moreover, we explore the diagnostic performance of dynamic data in the detection of LNM and distant metastases compared to standard static PET scans at 60 min p.i. First, methodologically, we demonstrate the reliability of dynamic whole-body PET/CT acquisition in a multi-bed–multi-timepoint technique with continuous table movement in the clinical routine on a conventional PET scanner. Second, we confirm that the quantified metabolic rate of [^{18}F]FDG (MR-FDG) seems to be at least as accurate in distinguishing malignant from benign findings as the state-of-the-art semiquantitative SUV measurement using 60 min p.i. static scan.

Parametric data from MR-FDG and Patlak Ki correlated strongly with the established SUVmean measurements and had comparable AUCs for the classification of lung lesions. However, a closer look at the ROC indicated a slightly higher specificity in the mid-high sensitivity range for MR-FDG. This finding may indicate that MR-FDG and Ki are slightly more robust than SUV, which is in line with the results of the virtual clinical trial by Ye et al. [17]. In that study, the Ki was found to be superior to the SUV in the detection of NSCLC and more robust in the case of significant count rate reductions. However, the findings were validated only on a small sample size [17].

The parametric whole-body dynamic [^{18}F]FDG PET measurements of our trial were consistent with the limited data available from previous studies [18]. In direct comparison to single-bed dynamic PET measurements published by Yang et al., our results demonstrate slightly higher SUVs in the primary tumor (M0: SUV$_{mean}$ 5.73 vs. 5.23; M1: 10.33 vs. 8.41), and considerably lower Ki values (M0: 0.0169 min^{-1} vs. 0.026; M1: 0.032 min^{-1} vs. 0.050) [6]. Similar results were also found for LNM, whose uptake was also shown to be dependent on the presence of distant metastases (SUV$_{mean}$: M0: 3.89 vs. 4.22; M1: 13.49 vs. 5.57) [6].

While SUV$_{mean}$ measurements are generally accepted in the clinical setting, the use of Ki$_{mean}$ is not validated yet. Here, the MR-FDG values of the lung tumors differed up to a factor of two compared to the dynamic single-bed measurements at comparable SUV$_{mean}$. This effect was more emphasized and indeed dependent on the presence of distant metastases (Patlak Ki$_{mean}$: M0: 0.0063 vs. 0.016 min^{-1}, M1: 0.031 vs. 0.033 min^{-1}) [6]. Notably, our data showed a significantly stronger correlation between SUV$_{mean}$ and Patlak Ki$_{mean}$ (r: 0.93–0.97 vs. 0.76–0.88) compared to the data published by Yang et al. [6]. Such varying strength of correlation between two parameters, which were calculated at one site each, indicate that the Ki values may depend on the calculation method. However, this must be further investigated.

In addition, it is also important to consider that although the magnitude increments of SUV$_{mean}$ and Patlak Ki$_{mean}$ or MR-FDG$_{mean}$ are quite similar, they represent different physiological information. SUV$_{mean}$ is the sum of metabolized [^{18}F]FDG-6P trapped in the compartment and un-metabolized [^{18}F]FDG, while MR-FDG solely reflects metabolized [^{18}F]FDG-6P activity [18].

Furthermore, data on our DV-FDG measurements, which represents the combined distribution volume of free [^{18}F]FDG in blood and tissue (reversible compartment), also revealed strong correlations with trapped [^{18}F]FDG measured within MR-FDG and Patlak Ki$_{mean}$ (irreversible compartment) [18]. Interestingly, the only hepatic metastasis in our cohort was visually more distinct and focal in the parametric DV-FDG image, compared to the other parametric parameters. Furthermore, this lesion presented with a remarkably higher DV-FDG value, when compared to the lung or bone metastases. One potential explanation for this effect in the liver metastasis is a previously reported increment of dephosphorylation of the trapped [^{18}F]FDG-6P in liver tissue [18]. High dephosphorylation activity would result in less irreversible trapping and significant efflux of the initially trapped [^{18}F]FDG-6P via the bidirectional GLUT (esp. GLUT 1) transporter out of the cell and back into plasma [18]. This would result in higher DV-FDG values since the reversible compartment also includes both free [^{18}F]FDG in blood and tissue as well as some [^{18}F]FDG-6P [18]. Even if the value of DV-FDG has caused some controversy [19], our data are supportive of investigations evaluating DV-FDG as a potential imaging biomarker for liver metastases.

Interestingly, in our cohort, the diagnostic performance of Patlak Ki_{mean} and MR-FDG seems to achieve at least equal or higher discriminatory power in the detection of mediastinal LNM when compared to the dual-time-point (DTP) dynamic PET using an SUV retention index (RI-SUV) between 1 h and 2 h p.i. by Shinya et al. [9] or the DTP data presented in the largest meta-analysis by Shen et al. [7] (AUC 0.958 vs. 0.794 and 0.9331) on lesion-based analysis. In detail, our MR-FDG$_{mean}$ quantifications presented with higher sensitivity of 92% vs. 74% at a defined specificity of 76% and higher specificity of 89% vs. 76% at a defined sensitivity of 74% compared to the DTP-based RI-SUV estimation published by Shinya et al. [9].

Regarding the performance of dynamic parameters for the detection of distant metastases, there are still insufficient data in the literature. The parametric [^{18}F]FDG dynamic data presented in this study, however, provide the largest published cohort with histologic validation. MR-FDG was shown to be a robust parameter with a very strong correlation to SUV$_{mean}$ regardless of the histology of the primary tumor or location of metastasis (bone, lung, or liver).

Limitations

There are several limitations in this prospective pilot study. First, the sample size of LNM and distant metastases is relatively small, even though it represents one of the largest published collectives. However, due to large effect sizes, the data presented are significant and, therefore, might enable a pre-conclusive analysis.

In addition, some of the lesions could not be confirmed by biopsy; thus, the diagnosis had to be confirmed based on the conclusion of the interdisciplinary tumor board, as is the gold standard for many lesions.

Data acquisition was performed within a single-center study setting; thus, the inter-comparability of measurements between different PET scanners cannot be evaluated.

5. Conclusions

The dynamic whole-body acquisition of [^{18}F]FDG using the Patlak plot was shown to be a stable method for the determination of whole-body glucose metabolism dynamics that operates well in routine clinical practice even on a standard PET/CT scanner. The quantification of the MR-FDG detects malignant lung tumors, LNM, and distant metastases with at least comparable accuracy as the established SUV$_{mean}$ or time-consuming dual-time-point PET scans. In contrast to MR FDG, which correlates strongly with SUV, the distribution volume (DV) of [^{18}F]FDG was considerably higher in liver metastases, indicating a potential additional benefit for the Patlak parameter DV-FDG in detecting hepatic metastases.

Supplementary Materials: The following supporting information can be downloaded at: https://www.mdpi.com/article/10.3390/jcm12123942/s1. Table S1: Extended AUC values of pulmonary lesions (n = 32, prevalence: 52.4%). Table S2: Extended AUC values of thoracic lymph nodes (n = 65, prevalence: 18.5%).

Author Contributions: Conceptualization, C.l.F., H.D., M.W. and K.N.; methodology, C.l.F., M.W. and H.D.; software, S.C.-V. and S.V.B.; validation, M.E.C., A.M.S., C.l.F. and H.D.; formal analysis, M.W. and C.l.F.; investigation, M.A., L.Z. and H.D.; resources, K.N. and C.l.F.; data curation, M.A., W.S. and M.W.; writing—original draft preparation, M.W., S.V.B. and C.l.F.; writing—review and editing, F.S., A.M.S., M.E.C. and H.D.; visualization, M.W.; supervision, L.Z., C.l.F. and K.N.; project administration, L.Z., W.S., C.l.F. and K.N.; funding acquisition, C.l.F. and K.N. All authors have read and agreed to the published version of the manuscript.

Funding: Funded by the Deutsche Forschungsgemeinschaft (DFG, German Research Foundation, Kennedyallee 40, 53175 Bonn) under Germany's Excellence Strategy (EXC 2180–390900677).

Institutional Review Board Statement: This prospective trial was approved by the institutional review board (registry No. 333/2019BO2) and is listed in the German Clinical Trial Register (DRKS-ID: DRKS00017717). All patients signed an informed consent.

Informed Consent Statement: Informed consent was obtained from all subjects involved in the study.

Data Availability Statement: The data presented in this study are available on request from the corresponding author. The data are not publicly available due to data protection regulations.

Acknowledgments: We acknowledge support from the Open Access Publishing Fund of the University of Tübingen.

Conflicts of Interest: Anne M. Smith and Michael E. Casey are full-time employees of Siemens Medical Solutions USA, Inc. The authors declare that they did not inappropriately influence the presentation or interpretation of the research results. The authors declare no further conflict of interest.

References

1. Barta, J.A.; Powell, C.A.; Wisnivesky, J.P. Global Epidemiology of Lung Cancer. *Ann. Glob. Health* **2019**, *85*, 8. [CrossRef] [PubMed]
2. Wankhede, D. Evaluation of Eighth AJCC TNM Sage for Lung Cancer NSCLC: A Meta-analysis. *Ann. Surg. Oncol.* **2021**, *28*, 142–147. [CrossRef] [PubMed]
3. Postmus, P.E.; Kerr, K.M.; Oudkerk, M.; Senan, S.; Waller, D.A.; Vansteenkiste, J.; Escriu, C.; Peters, S. Early and locally advanced non-small-cell lung cancer (NSCLC): ESMO Clinical Practice Guidelines for diagnosis, treatment and follow-up. *Ann. Oncol.* **2017**, *28*, iv1–iv21. [CrossRef] [PubMed]
4. Kalemkerian, G.P.; Loo, B.W.; Akerley, W.; Attia, A.; Bassetti, M.; Boumber, Y.; Decker, R.; Dobelbower, C.; Dowlati, A.; Grecula, J.C.; et al. NCCN Guidelines Insights: Small Cell Lung Cancer, Version 2.2018. *J. Natl. Compr. Cancer Netw.* **2018**, *16*, 1171–1182. [CrossRef] [PubMed]
5. Coello, C.; Fisk, M.; Mohan, D.; Wilson, F.J.; Brown, A.P.; Polkey, M.I.; Wilkinson, I.; Tal-Singer, R.; Murphy, P.S.; Cheriyan, J.; et al. Quantitative analysis of dynamic (18)F-FDG PET/CT for measurement of lung inflammation. *EJNMMI Res.* **2017**, *7*, 47. [CrossRef] [PubMed]
6. Yang, M.; Lin, Z.; Xu, Z.; Li, D.; Lv, W.; Yang, S.; Liu, Y.; Cao, Y.; Cao, Q.; Jin, H. Influx rate constant of (18)F-FDG increases in metastatic lymph nodes of non-small cell lung cancer patients. *Eur. J. Nucl. Med. Mol. Imaging* **2020**, *47*, 1198–1208. [CrossRef] [PubMed]
7. Shen, G.; Hu, S.; Deng, H.; Jia, Z. Diagnostic value of dual time-point 18 F-FDG PET/CT versus single time-point imaging for detection of mediastinal nodal metastasis in non-small cell lung cancer patients: A meta-analysis. *Acta Radiol.* **2015**, *56*, 681–687. [CrossRef] [PubMed]
8. Nogami, Y.; Banno, K.; Irie, H.; Iida, M.; Masugi, Y.; Murakami, K.; Aoki, D. Efficacy of 18-FDG PET-CT dual-phase scanning for detection of lymph node metastasis in gynecological cancer. *Anticancer Res.* **2015**, *35*, 2247–2253. [PubMed]
9. Shinya, T.; Rai, K.; Okumura, Y.; Fujiwara, K.; Matsuo, K.; Yonei, T.; Sato, T.; Watanabe, K.; Kawai, H.; Sato, S.; et al. Dual-Time-Point F-18 FDG PET/CT for Evaluation of Intrathoracic Lymph Nodes in Patients With Non-Small Cell Lung Cancer. *Clin. Nucl. Med.* **2009**, *34*, 216–221. [CrossRef] [PubMed]
10. Karakatsanis, N.A.; Lodge, M.A.; Tahari, A.K.; Zhou, Y.; Wahl, R.L.; Rahmim, A. Dynamic whole-body PET parametric imaging: I. Concept, acquisition protocol optimization and clinical application. *Phys. Med. Biol.* **2013**, *58*, 7391–7418. [CrossRef] [PubMed]
11. Karakatsanis, N.A.; Lodge, M.A.; Zhou, Y.; Wahl, R.L.; Rahmim, A. Dynamic whole-body PET parametric imaging: II. Task-oriented statistical estimation. *Phys. Med. Biol.* **2013**, *58*, 7419–7445. [CrossRef] [PubMed]
12. Rahmim, A.; Lodge, M.A.; Karakatsanis, N.A.; Panin, V.Y.; Zhou, Y.; McMillan, A.; Cho, S.; Zaidi, H.; Casey, M.E.; Wahl, R.L. Dynamic whole-body PET imaging: Principles, potentials and applications. *Eur. J. Nucl. Med. Mol. Imaging* **2019**, *46*, 501–518. [CrossRef] [PubMed]
13. Dias, A.H.; Pedersen, M.F.; Danielsen, H.; Munk, O.L.; Gormsen, L.C. Clinical feasibility and impact of fully automated multiparametric PET imaging using direct Patlak reconstruction: Evaluation of 103 dynamic whole-body (18)F-FDG PET/CT scans. *Eur. J. Nucl. Med. Mol. Imaging* **2021**, *48*, 837–850. [CrossRef] [PubMed]
14. Patlak, C.S.; Blasberg, R.G. Graphical evaluation of blood-to-brain transfer constants from multiple-time uptake data. Generalizations. *J. Cereb. Blood Flow Metab.* **1985**, *5*, 584–590. [CrossRef] [PubMed]
15. Patlak, C.S.; Blasberg, R.G.; Fenstermacher, J.D. Graphical evaluation of blood-to-brain transfer constants from multiple-time uptake data. *J. Cereb. Blood Flow Metab.* **1983**, *3*, 1–7. [CrossRef] [PubMed]
16. Smith, A.M.; Spottiswoode, B.S.; Vijay, K.; Hu, J.; von Gall, C. *FlowMotion Multiparametric PET Suite—The Patlak Model*; Siemens Medical Solutions USA, Inc.: Princeton, NJ, USA, 2018.
17. Ye, Q.; Wu, J.; Lu, Y.; Naganawa, M.; Gallezot, J.D.; Ma, T.; Liu, Y.; Tanoue, L.; Detterbeck, F.; Blasberg, J. Improved discrimination between benign and malignant LDCT screening-detected lung nodules with dynamic over static (18)F-FDG PET as a function of injected dose. *Phys. Med. Biol.* **2018**, *63*, 175015. [CrossRef] [PubMed]

18. Dias, A.H.; Hansen, A.K.; Munk, O.L.; Gormsen, L.C. Normal values for (18)F-FDG uptake in organs and tissues measured by dynamic whole body multiparametric FDG PET in 126 patients. *EJNMMI Res.* **2022**, *12*, 15. [CrossRef] [PubMed]
19. Laffon, E.; Marthan, R. Is Patlak y-intercept a relevant metrics? *Eur. J. Nucl. Med. Mol. Imaging* **2021**, *48*, 1287–1290. [CrossRef] [PubMed]

Disclaimer/Publisher's Note: The statements, opinions and data contained in all publications are solely those of the individual author(s) and contributor(s) and not of MDPI and/or the editor(s). MDPI and/or the editor(s) disclaim responsibility for any injury to people or property resulting from any ideas, methods, instructions or products referred to in the content.

MDPI
St. Alban-Anlage 66
4052 Basel
Switzerland
www.mdpi.com

Journal of Clinical Medicine Editorial Office
E-mail: jcm@mdpi.com
www.mdpi.com/journal/jcm

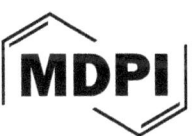

Disclaimer/Publisher's Note: The statements, opinions and data contained in all publications are solely those of the individual author(s) and contributor(s) and not of MDPI and/or the editor(s). MDPI and/or the editor(s) disclaim responsibility for any injury to people or property resulting from any ideas, methods, instructions or products referred to in the content.

www.ingramcontent.com/pod-product-compliance
Lightning Source LLC
LaVergne TN
LVHW070151120526
838202LV00013BA/914